D0212544

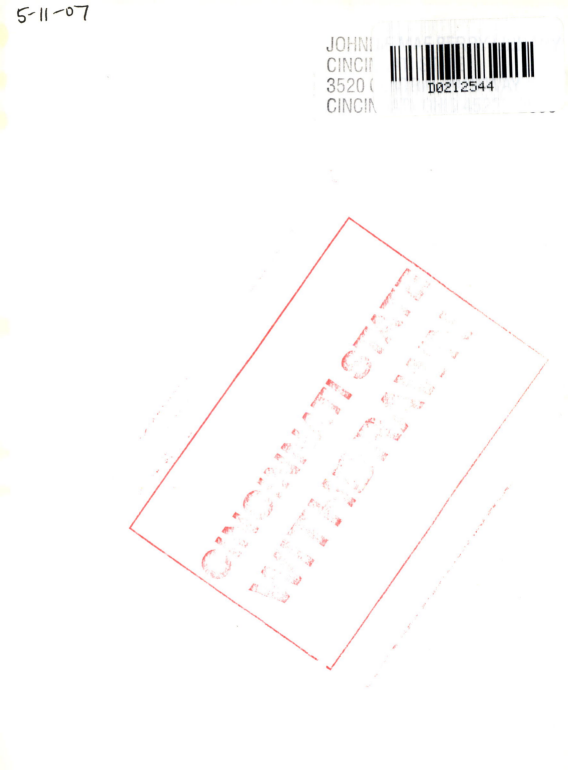

W. Marvin Davis, PhD

Consumer's Guide to Dietary Supplements and Alternative Medicines

Servings of Hope

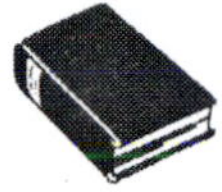

Pre-publication
REVIEWS,
COMMENTARIES,
EVALUATIONS . . .

"*Consumer's Guide to Dietary Supplements and Alternative Medicines* is the best that I have seen. It summarizes the good from the not-so-good based on the current status of science in this field and gives an enormous amount of information on the background of dietary supplements that is often difficult to find."

Norman R. Farnsworth, PhD
UIC Distinguished Professor
and Research Professor
of Pharmacognosy,
College of Pharmacy,
University of Illinois at Chicago

"This is a valuable and engaging source for health care practitioners and the general public alike. The greatest strengths of this book include the debunking of many widely held myths, the breadth and depth of the products detailed, the exhaustive list of peer-reviewed references, and the humor of the sophisticated author. I strongly recommend this book. I look forward to its use in my work and its presence on my bookshelf."

Robert D. Sindelar, PhD
Professor and Dean,
Faculty of Pharmaceutical Sciences,
The University of British Columbia

More pre-publication
REVIEWS, COMMENTARIES, EVALUATIONS . . .

"The days of patent medicines prior to 1906 were a dark chapter in American history, in which a host of unscrupulous companies preyed upon the public by promising fantastic cures for serious medical conditions, while delivering dangerous, addictive, and worthless remedies. Several federal laws stopped those abuses. However, through the machinations of a lobbyist-driven Congress and the resultant 1994 Dietary Supplement Health and Education Act for which it is responsible, American medicine has retrogressed to pre-1906 levels in regard to dietary supplements. In his new book Dr. W. Marvin Davis attempts to describe this situation for the consumer. The book provides clear and understandable explanations for the non-medically trained lay reader. For instance, it has an engaging discussion of the scientific method and the various precepts upon which it is founded.

The book spends a generous amount of time dissecting DSHEA. It deftly describes the war the FDA faces from a Congress that seems largely unconcerned about protecting the health of the American people but extremely concerned about meeting the desires of special interests, such as the supplement industry.

The book explodes many myths hawked by the supplement industry, such as anything that is 'natural' is safe; the FDA allows supplements because they are safe; botanicals don't pose any risks when used with prescription medications; and supplement users can trust the labels of supplements.

The book also covers fountain-of-youth formulas, antioxidant supplements, soy products, sexual supplements, cancer cures, and immunoenhancing supplements. It contrasts the role of DSHEA-authorized pseudosupplements with actual dietary components such as carbohydrates, proteins, vitamins, and minerals.

Dr. Davis writes with a friendly style that does not underestimate the intelligence of the reader. At the same time, he has a gift for summarizing and communicating complicated concepts. This book should have a prominent place in the library of every home in the United States."

W. Steven Pray, PhD, DPh
Bernhardt Professor,
Nonprescription Products and Devices,
College of Pharmacy,
Southwestern Oklahoma State University;
Author, *A History of Nonprescription Product Regulation*

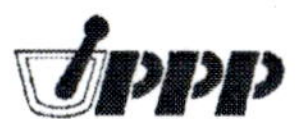

Pharmaceutical Products Press®
An Imprint of The Haworth Press, Inc.
New York • London • Oxford

NOTES FOR PROFESSIONAL LIBRARIANS AND LIBRARY USERS

This is an original book title published by Pharmaceutical Products Press®, an imprint of The Haworth Press, Inc. Unless otherwise noted in specific chapters with attribution, materials in this book have not been previously published elsewhere in any format or language.

CONSERVATION AND PRESERVATION NOTES

All books published by The Haworth Press, Inc., and its imprints are printed on certified pH neutral, acid-free book grade paper. This paper meets the minimum requirements of American National Standard for Information Sciences-Permanence of Paper for Printed Material, ANSI Z39.48-1984.

DIGITAL OBJECT IDENTIFIER (DOI) LINKING

The Haworth Press is participating in reference linking for elements of our original books. (For more information on reference linking initiatives, please consult the CrossRef Web site at www.crossref.org.) When citing an element of this book such as a chapter, include the element's Digital Object Identifier (DOI) as the last item of the reference. A Digital Object Identifier is a persistent, authoritative, and unique identifier that a publisher assigns to each element of a book. Because of its persistence, DOIs will enable The Haworth Press and other publishers to link to the element referenced, and the link will not break over time. This will be a great resource in scholarly research.

Consumer's Guide to Dietary Supplements and Alternative Medicines

Servings of Hope

Pharmaceutical Products Press®
Titles of related interest

The Millis Study Commission on Pharmacy: A Road Map to a Profession's Future edited by Dennis B. Worthen

Taking Your Medicine: A Guide to Medication Regimens and Compliance for Patients and Caregivers by Jack E. Fincham

Prescribed Medications and the Public Health: Laying the Foundation for Risk Reduction by William N. Kelly

Pharmacy Practice in an Aging Society by Jeannette Y. Wick

Patient Compliance with Medications: Issues and Opportunities by Jack E. Fincham

Consumer's Guide to Dietary Supplements and Alternative Medicines

Servings of Hope

W. Marvin Davis, PhD

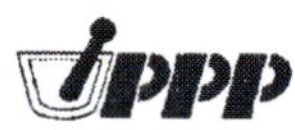

Pharmaceutical Products Press®
An Imprint of The Haworth Press, Inc.
New York • London • Oxford

For more information on this book or to order, visit
http://www.haworthpress.com/store/product.asp?sku=5698

or call 1-800-HAWORTH (800-429-6784) in the United States and Canada
or (607) 722-5857 outside the United States and Canada

or contact orders@HaworthPress.com

Published by

Pharmaceutical Products Press®, an imprint of The Haworth Press, Inc., 10 Alice Street, Binghamton, NY 13904-1580.

PUBLISHER'S NOTE
This book has been published solely for educational purposes and is not intended to substitute for the medical advice of a treating physician. Medicine is an ever-changing science. As new research and clinical experience broaden our knowledge, changes in treatment may be required. While many potential treatment options are made herein, some or all of the options may not be applicable to a particular individual. Therefore, the author, editor, and publisher do not accept responsibility in the event of negative consequences incurred as a result of the information presented in this book. We do not claim that this information is necessarily accurate by the rigid scientific and regulatory standards applied for medical treatment. No warranty, expressed or implied, is furnished with respect to the material contained in this book. The reader is urged to consult with his/her personal physician with respect to the treatment of any medical condition.

The development, preparation, and publication of this work has been undertaken with great care. However, the Publisher, employees, editors, and agents of The Haworth Press are not responsible for any errors contained herein or for consequences that may ensue from use of materials or information contained in this work. The Haworth Press is committed to the dissemination of ideas and information according to the highest standards of intellectual freedom and the free exchange of ideas. Statements made and opinions expressed in this publication do not necessarily reflect the views of the Publisher, Directors, management, or staff of The Haworth Press, Inc., or an endorsement by them.

Cover design by Jennifer M. Gaska.

The photo of Allison Hayes included in Chapter 1 is taken from Web article "The Real Allison Hayes" by Jackrandall Earles, found at http://www.horror-wood.com/allison.htm. Web site © 2006 by Joe "Renfield" Meadows. Every attempt possible was made to find the copyright holder for the photo itself, and all avenues have been exhausted.

Library of Congress Cataloging-in-Publication Data

Davis, W. Marvin.
Consumer's guide to dietary supplements and alternative medicines: servings of hope / W. Marvin Davis.
p. ; cm.
Includes bibliographical references and index.
ISBN-13: 978-0-7890-3040-5 (hard : alk. paper)
ISBN-10: 0-7890-3040-3 (hard : alk. paper)
ISBN-13: 978-0-7890-3041-2 (soft : alk. paper)
ISBN-10: 0-7890-3041-1 (soft : alk. paper)
1. Dietary supplements. 2. Alternative medicine. I. Title.
[DNLM: 1. Dietary Supplements. 2. Complementary Therapies. QU 145.5 D265c 2006]

RM258.5.D38 2006
615'.1—dc22

2006004220

DEDICATED
to the memory
of Sandra S. and Catherine L. Davis

IN HONOR OF
Emmanuel, who knew at the outset how much
that I would need this project

ABOUT THE AUTHOR

W. Marvin Davis, PhD, BS Pharm, MS, passed away in 2005. Dr. Davis was Emeritus Professor of Pharmacology at the University of Mississippi's School of Pharmacy. His career included 48 years of classroom teaching in schools of pharmacy. His research investigated ways that drugs affect the brain and behavior, with an emphasis on their neurochemistry and on the dependence-producing agents of chemical dependence and drug-seeking behavior. Dr. Davis's substantial research findings have been published in several research journals and as book chapters. His other writings include several dozen non-experimental professional papers, many of them supporting professional continuing education for pharmacists. He served as reviewer for the *Journal of Natural Products,* the *Journal of Ethnopharmacology, Phytotherapy,* and numerous other research journals in pharmacology, toxicology, and neuroscience.

CONTENTS

Foreword

It has been my privilege to have known, Professor Marvin Davis, as a mentor, professional colleague, and friend. In 1964 he was chosen as the founding member of the Department of Pharmacology in the School of Pharmacy at the University of Mississippi, and for nearly 40 years anchored the department, serving as its chair for 20 years. He taught thousands—students, pharmacists, and faculty colleagues—about this fascinating discipline of pharmacology. None who knew him can fail to remember him as a keen observer of nature and of life in all its aspects—physical, mental, social, and spiritual. He was a unique mix of keen intellect, vast experience, enthusiastic inquiry, healthy skepticism, and a wry humor set in a robust faith, a quiet resolve, and a compassion for others.

It is a special perspective, therefore, that he brought to this book, *Consumer's Guide to Dietary Supplements and Alternative Medicines.* Dietary supplements are timely subjects, and objective, reliable, factual information is dwarfed by a deluge of marketing schemes and testimonials. Several works have appeared in recent years informing, cataloging, promoting, "debunking," praising, and warning about these trends and fads in "natural remedies." Patients as well as medical professionals considering these supplements can find it difficult to discriminate between help and hype or the innocuous and the outright harmful. Professor Davis wove together in this volume an insightful commentary that is critical but balanced: part science, part history, part societal analysis, and part common sense, with a touch of his own spiritual outlook.

A fundamental theme, the need for application of sound scientific approaches in the assessment of the promise and the pitfalls of botanical remedies, is addressed early in the book. In order to develop clear answers, many carefully controlled studies using well-characterized products in various populations and disease states are needed. Nobel laureate Dr. Alexis Carrel advised, "A few observations and much reasoning lead to error; many observations and a little reasoning to truth" (Enerson, 2001). In particular for safety studies, it may be many years and many thousands of doses later when a toxic effect appears. Professor Davis cites examples wherein unan-

Consumer's Guide to Dietary Supplements and Alternative Medicines

doi:10.1300/5698_a

ticipated and unacceptable toxicities developed only after years of exposure to a "natural, therefore safe" supplement.

The subsequent chapters guide the reader through a careful consideration of many myths that are all too prevalent in the field of dietary supplements, e.g., the supposition that "natural" implies "safe" and the presumption that potentially harmful herbal products are barred from the market by current regulations. These fallacies are illustrated with historical examples and pointed, often humorous observations. Davis highlights the fantastic claims that help to create seemingly insatiable consumer markets, especially in the areas of weight loss, antiaging, sexual or athletic performance enhancement, and cancer cures, and provides advice for evaluation of such pitches.

Dr. Davis is also careful to keep the discussions in perspective. He notes that the record for prescription pharmaceuticals has certainly not been pristine. Even with the extensive safety testing—preclinical and clinical—many serious and even life-threatening adverse effects have appeared with broader use after marketing. By comparison, with a few exceptions, herbal remedies have been to date relatively free of such devastating events. However, with broader and indiscriminate use of relatively unregulated products the potential for such occurrences becomes quite high. He also reminds us that many botanicals were once the mainstays of medicine and pharmacy; indeed, some of them are still foundational to our modern therapeutics. A brief synopsis of some of these wonders is provided, with commentary on their impact in medicine and pharmacology. He describes the critical roles for many vitamins, minerals, and metabolites from plant sources and highlights their known and potential health benefits.

In the final section, Professor Davis reviews developments in the field of complementary and alternative medicine and some of the current studies underway to establish the potential efficacy and safety of botanical remedies. The future scenario for the field of herbal remedies is discussed, outlining likely changes in the industry and regulatory environment. A major focus is the importance of behavioral and lifestyle choices, emphasizing moderation, responsibility, and emotional and spiritual aspects.

All who read this book will sense Dr. Davis's love of sound science, his grasp of the discipline of pharmacology, and his commitment to ethical principles. Here is a dose of realistic assessment on dietary supplement myths, tempered with an appreciation of the proven (and potential) value, medicinal and otherwise, of many marvelous designs in the fabric of our natural world.

Larry Walker, PhD,
Director, Thad Cochran National Center
for Natural Products Research,
University of Mississippi, Oxford Campus

Preface

Hope in a Bottle

> It was the best of times, it was the worst of times, it was the age of wisdom, it was the age of foolishness, it was the epoch of belief, it was the epoch of incredulity, it was the season of Light, it was the season of Darkness, it was the spring of hope, it was the winter of despair, we had everything before us, we had nothing before us, we were all going direct to Heaven, we were all going direct the other way. . . .
>
> Charles Dickens, *A Tale of Two Cities*

Charles Dickens gave us a memorable description of a time of struggle, turmoil, and ferment, a time of paradoxes and contrasts that could in many respects also apply well to the end of the twentieth century and beginning of the twenty-first. The degree to which this description applies to current self-efforts by many persons for health maintenance and restoration and/or their resorting to health care practitioners of "natural medicine" or complementary and alternative medicine (CAM). Specifically, we will contrast the use of dietary supplements with the conventional practices and "conventional wisdom" of Western mainline or conventional medicine that are directed in many instances, but not always, toward the same goals (Eisenberg et al., 1998).

A contemporary illustration of this paradox is the following ironic commentary on changes of our times that has been making the rounds for several years in various print media and e-mail messages:

> **A Brief History of Medicine**
> *I have an earache. What can I do?*
> 2000 BC—Here, eat this root.
> AD 1000—That root is heathen; say this prayer.

Consumer's Guide to Dietary Supplements and Alternative Medicines

doi:10.1300/5698_b

AD 1850—That prayer is superstition; drink this potion.
AD 1930—That potion is snake oil; swallow this pill.
AD 1980—That pill is ineffective; take this antibacterial.
AD 2000—That antibacterial is *synthetic!* Here, eat this root.

It is remarkable that two important themes have prospered in recent decades—one being a trend for the public to be widely accepting of alternative therapies, and another has been an increasing pursuit of "scientific-evidence-based" practices by much of Western medicine. These trends stand in remarkable contrast. Most striking in this respect is a wide renaissance of herbal remedies as well as a tremendous burgeoning of other nutritional supplements (Eisenberg et al., 1998). For a majority of these minimal, if any, scientific validation exists. One physician expressed it very aptly:

> It is ironic that patients want the best and most scientifically proven therapy when they are ill with serious diseases, yet trust their health to salespeople at the local health food store, magazines, newspaper, radio and television testimonials or commercials, recommendations from "alternative medicine authorities," and some health resorts. (Ewy, 1999)

Simultaneously with the late-twentieth century renaissance of herbal remedies the contemporary practice of scientific medicine was becoming much more focused on the advent of "evidence-based" therapeutics. This new phrase, which dates from the early 1990s, describes a school of thought that demands strong evidences (by new and higher scientific standards than in former times) for the effectiveness/efficacy of every therapy, whether old or new, if it is to be endorsed as worthy of general acceptance by "mainline medicine."

The streams of attitude and behavior between the general population and the medical profession seem to be flowing in opposite directions. Resolving these conflicts is a problem of considerable dimensions. Persons who are inclined to be actively rather than passively oriented to their personal health issues need to be well-informed and need to give thought to such matters. Providing the essential basic information to facilitate critical consideration is an aim of this book.

This is not the book I began to write years ago in the past millennium. My research and writing started as a highly skeptical denunciation of the most obvious faults of the supplement sellers and their products. It was to be a warning for readers to flee the arena of self-therapy via dietary supplements and the self-deception encouraged by their physician promoters. The stimulus for my negative outlook was the aggravation arising from excessive direct-mail advertising for supplements that seemed extremely misleading, inaccurate, and antiscientific. About that time, Wallace Sampson (1996) presented an analysis that attacked "antiscience" trends in the movement to alternative medicine using the anticancer fraud of laetrile as a typical case, which arguably it is not.

In short, many promotional materials seemed to cultivate a hope for benefits that the sources must have known could not be delivered. The people responsible for deception of this sort became "hopemongers," seemingly a subtype of quackery. To my view an especially reprehensible aggressive targeting of older Americans, with their burden of age-related maladies, occurred. Many of them have failed to obtain much if any benefit through the current mainline medical therapies. It seemed that such people frequently were being promised hope in a bottle, but with the bottle containing only the deception of false hope instead of truth.

The crucial importance of hope was appreciated long ago: "The miserable have no other medicine, but only hope" (William Shakespeare, *Measure for Measure,* act III, scene I).

And it surely is true yet today:

> In terms of money, $13.7 billion was spent on these unconventional therapies, of which $10.3 billion was out of pocket (not covered by insurance). When this amount of time, money and hope is spent on "alternative" approaches to therapy, it is clear that scientific medicine is not giving a significant number of people everything they want . . . Without very much reflection, curing replaced caring as the dominant ideology of this new technology-driven medicine. We are slowly realizing that most people want both. (Golub, 1997, p. 215)

Thus, although we think of our taking of either natural remedies or modern synthetic pharmaceuticals as a material action, a nonmaterial aspect, our hope for benefit, also exists, which may be a factor in the outcome of the therapeutic process. A simple major reason for people turning to unconventional remedies is that the promoters and vendors of such items are offering hope for areas of life in which conventional medicine offers little or none. The importance of hope for success in fighting an illness has been greatly expounded by the writer Norman Cousins (1989) in his book titled *Head First: The Biology of Hope.* The converse is also described as the disastrous effect that can result when the physician's statement of prognosis removes all hope.

The following list of conditions includes many for which dietary supplements are touted as being able to give benefit where prescription pharmaceuticals cannot:

Aging-related problems—of the brain, digestive tract, neuromuscular system, skin, bones
Alzheimer's or other dementias
Back pain
Cancers
Chronic fatigue syndrome
Chronic headaches
Deficient libido (low sex drive)
Erectile dysfunction (impotence)
Fatigability, low energy
Fibromyalgia
Memory problems
Multiple chemical sensitivity
Multiple sclerosis
Obesity
Osteoarthritis
Paresthesias/peripheral neuropathy
Poisonous chemicals
Sleep disorders
Tinnitus

Whereas unconventional remedies can be found that promise significant help against all of the listed conditions, rather few conventional medicines are found to promise the degree of benefits that people desire against any of them. One exception to this exists: sildenafil (Viagra), a major advance toward the solution to the problem of impotence (erectile dysfunction).

The value of conventional medicine for cancer therapy is often described pejoratively by "the other side" as merely "cutting, burning, and poisoning" that may prolong survival, but at the cost of all quality of life. Granted, the conventional physicians will reply that they deal in truth rather than in fictional promises that can't be fulfilled. The unconventional practioners will say that they are open-minded to practicing the principles of health promotion and maintenance that Medicine with a capital M is too busy making money to bother about. It is a time of ferment indeed.

THE NEW THERAPEUTIC SCENE

When I was first studying pharmaceuticals in mid-twentieth century, prior therapies that consisted of multiherbal combinations were contemptuously described as "shotgun medicine." That approach had been suited for an earlier era, but was no longer so in an era having the specific goal of "one disease, one drug" via scientific medicine. Medical practice had advanced into a more focused therapy. Thus, when 50 years later we saw a return to herbals in the former "shotgun" pattern, it was quite disconcerting.

More frequently than not individual botanical remedies are yet to be validated; thus, combining them only multiplies our ignorance of potentially crucial facts regarding their safety, and this without any solid assurance of gaining a greater efficacy. Moreover, only a small minority among the hundreds of botanicals currently in use seem likely ever to be validated through adequate clinical testing under current standards of the Food and Drug Administration (FDA) because of the 1994 Dietary Supplement Health and Education Act (DSHEA) legislation. That is because of the extreme expense to meet the currently prevailing requirements of the FDA for new drugs, and because the DSHEA legislation exempted supplements from having to meet them by calling them all "foods." Thus, such expenses will seldom be borne voluntarily by manufacturers.

However, my initial level of extreme skepticism toward supplements, and especially botanicals, has been tempered by a broad process of literature research and some significant firsthand experiences of the benefits of dietary supplements. I must concede that these have reduced my negative bias toward the idea that alternative therapy via dietary supplements may indeed prove beneficial. In the course of research, my goal became to provide the reader with balancing doses of "facts" on both sides of the issues. Admittedly, some information still is intended to serve as an antidote to what yet seems nearly poisonous over-reaching and exaggeration—the hyperbole, or "hype," that composes too much of the current supply of "information" on dietary supplements, especially the nonnutrients. One of my continuing objectives is to convince readers that they should exercise concern and caution for their safety when using dietary supplements akin to what is needed in taking prescription or nonprescription pharmaceuticals. This care and concern involves obtaining the best possible information by means of which to differentiate between the good, the bad, and the ugly.

Indeed, the good among the supplements, as among pharmaceuticals, do have quite remarkable and marvelous properties. I prefer describing them as marvelous rather than miraculous—as their proponents are overly prone to do. Misusage of the term *miracle* has rather degraded it from its basic implication of a supernatural basis for benefits, or, alternatively, of a magical basis, which hardly befits our twenty-first century scientific age. That actions to be found in familiar plants deserving to be dubbed *marvelous* if not *miraculous* was proven to me long ago when I first applied a fresh broken surface from the stem of an aloe cactus to my skin where it had just been accidentally burned. The pain was soothed so completely and instantly it was marvelous, even magical! Indeed, if all or even many of the claims made for dietary supplements were confirmed as true I would be highly delighted. However, we must also deal with the bad and the ugly, which occur altogether too often within the broad dietary supplement scene.

My initial interest in this general topic was provoked in no small part by my reading a fascinating, remarkable, and tragic story from a 1977 *Journal of the American Medical Association* article titled, "Lead-Contaminated Health Food: Association with Lead Poisoning and Leukemia" (Crosby, 1977). The story, one of a real-life Hollywood tragedy that stemmed from a "food supplement," is told in the introductory chapter (Chapter 1). This article brought a realization that dietary supplements could be professionally meaningful to an academic pharmacologist-toxicologist.

Additional beginnings of my concern for nonpharmaceutical remedies date to my writings for the continuing education of practicing pharmacists. Beginning in the early 1980s I increasingly compared the benefits and risks of using dietary supplements. In 1983 I wrote about a controversial pseudovitamin, calcium pangamate (vitamin B15). A 1991 topic was the use of amino acids in neuropsychopharmacology. Dietary supplements appeared in my other writings, e.g., in writings regarding antiaging approaches and alternative osteoarthritis therapies, but a 2001 work hit directly: "Dietary Supplements: Are They Safe and Reliable?" (Davis, 2001).

For many maladies I retain a distinct bias in favor of the utilization of conventional pharmaceuticals versus supposedly effective alternative remedies. For example, I am unaware of botanicals that truly can substitute reliably for the synthetic pharmaceuticals employed to control epilepsy. However, having taught classes of pharmacy students for nearly five decades, with a focus mainly on prescription drugs, I am keenly aware of their hazardous aspects in addition to their great benefits.

The disturbing behaviors of dietary supplement promoters were also the behaviors of the mainline pharmaceutical industry in the past and would be still if the pharmaceutical industry were not subject to federal regulations intended to restrain abuses and misbehavior. I find the mainstream pharmaceutical industry's current direct-to-consumer advertising and their "physician education" practices as repugnant as the ugly aspects of the supplement scene. I am persuaded by some severe contemporary criticism that the giant pharmaceutical multinationals did well to drop their former self-description of being part of the "ethical pharmaceutical industry." Such a title is less justified now than it was 50 years ago.

I confess a positive bias favoring biochemical/nutrient products (except for multivitamin and multimineral products) and a negative bias toward even the single-component botanical extracts since they usually are intrinsically a highly complex mixture. From my laboratory experience in experimental pharmacology I know that it is quite difficult to obtain "clean" experimental data when examining a "dirty" subject item, i.e., one that contains multiple constituents. This may be as true for a synthetic compound that has not been very well purified by the chemist supplying it as it is for a plant extract having a composition that can be variable, depending on multitudinous factors of growth, harvesting, and preparation.

Reinforcing my negative bias toward botanical marketers is their accelerating use of the regressive practices of the past or seemingly following a pattern of TCM (traditional Chinese medicine) of combining large numbers of poorly characterized natural agents. Recently they began to add biochemical and nutrient components. My view is that combining multiple botanical components serves as a multiplying of factors of uncertainty that causes me to doubt that such situations could be supported by any sound science.

Nevertheless, the consumer has a need to be as well-informed as possible about the scientific standing of dietary supplements. One of the ferments of the present scene concerns the means of becoming and remaining informed. Recently it has been declared that the Internet lets medical information out of the doctor's bag. However, correctly utilizing either Internet or conventional published medical sources requires a background that most persons lack. This book seeks to prepare the consumer to succeed in his or her pursuit of better understanding of their health issues and to start the reader on that road. It should already be apparent that the importance of hope (or its absence) for persons experiencing illness will be emphasized.

Acknowledgments

For their assistance and encouragement I owe a debt of gratitude to my colleagues at the University of Mississippi: Rachel C. Robinson, Clinical Assistant Professor and Director of Drug Information Services; Professors Wade Waters, Robert Speth, and Dennis R. Feller of the Department of Pharmacology; and librarians Nancy F. Fuller and Sherrie Sam Rikard of the Science Library.

Much appreciation is also expressed to Brian L. Davis, Bob England, Mary Alice Beer, and Betty Streett for information, suggestions, and encouragement received and for their reading of sample chapters.

Shirley Davis (Mrs. W. Marvin Davis) would like to acknowledge Wade Waters for his work on this book after the author's life ended.

Consumer's Guide to Dietary Supplements and Alternative Medicines

doi:10.1300/5698_c

Reviewer's Acknowledgments

To you from failing hands we throw
The torch; be yours to hold it high.
If ye break faith with us who die
We shall not sleep, though poppies grow
In Flanders fields.

"In Flanders Fields"
Lt. Col. John McCrae

At the time of Dr. Marvin Davis's passing, much work remained to be done to complete this book. Dr. Wade Waters took up the torch and held it high to assure this book's completion. Wade reviewed more than half of the chapters and painstakingly responded to the editorial requests for verification of quotations or to provide suitable alternatives. The dedication and commitment that Dr. Waters has made to this book is nothing less than heroic, and does great honor to the memory of Dr. Davis.

Dr. Waters was assisted in his efforts to bring this book to completion by several faculty of the School of Pharmacy at the University of Mississippi. Drs. Larry Walker, Charlie Hufford, Alice Clark, Tony Verlangieri, Dennis Feller, and Bob Speth also reviewed chapters to bring them to their final versions. We owe a debt of gratitude to these individuals who spent considerable time in this effort, with no expectation of reward, other than the satisfaction of knowing that they helped to bring this outstanding treatise to the consciousness of the readers to whom Dr. Davis wished to provide his Servings of Hope, tempered with the wisdom of science.

Bob Speth, PhD
May 25, 2006

Consumer's Guide to Dietary Supplements and Alternative Medicines

doi:10.1300/5698_d

Abbreviations and Acronyms

Some readers may already be familiar with these items, but a review of this section (along with the Glossary) will for many readers be helpful and facilitating.

5HT	5-hydroxytryptamine
17HP	17-hydroxyprogesterone
AA	amino acids
ACAM	American College for Advancement of Medicine
ACE	angiotensin converting enzyme
ACh	acetylcholine
AD	Alzheimer's disease
ADHD	attention-deficit/hyperactivity disorder
ADR	adverse drug reactions
ALA	alpha-linolenic acid
alpha-LA	alpha-lipoic acid
AMA	American Medical Association
AMD	age-related macular degeneration
AOAC	Association of Official Analytical Chemists
APPROVe	adenomatus polyp prevention on Vioxx
AREDS	Age-Related Eye Disease Study ARG arginine
ASPET	American Society for Pharmacology and Experimental Therapeutics
ATP	adenosine triphosphate
BCAA	branched-chain amino acid
BMI	body mass index
BMJ	*British Medical Journal*
BPH	benign prostatic hyperplasia
BPM	beats per minute
BSE	bovine spongiform encephalopathy

Consumer's Guide to Dietary Supplements and Alternative Medicines

doi:10.1300/5698_e

CAM	complementary and alternative medicine
CCD	colon-cancer derived
CDC	Centers for Disease Control
CDHS	California Department of Health Services
CFS	chronic fatigue syndrome
cGMP	cyclic guanosine monophosphate
CHD	coronary heart disease
CHF	congestive heart failure
CJD	Creutzfeldt-Jakob disease
CLA	conjugated linoleic acid
CNS	central nervous system
COX	cyclooxygenase
CP	chromium picolinate
CSF	cerebral spinal fluid
CT	computerized tomography
CV	cardiovascular
CYP	cytochrome P450
DC	doctor of chiropractic
DEA	Drug Enforcement Administration
DDT	Dichlordiphenyltrichloroethane
DGL	deglycyrrhizinated licorice
DHA	docosahexaenoic acid
DHEA	dehydropiandrosterone
DLPA DL	phenylalanine
DMBA	7,12-dimethylbenzanthracene
DMSO	dimethyl sulfoxide
DNA	deoxyribonucleic acid
DO	doctor of osteopathy
DSHEA	Dietary Supplement Health and Education Act (1994)
ED	erectile dysfunction
EEG	electroencephalograph
EFA	essential fatty acid
EGb	extract of ginkgo biloba
EGCG	epigallocatechin gallate
EMS	eosinophilia myalgia syndrome
EPA	eicosapentaenoic acid
ERB	estrogen receptor beta
EU	European Union
FA	fatty acid
FAD	flavin adenine dinucleotide
FDA	Food and Drug Administration
FHF	fulminating hepatic failure

FM	fibromyalgia
FTC	Federal Trade Commission
GABA	gamma-aminobutyric acid
GAS	general adaptation syndrome
GERD	gastroesophogeal reflux disease
GHRH	growth-hormone-releasing hormone
GLA	gamma-linoleic acid
GI	gastrointestinal
GIT	gastrointestinal tract
GM	genetically modified
GMP	good manufacturing practices
GNC	General Nutrition Center
GPC	glyceryl phophorylcholine
GSE	grapefruit-seed extract
GTF	glucose tolerance factor
GWS	Gulf War syndrome
HCA	hydroxycitrate
HCV	hepatitis C virus
HDL	high-density lipoprotein
HERS	Heart and Estrogen/Progestin Replacement Study
HGH	human growth hormone
HHS	Department of Health and Human Services
HIV	human immunodeficiency virus
HMG-CoA	3-hydroxy-3-methylglutaryl coenzyme A
HMO	health maintenance organization
HNRC	Human Nutrition Research Center on Aging
HOLOTC	holotranscobalamin
HRT	hormone replacement therapy
HSDD	hypoactive sexual desire disorder
HSO	homeostatic soil organisms
IAT	immunoaugmentive therapy
ICD	implantable cardioverter defibrillator
ICE	intracardiac echocardiograph
ICSH	interstitial cell stimulating hormone
IDDM	insulin-dependent diabetes mellitus
IND	Investigational New Drug (application)
IOC	International Olympic Committee
IR	immediate release
IU	international units
IV	intravenous
JAMA	*Journal of the American Medical Association*
LDL	low-density lipoprotein

L-DOPA	L-dihydroxyphenylalanine
LH	luteinizing hormone
LTP	L-tryptophan
MAO	monoamine oxidase
MAOI	monoamine oxidase inhibitor
MCP	modified citrus pectin
MCS	multiple chemical sensitivity
MCV	mean corpuscular volume
MD	doctor of medicine
MDMA	methylenedioxymethamphetamine
MDR	minimum daily requirement
MI	myocardial infarction
MMA	methylmalonic acid
MRI	magnetic resonance imaging
MSG	monosodium glutamate
MSM	methylsulfonyl methane
NAC	N-acetylcysteine
NAD	nicotinamide adenine dinucleotide
NCAA	National Collegiate Athletic Association
NCCAM	National Center for Complementary and Alternative Medicine
NCI	National Cancer Institute
ND	doctor of naturopathy
NDA	New Drug Application [caps correct]
NF	National Formulary
NFL	National Football League
NHLBI	National Heart, Lung, and Blood Institute
NIDDM	non-insulin-dependent diabetes mellitus
NIH	National Institutes of Health
NNFA	National Nutritional Foods Association
NO	nitric oxide
NSAID	nonsteriodal anti-inflammatory agent
NSFI	National Sanitation Foundation International
NTF	non-tumor-forming
ODS	Office of Dietary Supplements
ORAC	oxygen radical absorbance capacity
OTC	over-the-counter
PBMC	peripheral blood mononuclear leukocytes
PCHRG	Public Citizen Health Research Group
PC	prostate cancer
PD	Parkinson's disease
PDE-5	phosphodiesterase type 5
PETA	People for the Ethical Treatment of Animals

PMS	premenstrual syndrome
PN	peripheral neuropathy
POCD	postoperative cognitive dysfunction
POH	perillyl alcohol
PPA	phenylpropanolamine
PS	phosphatidylserine
PSA	prostate-specific antigen
PSC	posterior subcapsular
PUFA	polyunsaturated fatty acids
RBC	red blood cell
RDA	recommended daily allowance
RDI	recommended daily intake
ROS	reactive oxygen species
RPE	retinal pigment epithelial (cells)
Rx	prescription
SAMe	S-anedosylmethionine
SARS	severe acute respiratory syndrome
SH	sulfhydryl
SJW	St. John's wort
SOD	superoxide dismutase
SPS	soy phosphatidylserine
SR	sustained release
SSRI	serotonin reuptake inhibitor
STD	sexually transmitted diseases
TCM	traditional Chinese medicine
TDH	Texas Department of Health
TIA	transient ischemic brain attack
TIF	tumor-inducing factor
TNF	tumor necrosis factor
TNJ	Tahitian Noni Juice
TRT	testosterone replacement therapy
UN	United Nations
USPSTF	United States Preventive Services Task Force
USP	United States Pharmacopoeia
UV	ultraviolet
UVA	ultraviolet A
UVB	ultraviolet B
vCJD	variant Creutzfeldt-Jakob disease
VDL	very-low-density lipoprotein
VS	vanadyl sulfate
WBC	white blood cell
WHI	Women's Health Initiative

WHO	World Health Organization
WNE	West Nile encephalitis
WNV	West Nile virus
WS	Werner syndrome

Author's Note

This book is intended to be used as an information source and guide to many aspects of the subject of dietary supplements. It is not intended to be encyclopedic in coverage, nor is it intended to be a substitute for advice from a health care professional. It is aimed at stimulating and facilitating the reader's becoming well-informed about his or her health maintenance issues as well as their participation in therapies for illness. Although many possible interactions between botanical supplements and prescription drugs could occur, such potential hazards are not described exhaustively. This book emphasizes that self-diagnosis and self-therapy of serious diseases usually are rather foolish undertakings, and one should instead obtain counsel from the best qualified medical practitioner available. Upon obtaining initial diagnostic and therapeutic services, referral(s) may be appropriate and necessary.

Consumer's Guide to Dietary Supplements and Alternative Medicines

doi:10.1300/5698_f

Chapter 1

Introduction: A Cautionary Tale from Hollywood

Allison Hayes was a striking Hollywood beauty (Figure 1.1) who by 1962 had become a successful film and television actress. However, in this same year she began to be the leading lady in a real-life tragedy.[1] It started when she began taking an oral calcium supplement for treating dysmenorrhea at the direction of her Hollywood doctor. Unexpectedly, by 1964 she had developed another illness, showing episodes of dizziness and easy fatigability which progressed to outright muscle weakness and an unnaturally irritable mood. Miss Hayes's physician responded to the new problem by merely recommending that she *increase* her intake of the calcium supplement. Over the next several years her health deteriorated further until by 1967 she became unable to walk without a cane, which ended her acting career. She lost weight and her auburn hair turned dark brown, then black and began to fall out (Crosby, 1977). By 1968, when she decided to stop taking the supplement, her muscular weakness had become so profound that she was confined to a wheelchair. In total she consulted 22 doctors, none of whom were able to identify the nature or the source for her illness, with more than a few of them baldly passing it off as primarily a psychoneurotic problem!

In her despair Miss Hayes decided she must take one of three actions: get psychiatric help to "learn to live with the pain," accepting that doctors couldn't diagnose her disease; commit suicide; or succeed by her own efforts to discover the cause for her health loss. After being put on hold by the suicide-prevention line, she chose the third option. After much searching in the UCLA Medical School library, she discovered a textbook on the toxicology of industrial metals. Miss Hayes found a description of a metal poisoning of factory workers that she said "fit her history like a glove." Convinced that she had been poisoned, she consulted by telephone a forensic toxicologist. After many questions, he asked that she send samples of both her hair and the calcium supplement.

Consumer's Guide to Dietary Supplements and Alternative Medicines

doi:10.1300/5698_01

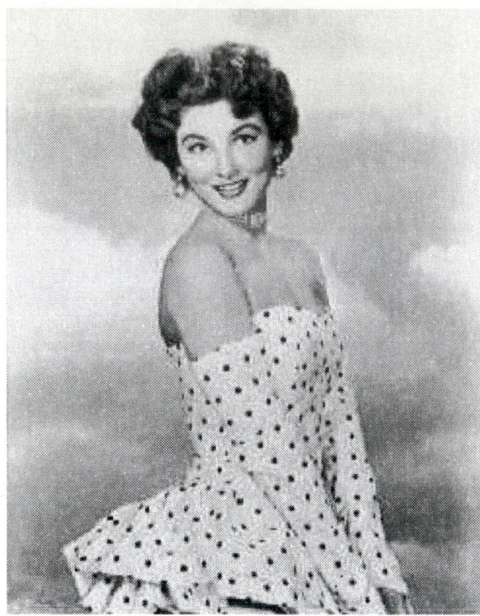

FIGURE 1.1. Allison Hayes
Source: Earles (2000).

His analyses revealed toxic levels of lead in her hair that indeed reflected a poisonous exposure. Analysis also detected sufficient lead in the supplement she had taken daily for six years for it to have been the source of her poisoning. As a result very high levels of lead had accumulated in her bones, nerves, muscles, and other organs by the time she first became ill in 1964. Removing herself from the lead exposure, by 1968 her strength improved, although it never approached full recovery. In 1976 she was diagnosed by the reporting physician, Dr. William H. Crosby, to have leukemia, which ultimately took her life. However, the cause of this illness was not necessarily the lead poisoning. Dr. Crosby speculated that the cause may have been the more than 300 diagnostic X-rays she endured at the recommendation of the 22 ineffectual physicians she consulted. Miss Hayes filed suit against the prescribing physician but dropped it at his pleading, and he died soon thereafter. However, she did win a settlement of $50,000 against the Los Angeles distributor of the calcium supplement.

The response of the Food and Drug Administration (FDA), as related by Dr. Crosby (1977),[1] was that when informed of the facts of the case an FDA source said that the calcium supplement product was neither a food nor drug and thus was not within the purview of the agency. Moreover, had it been treated as a food, no standard existed at that time for a maximum-permitted lead content in a food product. How disillusioning! The situation began to change when the FDA later wrote to her, saying, "We are incorporating 'health food' issues into our FY 77 and 78 compliance programs, including the bone-meal-and-heavy-metal matter. Your case is a key stimulus for so doing" (Crosby, 1977, p. 2629). Unfortunately, by the time of that letter Miss Hayes had already died prematurely at the age of 46 on February 27, 1977.

The case clearly was one of neurotoxic lead poisoning resulting from overuse of a bonemeal product that was contaminated by an excessive content of lead. According to Dr. Crosby, the product was manufactured from bones of aged horses (30 years old), of "metropolitan" carriage horses sent to a glue factory in the United Kingdom, from whence the bonemeal product was exported to the United States. This was before the era of unleaded gasoline, so in their urban life the horses were highly exposed to lead-filled dust and/or vapors that came from the exhaust systems of vehicles burning leaded gasoline. As a result, the horses' bones had accumulated large amounts of lead, which tends to be distributed and stored similarly to calcium.

Besides detailing Miss Hayes's case, Dr. Crosby reported on what she had learned of three other patients who had taken bonemeal prescribed by the same Hollywood physician. The most fortunate became ill during a trip to Paris, where she was correctly diagnosed and effectively treated, to the credit of the French physicians. Another, not so fortunate, had a similar illness but died without a diagnosis of lead poisoning. The third had an illness that included mental derangement, which led to a brief psychiatric hospitalization, where she recovered when no longer taking the bonemeal supplement.

This story had a lasting impact on my thinking about the safety of food supplements and the inadequacy of the governmental regulation of their marketing in the United States. It also carries lessons that are still valid, the main one being that the FDA was not then and is not now delegated to precertify the purity, safety, or efficacy of dietary supplements. One cannot assume with full confidence that any one of these—purity, safety, or efficacy—has been adequately established for any product of the dietary supplement class. Clearly, this tragic story would have been avoided if reasonable and basic quality-assurance standards had been applied to the product by its manufacturer.

You may be thinking, "That was 40 years ago, and FDA now has appropriate limits on lead content of foods and food supplements, so I needn't worry about such a thing happening now." Wrong! Although the FDA and others have indeed established standards, they do not have a mechanism for assuring that manufacturers are observing them. In early summer of 2003, a nongovernmental testing program operating under the name ConsumerLab reported that their study of calcium products revealed that two out of 15 products tested had an excessive content of lead. Moreover, one of the two exceeded the state of California's "no significant risk" level, which requires a warning label. This product, one of the "coral calcium" products highly touted via television infomercials (and against which the Federal Trade Commission [FTC] has warned consumers and producers of false advertising), did not bear such a label.

Thus, even now the application of reasonable purity standards by the FDA for lead in supplement products is *assumed* and *expected,* but the compliance with such standards depends on the knowledge and integrity of the producers. This book will supply evidence for deficits of either knowledge, integrity, or perhaps both. We will find instances parallel to but with even broader tragic consequences than those of Miss Hayes's story.

One lesson from this account concerns the making of a diagnosis when poisoning is involved: physicians are not accustomed to thinking of a poison as the source of their patients' problems, and a diagnosis not thought about will not be made. Other cases of poisoning from lead or other metals arising from their presence in remedies or cosmetics will be reviewed in Chapter 20.

Another lesson comes from the inappropriate prescribing of a supplement product for Miss Hayes. A calcium supplement (then or now) should not be expected to be an appropriate therapy for her diagnosed condition. This case refutes the dictum that "if a supplement doesn't help, at least it won't hurt." Equally distressing is that many other physicians were unable to make the correct diagnosis of her subsequent poisoning. This illustrates that the best doctor you can find may not be good enough." An older saying among physicians applies also when nonmedical persons undertake self-diagnosis and self-medication of a very serious condition: "The physician who treats himself has a fool for both doctor and patient."

PART I: Basic Scientific Principles of Using Natural Products to Maintain and Improve Health

Our crisis in health care . . . comes in part from making science a secular religion and then expecting miracles from it.

Edward S. Golub, PhD (1997)

Formerly, when religion was strong and science weak, men mistook magic for medicine; now, when science is strong and religion weak, men mistake medicine for magic.

Thomas Szasz, MD (1973)

Chapter 2

Do We Really Want Scientific Medicine, or Do We Want Magic?

> Anything can be made to sound logical. It is easy to become so entranced with miracles or magic that one casts aside weighty, cumbersome scientific principles. But scientific principles must apply to evaluating the unknown, even placebos and the plausible.
>
> Howard M. Spiro, MD (1998)

In the past two decades a broad and remarkable trend has developed among the U.S. population: the embracing of unconventional approaches to improving or maintaining health or for achieving relief from certain illnesses. The implied contrast of calling them "unconventional" is with respect to the "conventional" medical practices being taught as Western medicine, especially in the United States and Europe, that prevailed in the second half of the twentieth century. These approaches and remedies are known by various phrases. Some have a new and sophisticated sound, e.g., holistic, complementary, or orthomolecular medicine as well as nutraceutical therapy. Some of these and others are clearly not new at all but merely revived from the nineteenth century, as in the case of the American and European practices using homeopathic or indigenous herbal medicines. Others are natural medicines imported from Asia as ancient traditional medicines, especially India's ayurvedic medicine and China's TCM (traditional Chinese medicine). Some physical treatments, rather than the use of chemicals, also have flourished as seen in the form of acupuncture (also from China) and the supposed therapeutic effects of magnets or wearing of copper bracelets.

Consumer's Guide to Dietary Supplements and Alternative Medicines

doi:10.1300/5698_02

MAGIC OR MEDICINE? SUPERNATURAL OR SCIENTIFIC?

Magic, as employed in this chapter, refers to the idea that such unconventional therapeutic practices possess exceptional capabilities. In its long history, magical thinking has interpreted or explained events as occurring by means of extraordinary or even supernatural mechanisms. Thus, in the minds of some people a connection exists between herbal medicine and magic. A magical mode of thinking was initially decried by Varro Tyler in 1978 in the first edition of his book *The Honest Herbal* (Tyler, 1999). He refuted the idea that the "healing powers" of a compound produced by a plant through its natural biosynthesis exceeds the potential of the identical chemical molecule produced by human laboratory synthesis. Moreover, he indicated that magical thinking also occurs on the other side of the coin: "Particularly insidious is the myth perpetuated by these promoters that there is something almost *magical* about herbal drugs which prevents them—in their natural state—from inflicting harm on living organisms."

A recent example would be the inclusion of an extract of an animal organ in a formulation that is designed to "support" better function of that organ. Specifically, the addition of a bovine prostate extract to a saw palmetto product appears to have no scientific rationale and smacks of magical thinking as a means for helping men with the problem of benign hyperplasia of the prostate (a nonmalignant enlargement that can cause urgency and/or difficulty of urination). Directly making an appeal to magical thinking are some sales pitches that say something such as "The magic weight loss ingredient in this formula . . ." Dr. Tyler would be no less disturbed by today's marketing milieu.

Magic Is Again Timely Today

For anyone who thinks that magic is less appealing in current times, let them consider the centrality of magic and witchcraft in the Harry Potter books that have experienced an overwhelming popularity in recent years. Harry is an enrollee of an institute of magic and sorcery in which one required course herbology. One of the major herbs essential to the practice of magic is mandrake *(Mandragora officinarum),* which has a long and fabled history of magical properties. In Book II, *Harry Potter and the Chamber of Secrets* (Rowling, 1999), the young wizards and witches are taught the very special craft of transplanting mandrakes, but only after donning earmuffs to stifle the plants' outcries! As a magical plant, mandrake has an extraordinary, unequaled place in European folklore. It is traditionally regarded to be an aphrodisiac and is closely associated with witchcraft. The present tense is used to convey contemporary practices, which can be readily seen from a survey of Internet Web sites. An iconic connection of mandrake and the religion of Wicca is still extant. Being known both for its toxicity and its assumed medicinal properties, the "real" mandrake commanded the fear and respect of Europeans throughout the Middle Ages and earlier. Its folk uses and attributes may have arisen because of its anthropomorphic root, i.e., its having a physical resemblance to a human form. Thus, mandrake has played an important role in magic and witchcraft, which author J.K. Rowling indeed recognizes thoroughly in her Harry Potter stories. She and Harry have become the subjects for a great many fan Web sites as well as a few opposing the religious impact of witchcraft/sorcery tales.[1]

The beginning of humankind's use of natural remedies predates our most ancient historical records. All that can be said about the earliest origins is speculation based on archeological and paleontological researches, extrapolations from the earliest written records, and many educated guesses. In other words, the initial use of natural materials as remedies is hidden from certain view by the proverbial mists of times past. However, we can say with considerable confidence that the early history of this topic is intertwined with the realm of magical practices and beliefs. The oldest medical writings from ancient Egypt reflect this magical bent, as witnessed by the fantastic (to us) nature of their components. "Natural substances" in that age included, for example, various unpleasant animal components such as camel dung, the water (aqueous humor) contained in the eyes of pigs, animal blood and human urine, as well as the more expected plant materials. The discovery of the 5,300-year-old mummified body of Oetzi, the "iceMan of the Alps," in 1991 was of great interest in many respects, not least of these was that his gear included a leather pouch containing herbaceous material that has been interpreted to be his herbal medicine stock; if true, this would likely be the most ancient such discovery.

Root Meanings and Roots

The supernatural status of remedies/drugs/medicines in ancient times also is to be found in Greek mythology and other sources. The root word, "pharmaco-" has the meaning in English of "a drug or a medicine." This term in Greek does indeed have the first meaning of "drug," both for its action and use as a remedy or as a poison. However, it has another, older meaning of "an enchanted potion or philtre," hence "having an association with a charm or spell," i.e., magic!

It seems as if a deeply-rooted, unconscious hope exists that a drug product will display the magical properties of an enchanted potion to heal the one who believes and expects it will do so. Perhaps this is why promoters of remedies in previous times as well as more recent have found reason to describe their remedies, whether pharmaceutical or botanical, as miracle drugs, or to come very close to that sort of unsupportable claim. Because *miracle* implies that an agent has supernatural benefits, I will avoid using this word for remedies and instead refer to remarkable benefits by using the term *marvel* or *marvelous.*

Perhaps the reason for the power exerted on human behavior by natural products as remedies or medicines is related to the ancient origins of pharmacotherapy—in the idea of finding a supernatural solution to one's problems by using a magical remedy. A picture of this can be found in the episode of bitter water from a story in the Torah that describes the ancient Hebrews' exodus from Egypt (Exodus 15:22-27, King James Version). The people were very angry at being led into a desert place where the only available water was too bitter to drink, likely because of an excess content of alkaline salts. Their attitude about the water may have reflected not only their bitterness at their general circumstances but also their fear of being poisoned. The Lord showed their leader, Moses, a tree that he should throw into the water to cause it to become "sweet," which he did indeed with the desired change resulting. Commentators have connected this miraculous divine provision with the idea of magical properties. Many of the Hebrews were not only unfamiliar with but also uncomfortable with the God of Moses, as later demonstrated by their preferring to worship a golden image of a calf. They may have more easily perceived the event as resulting from a magical property inherent in trees. However, the divine use of the image of trees, leaves, and healing recurs at the very end of the New Testament. Revelation 22:2 speaks of the heavenly realm containing the tree of life the leaves of which were for the healing of the nations.

FUNDAMENTAL SCIENTIFIC CONCEPTS: WHAT IS SCIENTIFIC?

> The scientific mind does not so much provide the right answers as ask the right questions.
>
> Claude Levi-Strauss, French anthropologist (1983)

Science is a systematic search for understanding of the way things are, how they got to be that way, and how they work. Clearly science is based on the idea that the world is knowable, but knowing/science is not static but rather is a continuing process of gaining an ever more precise knowledge and understanding of a certain phenomenon. At any particular time this knowledge and understanding must be seen as provisional, possibly incomplete, and subject to being improved with new information. Better understanding may come when new methods for research become available that provide a new means for improving our understanding. With each new discovery a more precise clarification of the basic "how and why" questions may exist. Technology is based on the idea that we can bring about purposeful change; it is scientific knowledge that is being applied.

The scientific method is a phrase that describes how science is pursued.[2] To fully explain this method exceeds the scope of the book, but a central feature is the descriptive and analytical phases, often described by the following list:

1. description of a particular phenomenon (e.g., physiological or pathological events);
2. construction of explanatory hypotheses (one or more "educated guesses" to explain the occurrence of the phenomenon being considered);
3. designing and performing experiments to confirm or refute the hypotheses;
4. drawing conclusions from such experiments and designing newly modified and improved (or entirely new) hypotheses; and
5. achieving over time a greater understanding and better explanations that are best supported by the total body of evidence.

A "good" hypothesis must meet certain conditions, the most basic being that it must be subject to being tested and "falsified," i.e., disproved. According to the view propounded by a distinguished twentieth-century philosopher, Karl Popper, a scientific hypothesis can never be verified; it can only be falsified. No matter how much evidence may be gathered to "prove" a point, the chance always exists that one crucial contrary evidence will be discovered. If a hypothesis is found to be unable to be tested, progress is not possible along that track. Testing of a hypothesis is nominally aimed at falsification, but in reality the researcher typically is hoping and anticipating that his or her hypothesis will be established as correct.

Essential Definitions

Bioavailability: This is a critical feature of all substances that are being tested for possible therapeutic activity. Bioavailability expresses the characteristics of a test agent with respect to its uptake upon administration, and its distribution to its intended site of action. An agent may show desirable in vitro activity, for example against HIV, but if it fails to gain absorption after oral administration, it is showing very poor bioavailability in vivo for an intended systemic action. It must be in vivo results that make the case for further development of a candidate therapeutic substance. Some supplements taken in tablet form have shown inadequate bioavailability because the tablet fails to disintegrate so as to allow the active ingredient to be effective. This would be a consequence of using poor pharmaceutical technology in preparing the product for marketing.

Dose-response relationship: This phrase speaks of the fundamental quantitative measure in both experimental pharmacology and toxicology that expresses the change in response with increasing levels of exposure ("dosage") to a drug or toxicant.

Drug: For those biomedical scientists focused on pharmacology (pharmacologists), any substance exerting a biological effect on living cells that serves for diagnosis, prevention, or treatment of disease rather than providing the basic qualities of foods (which are supplied by the fats, carbohydrates, proteins, vitamins, and minerals) is known as a drug. Thus, dietary supplements consisting of botanicals are serving as drugs when they are used in the prevention or alleviation of disease. Some nutrients or their metabolic products when administered in large doses may also display pharmacological rather than nutritional actions. It is merely playing with words to distinguish between "supporting the health" of an organ (as is usually done to describe the actions of dietary supplements) versus "preventing a disease" of that organ.

Mechanisms of drug action:

1. For many important drug substances their effects are exerted selectively through special structures called "receptors," which are located in the cell membranes. These effects may consist of receptor activation (by an "agonist") or may be a result of inhibiting receptor activation (as an "antagonist"), which causes alteration of the rates of specific cellular functions of the cells bearing the receptor.
2. For many other drug substances their effects are exerted selectively through hormonal receptors located at the nucleus within the cell. These effects occur through a change in synthesis and release of hormonal molecules, which change actions of cells and organs physically separate from the cell being acted upon.

3. For other important drug substances their effects are exerted selectively through enzymes, more often consisting of enzyme inhibition or less often of "induction," causing increased synthesis (or activation) of an enzyme.
4. Some drugs act as precursor biochemicals to elevate the production of active mediators of physiological actions upon specific receptors. This is called "precursor loading," and it applies to natural substances such as amino acids or certain fatty acids.
5. A significant category of drugs act via more general mechanisms, such as by their altering osmotic pressure or by a chelating action, which is binding of elements to aid in their excretion (as for toxic heavy metals such as lead and mercury).

Pharmacognosy: The science that deals with natural sources for medicinal substances, in contrast to chemical synthesis for obtaining medicinals, known as "medicinal chemistry."

Pharmacology: The science that deals with the effects of chemicals on living organisms. It is generally oriented to human benefits and is fundamental to the process of new drug discovery and development.

Toxicology: The science that focuses on the adverse or undesirable effects of chemicals (toxicants) on living organisms, regardless of origin or possible usage, that may thus be called poisons. Toxicology is essential to the development of drugs as well as nondrug chemicals having various economic applications in order to assess possible human risks in terms of the benefit-to-risk ratio for human usage.

Laboratory Animal Research: Necessary but Not Sufficient

For about two centuries biomedical researchers have utilized animals for the initial exploration of the effects of agents considered as candidates for a role as drugs. This became a very formalized requirement of the FDA in the twentieth century regarding new drug development. A considerable range of animal studies—both pharmacologic and toxicologic—must be completed prior to initial testing of chemicals in human beings. FDA regulations guiding the process apply to both prescription (Rx) and over-the-counter (OTC) pharmaceuticals, but they do not apply to a new botanical dietary supplement, which may be marketed on the basis that the provider has reason to believe it to be safe. However, they are not required to provide data to support the belief.

Thus, animal experimentation is a basic necessity in new drug development. The animal rights groups who would do away with all biomedical research and tests in mammalian species, who wish and campaign for science to be conducted without the grounding foundation of animal research and testing, ignore or disavow the fundamental benefits to human health that have accrued from such experimentation. They do not carry their principles so far as to decline to receive the benefits from medical advances that were possible only by virtue of laboratory animal-based research. Before the discovery and initial separation of insulin from the pancreas of dogs by Sir Edward Banting in the early 1920s, insulin-dependent, childhood-onset diabetes was a diagnosis with a certainty of a fatal outcome after the victim's short life expectancy.

However, there are limitations to what animal research can tell us. It can predict most but not all adverse responses to drugs. Some of these are due to the differences in the physiology of mice, rats, pigs, or dogs and that of human beings. Ultimately, a transition to testing in people must be made, both to confirm effectiveness and to detect adverse responses. It is especially difficult to anticipate adverse effects that stem from an unfavorable, unwanted immune system action. Also, it is not always possible to confirm a human benefit when extrapolating from animal data. The true, ultimate test is human research, which occurs in four phases that are defined and described in the following section.

An April 2004 publication (Egan et al., 2004) provides an illustration of the preliminary status of animal research. It reported that the genetic-based biochemical pathology of the disease cystic fibrosis is corrected by curcumin, a major component of a familiar plant product, turmeric. However, the results came from research first on human cells in vitro and second on a mouse model of cystic fibrosis. Both test situations giving positive results provides a fairly firm basis for anticipating a successful application in patients. However, until confirmation is attempted in a clinical trial, it would be premature to say that the cure for cystic fibrosis is at hand. Nevertheless, too often supplement compounds are touted in an even more premature fashion.[3] When reading the promotional information on a new "cure," please remember that animal researches are necessary but not sufficient to support therapeutic claims and predict safety.

CLINICAL RESEARCH ASPECTS

> Medicine has come to look with disdain on the purely anecdotal [observation]. Still, if something happens once, it can happen again . . . Observation is not explanation . . . Knowledge comes from classifying and testing hypotheses.
>
> Howard M. Spiro, MD (1998)

The nature of the test material must be appropriate for valid human testing to be accomplished. It would be futile to perform a clinical evaluation or study using a material that does not have adequate bioavailability. Moreover, a botanical preparation needs to be standardized in order for a study to be worthwhile. This means that one or more marker components must be established (usually, a presumed active constituent) so that it can be employed as a standard of strength for comparison over time and in different batches. Without such standardization there could be so much variability in activity that it would potentially undermine the quantitative measure(s) being obtained. Such variability arising from using nonstandardized test materials may explain some discrepancies in outcomes of different studies of *supposedly* the same material.

Types of Human Research

A very common nonexperimental research approach is that of epidemiology, which is the scientific study of the relationships between various factors determining both the frequency and distribution of a particular disease or condition in the human population. As a branch of medical research it is oriented to discerning the causes of injury, poisoning, or illness. It commonly requires gathering data from large numbers (thousands) of people over an extended period of time. By statistical analysis epidemiologists seek to demonstrate correlations between factors that might conceivably influence the rate of disease in a community. When a significant correlation is found, this can never alone confirm a cause-and-effect relationship, but it provides a basis for a prospective (before-the-fact) experimental investigation.

For example, a large sample of 50-year-old men may be observed and followed over a period of ten years to see whether they develop or show a particular disease, for example, prostate cancer. Other data are gathered as to their habitats, occupations, diets, and other health factors. It may be observed by analysis that a statistically significant difference exists (one large enough to be unlikely to occur on a chance basis) in the dietary intake of fruits and vegetables in the two groups—the nondisease group having higher intakes than those developing prostate cancer. This may indeed be in accord with a suspicion that the experimenters had at the outset. However, it does not confirm the idea that fruit and vegetable intake is protective against prostate cancer. Too often such findings are presented to the public as if they establish a cause-and-effect relationship. The rules of science say that such an outcome provides a good hypothesis for experimental testing, but nothing more.

After arriving at such a significant correlation it is necessary to construct a before-the-fact test of the hypothesis that may involve an intervention—arranging a comparison between randomly selected groups (two or more) that receive or do not receive a "treatment," which in this case would be the addition or not of a fruit-and-vegetable condition on one group and a subsequent comparison to another group without the dietary condition. Does that sound like a difficult situation to set up? Yes, indeed it would be. In some respects it would be easier to make the intervention a dosage form that provides the sort of nutrient components of fruits and vegetables that are suspected of being capable of producing such a benefit as lowering the rate of cancer. Indeed, that would provide a cleaner approach because one group may receive a real nutrient formulation while the other receives a simulated one, which in research parlance would be dubbed the "placebo." This will be explained further on following pages. The important take-home message is that epidemiology prepares the way for experiments that are called "clinical trials."

Human (i.e., clinical) trials intended for submission to the FDA for approval of a therapy are classified into one of four phases, Phase I, II, III, or IV as defined by the FDA in the Code of Federal Regulations.[4] These clinical trials are designated, based on the type of questions that a study is seeking to answer, as the following:

- *Phase I:* Researchers test a new drug or other treatment in a small group of healthy people (20 to 80) for the first time to evaluate its safety, to establish the safe dose range, and to identify prominent or frequent side effects.
- *Phase II:* The study drug (other treatment) is given to a larger group of patients (100 to 300) to further evaluate its safety and also its therapeutic effectiveness.
- *Phase III:* The study drug (or other treatment) is given to large groups of people (1,000 to 3,000) to confirm its efficacy, monitor side effects, make comparisons to therapies already in use, and to collect data that allow a treatment to be used safely.
- *Phase IV:* The post-marketing period during which attention is paid to possible "signals" of a previously unrecognized adverse response to the agent. This must depend on reporting of adverse events by physicians. Studies during this period often are comparisons to existing products that may serve mostly commercial aims, which has recently brought criticisms in that direction (e.g., Warner, 2004).

The first three phases of study for a new agent (or procedure) are required as the basis for a New Drug Application (NDA) submitted for review by the FDA. If an NDA is approved, a fourth phase occurs, which consists of "postmarketing surveillance." Whereas this is a standard process after introduction of all prescription drugs, it is not required for dietary supplements, nor are the initial three phases. It is known that some responses of patients are likely to be discovered only during broadscale usage after the drug is marketed simply because of the rarity with which they occur. Unfortunately, it may not be possible to detect rarely occurring adverse effects prior to this stage, which means that some users of a new Rx product may experience fatal outcomes. If many such incidents occur it may provoke the withdrawal of a pharmaceutical after its marketing. Because monitoring comparable to that of Phase IV is not required for a new dietary supplement (owing to the logic used in the framing of DSHEA that such products are intrinsically nontoxic), no systematic basis exists for determining whether a new (or old) supplement agent is safe or may have an unrecognized toxicity. Neither will the benefit of their having undergone Phases I, II, and III exist.

SCIENTIFIC VALIDATION OF EFFICACY: THE "GOLD STANDARD"

By the latter decades of the twentieth century, the phrase "gold standard" had come to be applied to one mode of clinical testing for new therapies. This standard is described by the phrase "prospective, randomized, double-blind(ed), placebo-controlled clinical trial" (see www.jameslindlibrary.org). However, this gold standard was not yet established as recently as 1974, and many good or excellent drugs preceded it. Most drugs previously had been recognized as effective through after-the-fact gathering of data in human subjects, which is known as a retrospective (literally, "looking backward") study. This has most often been the style of data gathering that has occurred with supplements.

An unstated characteristic of research that meets the "gold standard" is that it must be based upon a rather large number of participants. A basic fact of statistical analysis pertains to a research needing to have a "large enough" number of participants (patients or subjects) to detect a difference between treated and control groups. The smaller the difference may be, the larger the number of subjects must be to detect reliably the effect. Also, when the number of subjects is small, the uncertainty of whether a seeming difference is a real one is increased. The high cost of running clinical trials depends to a great degree upon the need to use group sizes in the hundreds to thousands of participants. This expense factor has generally kept the supplement industry from attempting to achieve the same standard required of pharmaceuticals, especially since supplements were exempted from such by DSHEA. The bottom line rules. However, absence or infrequency of data on supplements from studies meeting the gold standard is a major reason that recognition is withheld by mainline medical authorities.

In order that another fundamental principle of statistical science be fully satisfied, all participants in a clinical (or laboratory) study must receive the assignment to different groups in such a random manner that all participants have an equal opportunity to receive assignment to all of the groups involved. If the assignments are so handled, the study qualifies *randomized.* Moreover, it is critical that the sample studied is actually fully representative of the whole population to which the results are intended to apply. If representative sampling is inadequate the resulting sampling error prevents the outcome from being valid for the full population. In 2002 it was discovered that sampling error had occurred in many earlier studies of the possible benefits of hormone replacement therapy and had invalidated the application of outcomes and conclusions from those samples. They can no longer be applied to the whole population of women in the United States. This example of the serious adverse impact of sampling error and faulty experimental design in research will be discussed further in Chapter 3.

What are these different groups to which assignment should be randomly decided? Obviously, two groups might exist for high and low levels of a treatment, drug, or otherwise. However, another group must be established that does *not* receive the treatment being tested; in the case of a drug, this would be a "zero-dose" group, which is known as a *control group.* Without such a group the study would be uncontrolled rather than controlled. Generally such a group must, however, be given a semblance of a treatment. If the actual treatment is an injected solution, then the control group must receive an injection of the fluid in which the drug is dissolved in exactly the same manner (volume, schedule, etc.) as the treated group(s). An alternative accepted in some instances is an "active control" group receiving a currently standard treatment for the condition.

To eliminate the possibility of a psychological bias influencing their response, the participant should not be told their group assignment, and preferably (in so much as is possible) should not be able to figure it out. Thus, they initially were described as "blinded," which generally became shortened to *blind.* Moreover, the persons running the trial and observing the participants (the medical and nursing staff) so as to record the response(s) should also be prevented from knowing who is in which group, lest that knowledge be allowed to exert an unconscious influence (bias) on their perceptions. In earlier times when only participants were unknowing, the study would be described as "single-blind." When it was appreciated that the observer's bias could lead to false conclusions, it became routine or standard for both sides to be blind(ed), and thus we arrived at the *double-*

blind condition as fundamental for clinical research studies. That leaves us to explain the final term from the gold standard phrase, *placebo-controlled,* which we will now do at greater length

THE USE OF PLACEBO CONTROL GROUPS IN HUMAN RESEARCH

Placebo is a word taken from Latin that means "to please." As used in medicine, the word initially meant an inactive substance knowingly prescribed with the intent of satisfying symbolically a patient's perception of their need (or at least desire) for drug therapy. A common view is that many (if not most) medicines dispensed at the turn of the nineteenth century to the twentieth could exert no greater effect than that of a placebo. Aside from ether and chloroform (the volatile anesthetics used in surgery), alcohol, opium (or morphine), quinine, bromides, and the arsenic-containing chemicals for treating syphilis, the available medicines were mainly undistinguished herbal concoctions. In later times little or no specific drug activity could be demonstrated for such herbal remedies when more scrupulous methods of testing were applied.

Later the contemporary definition of a placebo came into usage as meaning an inert dosage form employed as a control in human drug studies. Its purpose is in effect to define an untreated baseline condition to enable a comparative quantitative measure of the efficacy of a new medicinal substance or other therapy. But to avoid a negative bias that would occur if the persons received no treatment, the inactive (sometimes called "sham" or "dummy") treatment is administered in a similar manner as the actual one. Thus, persons taking the placebo provide a baseline to which the response of the same persons, or an independent group, must be compared via statistical analysis when evaluating the test therapy for improvement of the condition to be treated. Unless the test responses are found to be significantly superior by statistical procedures one cannot conclude that any benefit or value exists to the candidate product. Basic limitations of statistical analysis are such that they never allow an absolute conclusion concerning such comparisons. An element of doubt or uncertainty about the results of either laboratory or clinical test results always exists, as will be considered further in Chapter 3.

Thus, medical research has arrived at a standard that requires a randomized, double-blind, placebo-controlled clinical trial for valid scientific data to be obtained on the efficacy of both new and old pharmaceuticals. However, it must be recognized that this standard has been introduced progressively over merely the past one-third of a century in the United States.

Skepticism of physicians or medical scientists about botanicals and many nutritional supplements arises mainly from the general lack of data obtained through tests meeting this standard for a recognition as "evidence-based." Many dietary supplements have not been convincingly demonstrated to be superior to a placebo for the uses advocated for them. One major exception to the attitude of doctors that supplements are "unproven" is in the use of vitamins or minerals to correct well-defined deficiency diseases that arise from dietary insufficiency (malnourishment) or from an innate or acquired hindrance to their absorption and/or utilization by a patient.

Efficacy of a supplement generally must be shown in terms of one (or better, several) substantial quantitative or semiquantitative measure(s) that provide objective evidence for improvement of the condition being treated. Mere testimonials on behalf of any intervention reporting that persons feel better, function better, or show other sorts of positive changes in the condition being treated are not acceptable as scientific evidence. A major reason is that it is impossible to tell to what degree a placebo effect has caused or contributed to such changes.

Placebo Effects May Be Real, Not Just "In Your Head" or "Imaginary"

The concept implicit in the phrase "placebo effect" is a fundamentally important one to this discussion. Medicine has come to recognize that an inactive placebo dosage form (or other sham therapeutic procedure) can exert a quantifiable influence on a patient's symptoms. This often is in terms of feeling better but may also be negative in terms of feeling more ill or developing new symptoms. In at least some situations such feelings have been found to be paralleled by actual physical measurements. An illustrative example from the medical research literature is from tests to detect an antinauseant activity for a drug to oppose nausea and emesis (vomiting). In human studies of a new antinauseant-antiemetic a placebo was found to exert a significant favorable effect. Some persons believing that they had received an active agent for this purpose not only reported a reduction of nausea but also showed a diminished level of a type of stomach contractions that are associated with nausea and that precede vomiting.

The important area of pain relief is remarkably subject to the placebo effect. Not everyone shows this pain relief from a placebo equally, but a great many persons will report roughly a one-third reduction in their symptoms, whether pain, nausea, or various other states. For this reason, the randomized, nonsystematic assignment of persons to the test or placebo group can be a critical factor. A nonrandom assignment of participants might lead to more "placebo responders" in a treatment or control group. This would prevent a statistical analysis from being valid. The placebo effect requires that for a therapy to be validated it must exert an effect significantly superior to the responses to a placebo in the same or another suitable group of patients. For this reason a major component of scientific validation tests for any remedy must be the inclusion of a placebo control group along with random assignment to the experimental groups.

That a candidate agent must show superior benefit in a therapeutic trial to a response occurring when the placebo is taken seems a straightforward, minimal expectation for the validation of new therapies. However, this expectation is not always fulfilled. Davis et al. (2001) showed that results may sometimes indeed be contrary. Women who had required therapy for troublesome menopausal symptoms were treated with a combination of 12 herbs reputed to be of value for this condition. However, the combination proved to be significantly less effective than a placebo. The authors concluded that women should choose estrogenic hormone therapy for relief of menopausal symptoms rather than experimenting with such herbal treatments.

Recent advances in clinical neuroscience research include some that bear on the reality of the placebo effect (Holden, 2002). Much new research involves use of modern imaging technics that enables visualization of the brain "in action." These "functional" methods include MRI (magnetic resonance imaging) and PET (positron emission tomography) scanning as the basis for many significant new modes of diagnosis, e.g., routine MRI of the spine for detection of ruptured discs and of the brain for detecting multiple sclerosis, tumor growths, or blood vessel defects in a stroke. These are also very effective research tools of basic neuroscience. A remarkable report by Petrovic et al. (2002) showed great similarity of the functional PET scan after an active opioid (morphinelike) analgesic and after a dose of a placebo. Intravenous injections of both the real analgesic solution and a placebo solution were followed by an image-activation representing an increase of blood flow to an area of the brain known for its association with receptors for endogenous opioid peptides. Those who responded with the greatest pain reduction from the placebo solution also were the ones who showed the most activation of the PET scan.

Ethical Status of Research Using a Placebo Control Group

It has been questioned whether medical researchers may ethically use a placebo as a control rather than an active agent believed to provide some benefit for some serious disease condition. For example, it was questioned whether using a known-to-be inactive placebo control for studies on Alzheimer's disease (AD) is still ethically proper after benefits of donepezil and vitamin E to such patients had been established (Karlawish and Whitehouse, 1998). The query relates to a rather lengthy treatment-observation period needed to test whether a new therapy might slow the progression of a loss of brain functions. In AD it is no longer permissible to use a placebo control because no accepted active therapies exists. To do so now means that patients receiving a placebo are being deprived of a probable benefit. This principle has been applied already for some clinical researches, e.g., therapies for cancer and epilepsy, wherein new therapies may be tested as add-ons for their ability to increase significantly the benefits from prior-accepted medicines.

META-ANALYSES OF CLINICAL PHARMACOLOGIC INTERVENTIONS: USEFUL BUT NOT PERFECT

A meta-analysis is a method for the quantitative synthesis of two or more research studies concerning the same outcome measure with the same treatment. Meta-analyses are key components of decision making in the pursuit of an evidence-based standard for a particular therapy. This is the main means for handling the data when the results of different studies are discordant or contrasting. As with other modes of statistical analysis, a well-conducted meta-analysis may be quite valuable, but a poorly conducted one may lead to false conclusions. It has been stated recently that the science of meta-analyses is imperfect. Detecting the weaknesses or fallacies in an analysis of research data is often difficult even for workers in the area of research unless obvious violations of proper methods are involved. The point to be made is that the reader may need an awareness of this means of analyzing multiple researches on a topic, all of which will not give identical outcomes, so as to arrive at a comprehensive answer to the question being pursued.

Meta-analysis has the ability to pool the findings from a number of smaller studies so as to derive a more precise and reliable conclusion than was achieved by any single study. In one actual example, eight different randomized trials were individually underpowered (i.e., having too small a number of patients in each) to detect reliably any reduction in mortality when streptokinase was administered to patients with acute myocardial infarction (heart attack). But when the data from all eight were pooled via meta-analysis, a more precise and reliable estimate for the value of using streptokinase was obtained—a 20 percent reduction in mortality. Without available data being from multiple studies on a question, the results of which have been submitted to meta-analysis, persons who are strongly committed to an evidence-based approach will not acknowledge that any evidence exists in favor of or supporting usage of a particular treatment (Anonymous, 1992). It is only a rather small fraction of all dietary supplements for which enough "acceptable" research studies have been done to demonstrate efficacy by the process of meta-analysis.

BIASES OF MEDICAL-RELATED PROFESSIONALS

A negative bias against alternative medical agents—botanicals and nutritionals—is unquestionably involved in their nonacceptance by many if not most contemporary health professionals. They would declare this to be based upon the lack of positive evidence for supplements having value. Few physicians, nurses, and even pharmacists now in practice were taught anything about dietary supplements in their professional curricula. In essence, because supplements were ignored, the students were taught to regard supplements, especially botanicals, as not "real" (i.e., not significant) agents for improvement or recovery of one's health.

An article by two physicians (Goodwin and Tangum, 1998) examined the sources of a negative bias of medical school professors toward nutrient supplements (*not* botanicals). They concluded that resistance to vitamin and other nutrients as therapies arises because support for nutritional therapies comes from outside of medical schools; i.e., opposition stems from a narrow prejudice against "truths" being supplied by "outsiders."

Physicians also have been actively led to think of botanicals, if they were attended to at all, as merely placebos. However, currently some movement is occurring toward revising and rethinking such prejudiced attitudes and expanding the knowledge of health care professionals in this area. This is largely a consequence of the pressure arising from the public's greatly enlarged acceptance and usage of herbals and nutritionals. This change is being promoted, for example, by medical schools introducing a new curricular aspect known as "integrative medicine," which represents an effort to incorporate those topics of CAM that are validated. How serious are such curricular changes? Some observers suspect them of being merely window-dressing, but that remains to be seen. With enlarged federal research funding toward CAM remedies it may be anticipated that some such remedies will cross over into an accepted status when enough positive evidence is obtained. However, it seems likely that the present dominant orientation to prescribing drug and ignoring nutritional medicine will not soon be greatly altered.

CONFLICT OF INTEREST

However, a bias of greater concern is that which may occur in the conduct of clinical studies to evaluate the efficacy and safety of both pharmaceuticals and supplements. In 2003, several state and federal judges handed down judgments against makers of ephedra-containing (or other) supplement products for false advertising. At question was the truthfulness or validity of their claims for clinical results supporting the weight-reduction benefits of the products against which charges were brought. An "expert" was quoted in the *New York Times* as saying that quality of research studies for supplement products is "somewhat notably less than for a drug study." Even a supplement industry spokesman acknowledged that whenever a desired outcome exists, the potential for bias exists.

By this he meant that a researcher financially supported by a supplement producer knows what sort of outcome is hoped for (or expected), and this may exert an influence toward that outcome. An old saying that may apply here is "Whose bread I eat—his song I sing." Indeed, a significant number of incidents have occurred in which the pharmaceutical industry supported an outside clinical investigator who played fast and loose with the data so as to satisfy his source of funding. A study published in the *Journal of the American Medical Association (JAMA)* (Als-Nielsen et al., 2003) was based on an examination of 370 randomized drug trials. It found that the clinical trials of candidate new drugs funded by for-profit sources tended to be more favorable than ones that were funded by nonprofit sources. Interpreting the trial results in a biased manner is one way that this contrast might occur, but it also could result from numerous subtle factors such as choice of where emphasis is placed among several alternative outcome measures or subgroups. In a celebrated case in the 1990s an investigator adamantly refused to "play ball" and comply with the sponsor's pressure to suppress her negative findings, which were clearly not what the sponsor expected or wished to receive. An Internet search on "conflict of interest" and "physicians" on January 19, 2004, obtained a very high number of hits.

Some critics feel that the FDA review process is not stringent enough to prevent market access to Rx drugs that will prove to cause a level of fatal adverse reactions. Studies required to meet FDA regulations for bringing a new drug to approval for marketing are much more than they were 40 years ago, but is the public being sufficiently protected even now? Since no clinical testing requirements for the supplement products exist, their producers clearly spend the money for clinical trials only if or when they expect that doing so will be rewarded by better sales. In short, it should be no surprise if biased results were to be reported from any developer-sponsored human trial, whether in evaluating a supplement or a pharmaceutical. Moreover, instances have occurred in which the clinical trials supported by a pharmaceutical company allegedly have been utilized selectively, i.e., to submit "good" trials and to suppress ones that do not show a favorable response, or show an adverse one, to the candidate drug product. This would appear to be a serious ethical lapse that should be made illegal for public safety.

The problem of conflict of interest among medical researchers who receive funding from industrial sources is increasingly being discussed in clinical and biomedical journals. In September 2001 the editors of 13 medical journals (including *JAMA, New England Journal of Medicine,* and *The Lancet*) co-authored a signed statement that highlighted their concerns about financial conflicts of interest in the development of medical devices and Rx drugs (Davidson et al., 2001). The former editor-in-chief of the *New England Journal of Medicine* has joined the ranks of physicians writing "exposés" on the contemporary health care system and the role of the pharmaceutical industry in the practice of medicine, with a large emphasis on conflict of interest (Angell, 2004).

Since the onset of the twenty-first century many revelations have been made that "financial transfers" that are potentially corrupting occur not only to physicians involved in drug tests but also to "run-of-the-mill" doctors whose prescribing practices might be influenced by benefits. These at times include travel to "medical meetings" dealing only with the sponsors' topics—their products—in very attractive vacation locales. One major medical journal dropped its requirement for a conflict-of-interest-free status for writers of their editorials (who usually are academics writing comments on an article) when it became evident that they could no longer find a sufficient supply of writers who were conflict-free and thus presumably unbiased. A medical school professor who published a strong critique (Bodenheimer, 2000b) presented an even more critical analysis on medical conflicts of interest via the Internet (Bodenheimer, 2000a).

Another point of concern of concern in the realm of conflicts of interest in the arena of medical research was directed toward even senior clinical researchers at the National Institutes of Health (NIH). In late 2002 and 2003 it became known, with first revelations coming from the *Los Angeles Times,* that NIH regulations had been loosened to allow NIH staffers to receive, but not to report, very generous consultant fees from pharmaceutical or related biotechnology companies. The question rising from this information is whether scientists' contracting with industry may lead to their not conducting impartial and objective research for the sole good of the American people.

PHARMACEUTICAL PRODUCERS LIVE IN GLASS HOUSES

The vested economic interests of the pharmaceutical industry and its academic clinical collaborators supply the industry with plenty of reasons to be negative toward CAM approaches, which extract money from the same pockets from which the industry reaps its profits. However, their own tactics are under question for the validity of the "promising new drugs" that the industry hypes via direct-to-consumer media blitzes (Warner, 2004). The appropriateness of much "me-too" marketing of multiple new members of the same action class is one practice criticized by a few stalwart physicians willing to go "against the flow."

From Australia has come a critical operation known as Adwatch, a Web-based analysis of "the logical, psychological and pharmacological tricks" of drug advertising (Sweet, 2003).

This also raises the point that members of the "in-group" of scientific medicine are on shaky ground when pointing fingers at the supplement situation when their own bailiwick of both premarketing and postmarketing drug testing of Rx drugs are being indicted for practices that clearly have economic rather than scientific justification uppermost. Indeed, attacks also have been directed at postmarketing misbehavior.

THE PROBLEM OF DELAYED EFFECTS: EXAMPLES OF LONG-TERM TOXICITY ISSUES

It is difficult enough to evaluate the early effects of a candidate drug, but it is very much more difficult and costly to document a possible delayed adverse response to a short-term exposure. Likewise, documenting a delayed benefit (e.g., reduced probability of developing a disease) or a delayed adverse effect of a nonnutrient supplement is a very daunting task. Inducing of a cancer, for example, or the reducing the risk for cancer cannot be determined for a single individual but can only be demonstrated as an increase or a reduction in the statistical probability of disease over a large sample of persons. This problem with a supposedly beneficial effect will be discussed at length in the next chapter.

Possible Genotoxicity (Genetic Damage)

An example from among many possible examples concerning the difficulty in evaluating the safety for chronic use of a dietary supplement relates to chromium picolinate (CP). This agent is sold and promoted for its supposed ability to reduce body fat and to help build muscle. It also has been suggested that CP may reduce the risk of cardiovascular disease by opposing the complications of diabetes, especially type 2 diabetes (non-insulin-dependent diabetes mellitus). It has become a common ingredient of products ranging from supplement formulations to sports drinks and chewing gum. Nevertheless, it is not known what may happen in the human body, or even whole laboratory animals, when CP is consumed on a chronic basis.

Feeding studies in rodents should last for one year or more to be definitive. Reproductive studies also would be another needed test to detect possible injury to the DNA of the sex chromosomes in the reproductive cells. Clearly, the current widespread use of CP by young people (e.g., in "power bars" and sports drinks) is of greater concern than their usage by older persons past the reproductive phase of life who are the main population at risk for type 2 diabetes.

Possible Induction of Cancer

The process of chemical carcinogenesis, the induction of cancer owing to exposure to a certain chemical, is fundamentally a long-delayed toxic consequence. It may be a response to only a limited-time exposure, from hours to days or weeks, or it may involve exposure for months to years. Subsequently, the person who experiences a potential carcinogenic exposure will not manifest a readily detectable response within merely weeks or months but years later. Moreover, it would be exceptional if the delay for human beings were merely several years or even less than a decade. In most known cases the delay is more likely to be two or three decades. This long interval between exposure and disease manifestation makes it quite difficult and unlikely for some sources of cancer induction to be recognized. This fact is a reason for criticizing the increasingly broad exposure to botanical supplements among children, adolescents, or even young adults. They will generally live long enough for delayed toxicity, such as carcinogenesis, to be manifested, whereas mature and older adults are less likely to have that liability.

A recent instructive example from the herbal product arena is the occurrence of kidney cancers that has been attributed to herbs of the genus *Aristolochia.* More precisely, the injury is attributable to their component known as aristolochic acid. An outbreak among western European women of kidney injury and failure came to be associated with exposures such that it was dubbed "Chinese herbal nephropathy." This epidemic of severe kidney injury focused attention on those women, many of whom required a kidney transplant for survival, otherwise it might not have been readily discovered that renal carcinogenesis (cancer induction) had also begun in some cases. More details of this story are supplied in Chapter 29. Three unanswered questions remain: (1) whether persons in the United States already were similarly affected before the banning of aristolochic acid-containing botanicals, (2) whether similar hazards from other botanicals exist that have not yet been recognized, and (3) how to ensure against accidental or intentional adulteration of botanical mixtures from other countries, which can be readily accessed via the Internet.

Chapter 3

The Uncertainty Principle in Medicine

Even after good research, no remedy can be known to be either safe or effective with 100 percent certainty.

One of the greatest difficulties that the general reader will encounter in this book is dealing with uncertainty, i.e., the gap between what we wish and need to know versus what we can and cannot know about the safety and effectiveness of a dietary supplement that we might take for any intended purpose. Readers likely wish to know for certain whether a supplement product will benefit him or her and whether the product is or is not safe. The flat, honest fact of the matter is that in many if not most instances we cannot answer these questions for certain. Although it applies broadly, this problem is less the case with immediate-onset (acute) effects and more the case for delayed-onset (chronic) effects. This is also true for prescription drugs in the U.S. market. Whether the degree of uncertainty differs between supplements and pharmaceuticals will be one of the significant issues to be considered through this book.

WHEN THE GOLD STANDARD CANNOT BE MET

Many drug evaluations at times encounter the one criterion that may be difficult or impossible to meet: blinding. Most dietary supplements have such characteristics that this problem is less likely to occur. When the dosage form is an oral tablet or capsule or an ointment or cream for cutaneous application, a placebo tablet or capsule or topical preparation may be made to look identical to the test agent. If the form is a colorless solution for injection, a placebo solution with no visible difference can be used. On the other hand, an oral liquid preparation is almost certain to have a taste that will require masking. Although difficult, the equating of a test agent in liquid form

doi:10.1300/5698_03

with a placebo may be possible. However, in all of these instances rapid-onset actions may exist consisting of a perceptible internal response that will cue the trial participants that they are getting an active agent rather than a placebo, and the blinding will have failed. This is more the case when the same participants at different times receive both active and placebo treatments, i.e., a "crossover design" in which they serve as their own control group. Without blinding of the subject, the use of a placebo in a control group becomes fruitless. Not being a blind comparison, the operation of bias can enter the trial and call into question the validity of the outcome. A certainty that bias has operated may not exist, but the presence of bias often cannot be excluded. Some human trials of dietary supplements were not conducted according to these standards. A strict interpretation will say that any "evidence" gathered in this manner is unscientific and unacceptable. Whether the test results might be correct rather than wrong is another question that cannot be settled. Uncertainty wins!

When the condition under treatment is life-threatening, an ethical problem exists concerning use of an inactive placebo. A solution to this has at times been for a test agent to be added to an existing active agent, while the control group receives a placebo plus the existing treatment. An example is for therapy of epilepsy. Although some oriental botanicals are claimed to benefit epileptic patients, their being tested in scientific manner seems unlikely to occur because of the expense involved. Tradition is the sole or main justification for the claim of benefit from using such traditional medicines. No real evidence exists to support or refute the claims. Again, uncertainty prevails.

THE PROBLEM OF VALIDATING DELAYED EFFECTS OF LONG-TERM THERAPY

The Postmenopausal Estrogen Saga

For the second half of the twentieth century, drug companies have tried with considerable success to convince physicians that estrogenic hormone was the key to keeping women eternally young by their taking it indefinitely from the beginning of menopause. Western medicine has mainly bought the story it was told and sold, and physicians have been encouraging women to initiate estrogenic hormone replacement therapy (HRT) from the onset of menopause and to continue it through the subsequent years of postmenopausal life, despite the fact that no scientific foundation existed for doing this. In prior centuries too few women lived much beyond menopause for data to be available about their physiological conditions in postmenopausal years.

Initially, HRT was motivated by women's desire for relief from various symptoms of discomfort characterizing the menopause, especially hot flashes, mood changes, and reduced lubrication (vaginal secretion associated with sexual arousal) resulting in vaginal dryness. Reversal of such symptoms is an early benefit of HRT that can be recognized readily and with a high degree of certainty by all women taking HRT for this purpose.

However, as time passed HRT came to be promoted for other supposed benefits, particularly a reduction of the risk for cardiovascular disease leading to heart attacks and for weakening of the bones (osteoporosis) leading to higher fracture rates in women's postmenopausal life. Moreover, HRT was also promoted not only with a view to reducing urinary incontinence and depression but also for a supposed lowering of the risk for Alzheimer's disease. All of these supposed benefits are not easily recognized and documented with statistical confidence. They are much more difficult to validate for the reason that they do not appear immediately as does repression of the menopausal symptoms. Also, rather than the outcome measure being cessation of a symptom, the endpoint for the desired effect in these cases is that a woman does not develop a disease condition, and the target conditions do not ordinarily occur in all women anyway. Thus, when after some years of HRT any woman does not develop osteoporosis it cannot be known whether she would have developed it or not without HRT.

After many years of their giving only equivocal support, HRT was finally endorsed in 1992 by the American College of Physicians and the U.S. Preventive Services Task Force. They recognized the existence of biologically plausible mechanisms of action for supposing that estrogen therapy could be protective against cardiovascular disease. Laboratory animal experimental data were supplemented by observational data in women suggesting that HRT did indeed confer cardiovascular benefits. This endorsement did not arise from prospective randomized clinical trials, but rather it relied almost exclusively on clinical experience, i.e., physicians' observational findings in the patients they treated, the sort of observational "data" that are denounced as totally inadequate grounds for accepting unconventional CAM therapies.

Moreover, those observational data were gained from studying self-selected, nonrandomized samples of women who chose to receive HRT at their doctor's suggestion or from their outright requesting it. This aspect immediately made the sampling to be biased and the conclusions to be applicable only to women having the same profile as those in this nonrandom sample. Looking backward, it came to be recognized that the women observed after receiving HRT over past years had features not representative of all women of that age group. They tended to be wealthier, healthier, and more health-conscious than the norm. In short, factors besides HRT were present that could have contributed to their more favorable long-term condition.

Unfortunately, such analyses of a database merely accumulated rather than being collected according to strict scientific guidelines cannot provide a scientific evaluation. In essence, the use of HRT for delayed benefits such as reducing the risks for heart attack, stroke, or osteoporosis problems was not at all "evidence based." Indeed, when outcomes of well-designed and well-conducted primary (and secondary) prevention tests via randomized clinical trials for opposing cardiovascular disease became available, they showed that women had an *increased* cardiovascular risk rather than a benefit.

2002 Bombshells and Reversal of HRT Evaluation

Long after their 1992 endorsements, expert members of the Committee for the International Position Paper on Women's Health and the Menopause issued a monograph that renounced the former belief that HRT (either estrogen or estrogen plus a progestin) reduced the risk for heart attack by 35 to 50 percent (Vastag, 2002). Findings of a study reported in February 2002 suggested that older women who were taking the two sex hormones for HRT, except for those who were still suffering hot flashes without estrogen, did not even show improvement in their emotional and physical well-being. For women who were not experiencing hot flashes, HRT may have actually worsened their level of physical functioning. The researchers called the results surprising and said they cast doubt on the widespread and popular belief, encouraged quite explicitly by HRT drug advertisements, that taking hormones after menopause can make most women feel more youthful, active, and vibrant.

In a large randomized, double-blind, placebo-controlled study, not only did HRT fail to reduce the risk of heart attacks and strokes, but it also significantly increased the occurrence rate for blood clots and gallbladder disease. The reason that findings and conclusions of the recent study differed from those of the prior studies is believed to be because the former studies had been obtained from a sample of women that was not representative of women in the general population.

Another clinical trial on HRT for heart disease concluded in 2002 also showed that HRT failed to reduce the rate of coronary attacks in women with established coronary disease (Hlatky et al., 2002). This was the Heart and Estrogen/Progestin Replacement Study (HERS), which administered conjugated equine estrogens, 0.625 mg/day, plus medroxyprogesterone acetate, 2.5 mg/day, in one tablet (Prempro). The placebo group consisted of 2,763 women having an intact uterus but who had an already-documented state of coronary heart disease (CHD) before randomization. The HERS finding of no overall effect with years on CHD, but rather an apparent increase in risk during the first year of therapy, was surprising in light of prior studies on HRT in women with CHD that had reported a favorable response (Hulley et al., 1998; Pettiti, 1998).

The Women's Health Initiative (WHI) study was a large randomized, placebo-controlled, primary-prevention trial that had been planned for a duration of 8.5 years. WHI included 16,608 postmenopausal women aged 50 to 79 years having an intact uterus at baseline. These women were recruited by 40 U.S. clinical centers during 1993-1998. They then had either the same regimen of estrogen plus progestin as in the HERS study (Prempro; 8,506 participants) or a placebo (8,102 participants). The primary anticipated positive measure of WHI that could be quantitated was incidence of CHD (nonfatal myocardial infarction) or CHD death, and a higher rate of invasive breast cancer was a primary anticipated adverse outcome (Writing Group, 2002). A global index summarizing the balance of risks and benefits included the two primary outcomes plus secondary endpoints consisting of rates for stroke, pulmonary embolism, endometrial cancer, colorectal cancer, hip fracture, and death from other causes. On May 31, 2002, after a mean of 5.2 years of follow-up, the data and safety monitoring board recommended also stopping this trial of estrogen plus progestin versus placebo because the test statistic for invasive breast cancer exceeded the preset stopping level for this adverse effect, and the global index statistic supported a conclusion that risks were exceeding benefits.

Other disturbing findings threw doubt on the ability of HRT to reduce the rate of fractures. Women in this trial who took HRT had a slightly *higher* rate of hip fractures than those taking a placebo, which was contrary to expectations. Moreover, indications of a significantly increased risk for blood clotting incidents and biliary tract disease existed. It was already widely accepted that "estrogen-only" HRT was likely to raise the risk for uterine cancer. This was the reason that estrogen plus progesterone had become the standard for HRT except for women who had already undergone removal of their uterus. However, the addition of progesterone is not believed to alter the belief that estrogen replacement increases the risk for breast cancer. Thus, the long-awaited evidence-based evaluation concluded that HRT not only failed to provide the expected primary benefits regarding cardiovascular health, but also lacked the assumed safety from adverse changes.

Negative News in 2005: Synthetic Estrogens Might Cause Urinary Incontinence

One of the benefits claimed for continuing estrogen replacement therapy was reduction of women suffering urinary incontinence. However, another analysis of the WHI study instead found the opposite. In the study of more than 27,000 women between ages of 50 and 79 years, those who took estrogen for one year were 53 percent more likely to develop urinary incontinence than those who took a placebo dosage form. Women whose treatment included both estrogen and progestin had a 39 percent greater risk. Women taking the estrogen more than doubled their risk for stress incontinence, and those taking estrogen and progestin had similar results. Risks were most severe for stress incontinence in which urine leakage is a result of increased pressure on the abdomen when sneezing, laughing, or coughing. The WHI study had previously found that HRT increased the risk of heart attacks, strokes, breast cancer, and dementia. Those findings caused millions of menopausal women to stop using the hormones. In fact, prescriptions for those medicines fell to 11 million in the first half of 2004 from 16 million in early 2002 after first results of the study were released.

THE SIGNIFICANCE OF IT ALL

The story of the HRT developments dramatically emphasizes the extreme difficulty and high cost in time and money of "finding the truth" *with certainty* about either the favorable or adverse effects of *any* treatment. The reasons for the halting of several of the largest and most carefully designed studies was because it was discovered that women taking hormones after menopause had a greater risk of breast cancer, heart attack, stroke, and blood clots. An adequate effort toward the goal of "finding the truth" requires thousands of patients who by random assignment receive either the agent to be studied or a placebo. Testing endpoints must be carefully defined beforehand, and they must consider both positive and negative outcomes. Even though the HRT example was chosen from among pharmaceutical interventions, the principle is equally true of dietary changes, nutritional supplement use, or long-term intake of even small amounts of herbal components that lately are being incorporated into foods and beverages. Without prior evidence from randomized, placebo-controlled, double-blind evaluations one does not have a scientifically valid basis from which to reach conclusions with a degree of confidence, much less with certainty.

This applies to either efficacy or safety and to both short-term and long-term intake of most dietary supplements. The HRT example is of special significance to us in light of the recent popularity among some women of using phytoestrogens as a "natural" alternative form of HRT. Moreover, it bears on the unintentional exposures to phytoestrogens from the widening use of soy derivatives among persons of all ages and both sexes. Such concerns about soy are discussed in Chapter 15.

In addition, CAM practitioners are pursuing an alternative hormone replacement therapy that is claimed to be more physiological because it utilizes the natural human steroids rather the equine steroids isolated from pregnant mare urine in the case of Premarin and Prempro. This approach has been dubbed "bioidentical" therapy, and it has been available through certain compounding pharmacies that conduct small-scale production of steroid hormone dosage forms.

This trend has not been ignored by pharmaceutical manufacturers. For example, in October 2004 BioSante Pharmaceuticals, Inc. announced its ongoing Phase III clinical trial of Bio-E-Gel, a "bioidentical estradiol transdermal gel" for the treatment of moderate-to-severe hot flashes and vaginal atrophy in menopausal women. This study to support a New Drug Application was on track to enroll all the needed subjects by end-of-year 2004, and it was planned to be completed by the end of the first quarter 2005. Bio-E-Gel Phase data for efficacy and pharmacokinetics data were presented at an October 8, 2004, meeting of the North American Menopause Society. All doses studied in the Phase II trial showed significant decreases in the frequency and severity of hot flashes versus baseline conditions. A Phase III trial being conducted in the United States and Canada was a randomized, 12-week, double-blind, placebo-controlled study of symptomatic menopausal women. BioSante also had in its developmental pipeline a product LibiGel consisting of a bioidentical testosterone gel for treatment of female sexual dysfunction (low libido), and Bio-T-Gel bioidentical testosterone gel for treatment of men with testosterone deficiency. Also being developed was a combination female hormone therapy gel product of estradiol and progestin.

WHAT IS A DIETARY SUPPLEMENT?

Are you aware that the same molecule may be classed as either a drug or a dietary supplement? To be a dietary supplement requires that the molecule be a naturally occurring one rather than one known only from a synthetic chemical process in the laboratory. Those natural molecules that are derived from plants are called "botanicals." Some (but not all) botanicals are rightly subclassified as "herbals." That is, all herbals are botanicals, but not all botanicals come from herbs. A botanical is not an herb unless it is derived from an annual plant. According to *Merriam-Webster's Collegiate Dictionary,* eleventh edition, an herb is "a seed-producing annual, biennial, or perennial that does not develop persistent woody tissue but dies down at the end of a growing season." Unfortunately, imprecise usage by persons owing to either ignorance or carelessness has a long time ago equated *herbal* with *botanical* in common usage. Both words mean a plant product having utility because of some benefit to health. It must be remembered that whether a molecule has become a drug or a dietary supplement, or perhaps both, depends upon "accidents" of the time, manner, and purpose of its coming into human usage and into the marketplace. A more recent term for supplement ingredients derived from plants is *phytopharmaceutical* (or phytochemical).

An example of the chemical and functional equivalence of some supplements and pharmaceuticals may be seen in a clinical study conducted in the 1980s. Two potential interventions that were tested for the ability to slow the progression of signs and symptoms of Parkinson's disease were evaluated. They consisted of either a vitamin, alpha-tocopherol (vitamin E), or the prescription pharmaceutical, selegiline (L-deprenyl). In either case a pharmacological benefit was the aim. It is instructive to discuss several other such examples of a single chemical bearing a dual identity.

Levodopa (Rx Drug) versus L-Dopa (Supplement)

This molecule is a natural amino acid, which immediately qualifies it for use as a dietary supplement. However, its first significant human usage, apart from its being ingested as an ingredient of various foods, was about 40 years ago when it became a medicinal agent for the management of Parkinson's disease (PD). That neurologic disease is a consequence of a person's losing about 80 percent of their dopaminergic nerve cells in motor control pathways of the midbrain. *Dopaminergic* means "acting by means of dopamine," i.e., the neurotransmitter molecule dopamine is released by the nerve ends to send forward a neural message. Such neurotransmitter molecules are synthesized from a precursor amino acid, L-dopa, within the dopaminergic neuron. It was found to be possible to overcome the deficient function of such neurons by means of a "pump-priming" action of giving a large dose of the amino acid. The technical phrase for such a strategy is "precursor loading." It was indeed found that through promoting a higher level of dopamine biosynthesis by the surviving remnant of dopaminergic nerve cells a more adequate dopamine output occurs and acts to alleviate symptoms of PD.

Twenty or so years after being marketed as levodopa for treating PD the amino acid began to be seen as a component of dietary supplement products. *Mucuna pruriens,* commonly known as velvet bean, serves as a source of L-dopa for supplement producers. It is commonly presented as a component of natural products supplying antiaging benefits through an ability to promote the secretion of human growth hormone (HGH). However, little published scientific data exists to validate this alleged action (see Chapter 13 for more details). At the other end of the age spectrum, young adult bodybuilders favor formulations that include L-dopa for producing energy and facilitating weight loss by "fat burning." Again, human data to confirm these alleged effects are not supplied.

What about safety of such self-directed uses of L-dopa? It has been written concerning the therapeutic use of levodopa by PD patients that the toxic effects of levodopa are considerable. (These are compiled in Exhibit 3.1.) The pharmaceutical manufacturer originating levodopa therapy of PD was responsible for gathering data concerning the adverse responses associated with their product after its marketing. Clinical researchers evaluating the therapy then presented quantitative data on both desirable and unwanted, adverse responses. From such sources something about the level and nature of unwanted effects in therapy can be determined. Who is responsible for gathering comparable data on the usage of L-dopa-containing dietary supplements? No one! Thus, a major uncertainty about the supplements is to what degree adverse responses are occurring. If an L-dopa-containing product is combined (as users are urged to do at Internet Web sites) with creatine, synephrine (an analog of adrenaline), and 4-androstenediol (a supposed testosterone precursor), adverse effects involving the central nervous system might be expected. Could the adverse response be attributed clearly to one or another of these components? Not at all likely: uncertainty results because the situation is "confounded."

The uncertainty resulting from a simultaneous operation of multiple factors is known in statistics and in experimental science as *confounding,* a condition much to be feared and avoided. All potential conclusions from a research study will be invalid when the confounding is not recognized and eliminated in advance or otherwise compensated for by elements of the experimental design.

Again, in the case of L-dopa we must be especially concerned about the long-term exposure of children or young people since few data are available that demonstrate safety of long-term exposure.

Lovastatin As Cholestin (Supplement) versus As Mevacor (Rx Drug)

The cholesterol-lowering product Cholestin, derived from a traditional Chinese remedy made from red rice yeast, was marketed in 1996. The prod-

EXHIBIT 3.1. Adverse effects of oral levodopa intake.

Physical Side Effects

Hypotension. Low blood pressure is a common problem during the first few weeks of use, particularly if the initial dose is too high. The patient should drink lots of fluids and possibly increase salt intake to maintain normal blood pressure.
Cardiac arrythmias. In some cases the drug may cause abnormal cardiac rhythms.
Gastrointestinal effects. Stomach and intestinal side effects are common. Taking the drug with food can alleviate nausea. however, proteins interfere with intestinal absorption of levodopa, and some physicians recommend not eating any protein until nighttime in order to avoid this interference. The drug can also favor gastrointestinal bleeding.
Effects in the lung. Levodopa can cause disturbances in breathing function, although it may benefit PD patients who have upper airway obstruction. The mechanisms of such actions are unclear.
Hair loss. Most rare. Cause not known

Psychiatric/Mental Side Effects

The major adverse effects of the drug are psychiatric. Patients taking levodopa can experience the following:

Confusion
Extreme emotional states, particularly anxiety
Vivid dreams
Visual and possibly auditory hallucinations. The drug may even unmask dementia that had not been previously noticed.
Effects on learning. L-dopa appears to have mixed effects on learning. It may actually improve working memory. However, evidence suggests that it impairs areas of the brain related to other learning functions.
Sleepiness and sleep attacks

uct was rather successful and effective, but it was later found to have lovastatin, a known chemical already marketed as an Rx pharmaceutical, Mevacor, by Merck, Inc., as an active ingredient. When this became known to pharmaceutical giant Merck a suit to stop marketing of Cholestin was brought against those responsible for the product. Moreover, the FDA acted against the company for making druglike claims (what a novelty!) and later banned any further sales of lovastatin as Cholestin because it had not been used as a dietary supplement before the marketing of lovastatin as Mevacor. First come, first served? What would have happened if the Cholestin had been on the market prior to Mevacor, with the lovastatin not known yet? Would the Rx still have trumped the supplement?

Acetylcysteine As Mucomyst (Rx Drug) versus As N-Acetylcysteine (Supplement)

Again in this case the molecule is a naturally occurring amino acid derived from one of the 20 basic amino acids. Its medical use was initiated about 30 years ago as the product Mucomyst, which was named for its solution being administered by inhalation as an aerosol (mist) solution for reducing the viscosity of the mucous secretions in the respiratory tract. When their viscosity is excessive a blockage of airway function for gaseous exchange—oxygen for carbon dioxide—in the lungs may occur. Solutions are now available in a generic form.

In later years these solutions were applied by clinical toxicologists to serve as a valuable protective agent against some poisons. This protection may occur not only by action of the molecule as such but also from its serving as a precursor in a heightened production of the important "endogenous antidote," glutathione. That compound is a tripeptide, consisting of the three amino acids cysteine, glutamate, and glycine. A capacity to promote higher tissue levels of glutathione would tend to reduce short-term toxicity of injurious environmental chemicals. Indeed, glutathione is essential to protect us against normal doses of a common OTC analgesic drug, acetaminophen (e.g., Tylenol). In the case of a deficient level of glutathione a user of this analgesic agent will be at risk for toxic effects on the liver of one metabolite of acetaminophen. This circumstance applies to a poorly nourished, chronic alcoholic person whose liver has a deficit of glutathione. Thus, an alcohol abuser may show the same degree of liver injury following a normal, proper dose of acetaminophen as nonalcoholic persons would show only after intake of a very large overdose.

Another recent application for N-acetylcysteine (NAC) solution is as a thiol-supplying chemoprotectant against the toxic effects of some cancer chemotherapy agents. It acts in the bladder to oppose the cystitis provoked by the toxic metabolite acrolein, which is responsible for cyclophosphamide and ifosfamide irritating the bladder and for cisplatin causing injury to the kidneys. NAC has been shown to reduce cisplatin-induced kidney toxicity by forming a complex with it. Similar to other antioxidants, it can protect against genetic toxicity induced by an antibiotic used as an anticancer agent bleomycin.

More recently, being patent-free, NAC has appeared as a dietary supplement. In that guise the molecule is depicted as having antiaging benefits from its ability to scavenge (tie up) oxidizing free radicals, of the reactive oxygen species (ROS). These are highly reactive forms of a molecule that act to injure cells of the vital organs and are regarded as having much to do with the aging-related changes regarding loss of organ functions. Moreover, an ability to promote higher tissue levels of glutathione would tend to reduce the damaging effect of long-term exposure to some environmental chemicals or physical agents such as the ultraviolet (UV) rays of normal sunlight, which contribute to aging of the skin.

More specifically, NAC has been proposed as a supplement that may benefit sufferers from peripheral neuropathy, with consequent neuropathic pain in the feet and hands. This occurs most commonly among diabetic persons. As so frequently is true, only animal and no human data exist to encourage this application. Diabetic adult rats may serve as a model of the neuronal defects that often develop in human diabetics. After two months of NAC feeding, the peripheral nerve conduction of such rats was restored toward normal. Clearly, it would be more desirable to have similar measures taken after NAC in human patients, but the point is the comparison between usage of the same molecule as a drug and as a dietary supplement.

A high interest in promoting more adequate tissue levels of glutathione is the major reason for interest in NAC. The great favor of glutathione toward health benefits are reflected in the recent swarm of books concerning glutathione, as witnessed by an Internet bookstore site full of them (www.healthy-profits.com/book_store.htm). Another approach to raising the levels of glutathione now available is an undenatured powdered whey protein isolate product, Immunocal. This is claimed to serve as a superior source for the amino acid cysteine, essential for making glutathione, but not well supplied by the proteins from common foods (www.ammunotec.com/).

Oral Ascorbic Acid (Supplement) versus Intravenous Sodium Ascorbate (Drug)

No molecule is more clearly classed as a vitamin, and thus a dietary supplement, than is ascorbic acid, or vitamin C. It was discovered in the nineteenth century to be a specific nutrient needed for prevention or treatment of a deficiency disease known as scurvy. A considerable difference of opinion has existed as to what level of dietary intake is necessary and normal. Undoubtedly this value is highly variable between individuals and within one person as prevailing conditions change. The action of stress to deplete the supplies of ascorbic acid (for example, from the adrenal gland) has been recognized for more than a half century. For many persons this would suggest a greater current need for an outside source of vitamin C than ever before (Levy, 2002). The availability of vitamin C in broad-spectrum vitamin supplements is clearly recognized as important. More controversial is the value of those single-agent products that may be used to supply high oral doses (e.g., up to 2 g per day or 2,000 mg per day), which are multiples of the recommended daily allowance. The value of a high level of supplement usage is poorly accepted by medicine in general. In contrast, those physicians who are oriented to nutrition and CAM hold that high-level supplementation with ascorbic acid to be among their basic tenets of practice. This approach was first championed and called to attention by an American chemist, Nobel Laureate Linus Pauling, in the late 1960s.

Pauling's collaboration with cancer clinician and researcher Ewan Cameron involved very high doses that required administration by injection in order to obtain extremely high tissue levels of ascorbic acid. In such cases, high intravenous doses of the more soluble salt, sodium ascorbate, are necessary and appropriate (Cameron and Pauling, 1973, 1976). Pauling and Cameron reported that many terminal cancer patients so treated showed retardation of tumor progression, many others showed a halt of progression, and a few showed tumor regression. Survival times were improved for terminal patients whose survival prospects were extremely poor—a condition of their being involved in such experimentation with "megadose" vitamin C therapy. Patient tolerance of the side effect of gastrointestinal upset, sometimes to the point of diarrhea, came to be employed as a dosage guideline.

Ephedra (Supplement) versus Ephedrine (Rx/OTC Drug)

A final example of dual identity (which is more fully developed in Chapter 8) concerns the Chinese plant *Ephedra cinensis* from which an alkaloid, ephedrine, was first isolated in 1887. This molecule became in the 1920s and 1930s a major Rx drug because it has properties similar to adrenaline, but longer duration. This made it useful as a therapy for asthma and other illnesses. After about a half century of importance, ephedrine faded away in favor of newer synthetic agents, but it still held some favor for use in OTC products. With the post-DSHEA era rise in popularity of botanical products, ephedra became a widespread favorite in dietary supplement products for weight reduction and heightened energy. The ephedrine alkaloids, responsible for the actions of ephedra, have been found subject to abuse for their producing stimulation and euphoria to such a degree that the FDA banned ephedra from being sold in the United States in April 2004. Ephedra came under attack as well for allegedly causing dangerous and even life-threatening toxicity, not only to those exposed to escalating dosages (misuse) but also for persons who followed the recommended level of intake. The FDA ban on ephedra was implemented because of the toll of injuries and deaths blamed upon it. However, in a recent court ruling a federal judge in Utah struck down the FDA ban, ruling that ephedra is being regulated by the FDA as a drug instead of as a food as it should be. The FDA maintains its original ban, but is currently evaluating the ruling (Thiessen, 2005).

Chapter 4

Who's a Quack? Conflict on the Current Health Care Scene

WHAT APPROACHES ARE LEGITIMATE?

> Medicine and quackery have always been close, if not compatible, partners. At times, they may appear to have separated, but sooner or later, in one place or another, they wind up reunited. The present area of greatest mutual attraction for them appears to be in the treatment of disease by the use of herbal remedies. More misinformation regarding the efficacy of herbs is currently being placed before consumers than at any time, including the turn-of-the century [20th] heyday of patent medicines.
>
> Varro Tyler (1981)

This chapter is supplied to orient the reader to broad aspects of contemporary controversy involving self-treatment and/or alternative medical care systems. The topic of great concern is the tension between conventional and unconventional practices. If a person chooses to use an unconventional approach for maintenance and/or recovery of their health they should be well aware of the possible risks involved, otherwise the goal of a rational application of dietary supplements cannot be realized. This consideration requires an awareness of risks associated with the conventional medical approaches.

A strikingly negative statement on the marketing of botanicals is the one at the head of this chapter by the late Varro Tyler, former dean of the Purdue University School of Pharmacy and Pharmacal Sciences, professor of pharmacognosy emeritus, and author of noteworthy books on herbal medications in the 1980s and 1990s. Although this quotation is from his first edition of *The Honest Herbal* in 1981, developments in subsequent years did nothing to change Tyler's analysis. His later writings expressed similar

Consumer's Guide to Dietary Supplements and Alternative Medicines

doi:10.1300/5698_04

strong concern about the unvalidated claims made for herbal remedies after they were classified as dietary supplements under DSHEA in 1994.

Indeed, Dr. Tyler was not friendly to or accepting of herbalist practices currently embraced by a minor but growing category of enthusiasts in the Western societies, nor was he a fan of those phytotherapy practices more common in Europe than in North America. Numerous books have been authored by less science-oriented writers than Tyler who are more accepting of folklore and are unconcerned about a scarcity or lack of clinical research validation. Some differ to the extent even of espousing that one should grow and harvest one's own herbal materials for use as remedies rather than utilizing botanical materials processed for the marketplace into pharmaceutical-like products.

IF IT QUACKS LIKE A DUCK, WHAT IS IT?

The colorful explanation for the derivation of the English term "quackery" and "quack," when not pertaining to ducks but to fraudulent diagnostic and/or therapeutic practices, is the Dutch term, *kwacksalver,* meaning anyone who babbles, brags, boasts, or chatters (i.e., "quacks like a duck") about his or her "salves" or other remedies. This term and its associated concept may be too neglected and in need of revival in light of some current trends of the U.S. market.

Thus, "quackery" at its essence is the promotion of either a known-to-be-false or an unproven health scheme for a profit. It is rooted in traditions of the marketplace, whereas scientific thinking and resulting standards of conduct underlie consumer protection laws and the standards of professionalism. William T. Jarvis, PhD (1999), School of Public Health, Loma Linda University, has declared that: "At the present time, commercialism has overwhelmed professionalism in the marketing of alternative remedies. Neither patients nor legitimate businesses that adhere to the standards of science and consumer protection are well served by a double standard."

This quote expresses discouragement concerning the current state of the dietary supplement marketplace. A large proportion of the commercial promotions for most herbal and nutritional products is done with the aid and comfort of persons bearing the doctor of medicine degree, and to their profit. Such medical endorsements clearly distract from the remedy not yet having attained standing as a scientifically validated procedure for the prevention or treatment of disease. The FDA requires that not only the packages but also any promotional literature specific to a supplement product bear these disclaimers: "This product is not intended to diagnose, treat, cure, or prevent any disease" and "This statement has not been evaluated by the Food and Drug Administration."

Considering the previous definition, it could be argued that the many physicians whose names and faces are seen on promotional materials bearing the FDA disclaimers have left the realm of legitimate medicine and embraced the practice of quackery. An important point emphasized by Jarvis (1999) is the degree to which safety and efficacy, both unproven, are nevertheless "established" for many unconventional agents by stout assertions and vague, unverifiable claims, especially with the sponsorship or support of "So and So," MD.

An analysis that was intended for circulation to the supplement industry (Mertens, 1999) was titled *From Quackery to Credibility: Unconventional Healthcare in the Era of High-Tech Medicine* and focused on alternative and complementary health products. The report advised that any serious company in the supplement arena must evaluate its products scientifically via placebo-controlled human trials using random assignment of patients, multiple replications for validating data, and proper statistical analysis of the data. Who can disagree that those actions are much desirable? However, the current federal legislation has not required nor have the economic factors encouraged that process.

Double Standard on "Quackery" Accusations?

A commonly accepted belief is that any practitioner promoting an unproven remedy or other therapy for profit is a quack. It is most frequently applied to those physicians who are heavily involved in alternative remedies and therapies, but what about those physicians who promote "off-label" (not FDA approved) uses for an Rx drug that has the FDA's approval for only one application? Pfizer Inc. has been under fire for supposedly promoting to physicians ten or more off-label uses for their product Neurontin. By definition, off-label indications are those that have not met FDA standards and are unproven uses for that agent. The "experts" who aid the manufacturers' desire for greater sales by endorsing the product for off-label usage do not do so as an act of charity; they are rewarded handsomely by the manufacturer of the drug for making their appearances before groups of doctors to promote their views and give their endorsements.

In stark contrast, active harassment to the point of prosecution for quackery by state medical boards has been pursued by a small element of conventional medicine. For example, a New York State physician was forced out of practice by economic sanctions for the "crime" of treating children who were diagnosed with ADHD (attention-deficit/hyperactivity disorder) through nutritional interventions, in a fashion approved by the child's parents, rather than by prescribing the usual therapeutic stimulants of Ritalin (having an action mechanism similar to cocaine) or amphetamine. For neither of these has long-term safety of their use in childhood been well substantiated. Indeed, one recognized adverse effect is a reduction of the user's secretion of growth hormone, for which intervals off of the drug are regarded as important.

On another front, the question has been raised recently whether the conventional treatments being prescribed for osteoarthritis patients constitute malpractice. Jason Theodosakis, MD, on his Web site (www.drtheo.com) suggests that widespread prescribing of Rx nonsteroidal anti-inflammatory agents (NSAIDs), as well as the more selective COX-2 (cyclooxgenase) inhibitors violates a doctor's Hippocratic tenet of "first, do no harm." He emphasizes the considerable track record of the NSAIDs for causing hospitalizations for gastrointestinal injury and more than 16,500 deaths annually (Wolfe et al., 1999), as well as a risk for kidney damage or failure and for cardiovascular problems that include heart attack and stroke. Meanwhile, such drugs do nothing to actually improve the condition but provide merely a palliative, and usually incomplete, relief of symptoms.

This would be excusable if no alternative having a more positive activity profile existed. However, for a number of years considerable evidence has suggested that many (not all) osteoarthritis sufferers can gain comparable symptomatic relief from using the OTC supplement products containing glucosamine and chondroitin without risking the adverse effects that characterize the NSAIDs and COX-2 inhibitors. Moreover, data (badly needing confirmatory efforts) supporting the view that supplements are available, such as glucosamine and chondroitin, that slow or reverse the disease process—i.e., they have a disease-modifying activity toward osteoarthritis. One way to consider the subject is that osteoarthritis patients should not be prescribed NSAID/COX-2 products unless and until they have failed to obtain adequate relief using glucosamine and chondroitin, perhaps along with methylsulfonylmethane (MSM), and with a less-threatening pain reliever, acetaminophen. Critical in this is a recognition that full onset of benefit for such therapy is delayed and may require one or two months to manifest.

The problem of prescribing an Rx pain reliever for arthritis patients that elevates their risk for heart attack or stroke came to the front page news in fall 2004 because of the withdrawal of Vioxx from the market worldwide. The so-called "voluntary withdrawal" is putting the best face on a bad situation, especially when data existed indicating the need for such action as long ago as 2001. It is arguable that neither the manufacturer nor the FDA deserve any medals for their service to the public welfare in view of that level of delay. The final irony is that of Vioxx returning to the market newly "sanctified" by a black-box warning to the consumer that its use could cause a fatal complication! So, the patient is now given an "informed choice:" debilitating or even crippling pain or the possibility for premature death.

Another approach to the rather common and troublesome knee osteoarthritis that clearly is superior to the NSAIDs is the injection of a high viscosity hyaluronate solution (Synvisc and others) into the knee-joint capsule. Such injections should be administered by an orthopedist, but for some patients they repeatedly give relief for six-month periods. How many generalist physicians prescribe an NSAID or COX-2 inhibitor and neglect to instead give a referral to an orthopedist for the patient with osteoarthritic knee joints?

A therapeutics newsletter by the Therapeutics Initiative of the Department of Pharmacology and Therapeutics at the University of British Columbia at Vancouver, Canada, highlighted the problem of COX-2 inhibitors increasing cardiac risks (Therapeutics Initiative, 2002). However, it was a review paper appearing in an August 2004 *JAMA* that brought the problem into focus (Fontanarosa et al., 2004). It analyzed a human data set arising from three studies on risks for adverse cardiovascular events among Vioxx users. The conditions monitored were myocardial infarction (heart attack), sudden or unexplained death, resuscitated cardiac arrest, ischemic stroke, and TIAs (transient ischemic brain attacks). Patients taking rofecoxib (Vioxx) were 2.38 times more likely to experience any of those events than were patients taking the NSAID naproxen (Aleve, Naprosyn).

The manufacturer responded to the earlier report by choosing to await more data to confirm (or not confirm) the finding, with the FDA approving the choice. This and other cases tend to support those who declare that the FDA is too focused on ensuring the drug companies' profits to "do the right thing" for consumer safety. Results of the larger ongoing study that brought the September 2004 decision to withdraw Vioxx were not significantly different from the results known three years earlier (Mukherjee et al., 2001). As might be expected, reports suggested a similar problem with another COX-2 inhibitor, Celebrex, in winter 2004-2005. Moreover, a third COX-2 inhibitor, Bextra, was removed from the market April 2005 because of its association with serious dermatologic reactions.

CONVENTIONAL MEDICINE AND THERAPIES

Conventional Medicine and Therapies describes those practices and therapeutic agents taught in recent times by standard allopathic and osteopathic medical schools that are routinely offered by physicians holding the

MD (doctor of medicine) or DO (doctor of osteopathy) degrees, respectively. Thus, conventional medicine is generally equated with allopathic medicine (allopathy), which is defined as "a system of therapeutics based on the production of a condition incompatible with or antagonistic to the condition being treated" *(Dorland's Illustrated Medical Dictionary).* Differences in osteopathic approaches became progressively minimal over the second half of the twentieth century. This conventional viewpoint excludes practitioners with training in naturopathic, homeopathic, or chiropractic methods of therapy as well as traditional ethnic medicines of the East and South Asia. Other supposed (i.e., unconventional) healing approaches are discussed in this chapter as well. However, individual medical schools now are deviating from their former patterns to some degree with a trend toward embracing integrative medicine, which is an amalgamation of what some persons find to be acceptable aspects of unconventional therapies, to complement the conventional practices of Western medicine before equal scientific validation of the former has been achieved.

One basis for this trend may be a desire to show "political correctness" and "open-mindedness" calling for respect toward the supposed therapeutic knowledge of another culture, e.g., Asian practices. This is despite such practices lacking the scientific foundation characteristic of Western medicine. In other words, the argument is that the traditions of other cultures should be automatically respected and accepted while some traditional as well as newer practices of Western medicine are being subjected to severe scrutiny and often rejection.

Conventional therapy also excludes some practices conducted by a minority of MD or DO physicians who claim to provide successful therapy for serious diseases by applying unconventional agents, devices, or procedures not recognized by the FDA (although they sometimes have been approved by similar agencies of other nations) for the disease in question because of not having been adequately validated as effective by scientific evidence. A prime example of exclusion would be the unconventional agents, devices, and procedures used as cancer "cures" that have arisen repeatedly over the past century. A physician practicing, promoting, and profiting from the application of either false or unproven health schemes is defined in the United States as "quackery" (by the British called "humbuggery"). These terms imply fraud, deception, or sham in the delivery of therapy. When they are used in an accusation an adversarial situation arises among those who bear equal degrees, licensure, and legal standing to practice medicine. Even more likely to be quite adversarial are relationships between conventional practitioners and those on the "outside," such as those qualified as ND (doctor of naturopathy), DC (doctor of chropractic), and unlicensed practitioners such as TCM doctors, herbalists, or massage therapists.

Evidence-Based Medicine

Evidence-based medicine is a relatively new phrase that applies to a movement within conventional medicine to upgrade it to a more thoroughly scientific medicine (Anonymous, 2002). This intent is pursued by demanding a rigorous scientific validation of every new or old therapeutic agent, device, and process. Thus, both new, older, and long-accepted therapies have been or are being exposed to critical analysis by teams of medical and statistical scientists. A basic precept is the necessity for data being strictly scientific in the sense of meeting the criteria that have developed since about the mid-twentieth century. As described in Chapter 2, this requires data to be collected in prospective, randomized, placebo-controlled, double-blind clinical trials. Moreover, replication (repetition) usually by several independent research groups is a basic expected feature. Data from repeated trials meeting such standards typically are analyzed collectively by the method of meta-analysis to enable definitive conclusions.

Presently, not all that is conventional in medicine is yet evidence based. However, the contrast with unconventional medicine is that none of the latter, by definition, is so based; rather, many physicians who practice alternative therapies ignore, deny, or even overtly reject the principle that only scientific evidence is valid and entirely desirable or necessary. If or when a treatment is recognized as "evidence-based" it will make the transition from unconventional to conventional.

UNCONVENTIONAL MEDICINE AND THERAPIES

It is instructive to contrast the characteristics of different approaches to seeking better health or a respite from illness. The term *unconventional* is applied to a broad range of therapies that have not been taught in allopathic and osteopathic medical schools and thus are not usually approved, recommended, or provided by such physicians.

Homeopathic Medicine

Homeopathy is a system of medicine that is based on "the law of similars." The basic aim is to stimulate the body to recover by itself after giving patients minuscule doses of some remedy that in large doses would cause symptoms similar to those of the illness that they are already experiencing. The theory behind this is that such a minute dose will stimulate the body's healing powers without exerting any adverse side effects. The remedies typically consist of dose units that have been diluted a great many times. Many scientists who have done appropriate calculations conclude that most homeopathic products are too diluted to still contain any of the original compound. Therefore, they declare that such remedies cannot possibly have a helpful effect. Despite such conclusions, some double-blind, placebo-controlled clinical trials have been reported in recent years to demonstrate beneficial effects of homeopathic preparations.

To counter the well-circulated view of scientists, advocates of homeopathy have put forward the idea that the water in aqueous preparations has been changed by the compound even though it is no longer present. This "imprinting" is said to be activated when a substance is dissolved in water and then diluted repeatedly until not a single molecule of the substance could remain. Not surprisingly, this is a view that has received an extremely skeptical response among chemists and medical scientists. It seems tantamount to a sort of magical thinking. A recent study has purported to show that solutions that have been extremely diluted still retain patterns of hydrogen bonds that enable such solutions to transmit some molecular information or "biological messages." However, homeopathic remedies are often dispensed as solids rather than solutions, so this hypothesis would have limited usefulness to explain the claimed effects of all homeopathic remedies.

Complementary Medicine and Therapies

Complementary medicine and therapies are unconventional therapies that both health practitioners and laypeople may use as adjuncts to conventional therapies. They frequently include nutritional regimens, supplemental nutrients (often in much higher doses than "usual"), botanical dosage forms, or drinking herbal teas.

Alternative Medicine and Therapies

Alternative medicine and therapies describes various unconventional therapies used in place of the conventional therapies. Unfortunately, the promotion of alternative therapy often involves very negative attacks on conventional therapies as "too toxic" and expresses a (seemingly) paranoid view that "entrenched interests" in medicine and in the drug industry are standing in the way of a major benefit to the public's health by their nonacceptance of the unconventional approach. An implicit, if not explicit, denial of the need for scientific validation of the alternative therapy by means of prospective, randomized, double-blind, placebo-controlled clinical trials often occurs.

Unscientific Medicine

Unscientific medicine is a phrase used by its critics to describe CAM, emphasizing that most CAM therapies are lacking definitive evidence of effectiveness (efficacy) and safety. Physicians' observations supporting a benefit often exist, or claims are made that clinical cases not from clinical trials adequately demonstrate value; these often have not been published, or at least not by a prestigious, reputable medical journal.

Therapeutic Differentiations Among CAM, As Generally Recognized by Various Sources

- Acupuncture/acupressure
- Aromatherapy
- Biofeedback/relaxation techniques
- Chelation therapy
- Chiropractic
- Detoxification
- Energy healing, including "therapeutic touch"
- Ethnic herbal therapies—ayurvedic, Japanese (Campo), traditional Chinese medicine
- Exercise therapy
- Homeopathic medicine
- Hypnosis
- Magnetism
- Massage therapy
- Naturopathic medicine, applying diet, nutrients, botanicals (sometimes homeopathic)
- Prolotherapy
- Self-selected dietary supplements—botanicals, megavitamins, and "new nutrients"
- Spiritual/faith healing

Consideration of the many alternative approaches besides those involving the use of dietary supplements is beyond the scope of this work. Discussion will be limited to uses of dietary supplements as remedies, either self-chosen or as directed by any sort of conventional or unconventional practitioner.

Naturopathic Medicine

Of the unconventional approaches previously listed, other than herbalism, naturopathic medical practice is most closely allied to the usage of dietary supplements. NDs may incorporate multiple unconventional approaches into their practice, which may include homeopathic and herbal remedies, nutrition counseling, lifestyle modification, exercise therapy, physical therapy, and manipulation of bony and soft tissues.

WHY COMPLEMENTARY AND ALTERNATIVE MEDICINE NOW?

Western medicine, as practiced through most of Europe and North America as well as in many other developed nations, arrived at its present status via a lengthy process of evolution, plus some occasional revolutions. The second half of the twentieth century was an especially rapid era of advancement not only for the actual discovery of new therapies but also in regard to the refining of processes of drug discovery and of validation of new candidate therapies. Legislation affecting this evolution is outlined in Table 4.1.

TABLE 4.1. History of relevant federal legislative regulation of therapies.

Year	Legislation
1906	Pure Food and Drug Act—Established that the Food and Drug Administration could enforce standards for strength and purity of drugs by the official compendia of the USP-NF (National Formulary), and prohibit any mislabeling or adulteration of drugs.
1938	Food, Drug, and Cosmetic Act—Required registration with the FDA of all parties involved in the manufacturing, sale, and distribution of drugs; required the adequate testing to prevent marketing of a possibly toxic substance. New drugs must be safe as well as pure, but proof of efficacy was not required.
1951	Durham-Humphrey Amendments—Separated more the drugs that required an Rx ("legend drugs") from the nonprescription/OTC/"nonlegend" drugs.
1962	Kefauver-Harris Amendments—Required submission of proof of efficacy (in addition to safety) to the FDA for new drug approval, and established guidelines for conduct of clinical trials.

Drug Discovery

Modern scientific drug discovery usually begins with a long sequence of laboratory researches before a new candidate drug is ready for testing in human beings. Ordinarily, some tests are done on small numbers of normal, healthy persons before the first trials in patients having the targeted disease. More rarely, e.g., for cancer chemotherapy and AIDS therapy, human testing may begin instead upon patients whose prior therapies have failed, so that the candidate agent is used as a "last resort" when no help or hope remains for benefit from available approaches.

Since 1962 the FDA has required for approval for marketing that pharmaceutical products provide evidence of their having shown adequate efficacy (effective for achieving the claimed benefits) and safety for application in the manner indicated by the sponsor. Four phases of this review process occur, all involving human data collection based on supportive results from nonhuman biological tests. When a new chemical molecule meets the requirements through Phase III it is approved by the FDA for marketing within a strictly drawn set of conditions. However, the fourth phase of gathering data on human responses to the new agent, especially concerning safety, continues for months or years.

Sad to say, the need for this Phase IV review has been all too clearly evident in the past decade. Several pharmaceuticals that were undoubtedly providing favorable benefits to multitudes of patients were required to be removed from the market because of an unexpected level of adverse responses that may have been life-threatening or outright fatal in a small fraction of all exposed patients.

The beginning of the twenty-first century seems to be a time of unprecedented mistrust between the medical profession, the public, and the media. Furthermore, among devotees of CAM, a strong mistrust of the pharmaceutical industry and many of its products exists. The promoters of dietary supplements for CAM also tend to promote antagonism and suspicion toward the pharmaceutical industry. The ferment in the economics of health care in the past few decades has contributed much to the mistrust of physicians, as the assembly-line rapidity of their seeing patients has worked to deprive them of a formerly high level of respect.

Contrariwise, the regard of the public for alternative practitioners and modes of health care has been rising steadily. This book addresses as a major concern, among the varied aspects of the full CAM scene, the recent, explosively increased acceptance of herbal remedies and other aspects of the dietary supplements. To what extent is this a result of the public finding greater satisfaction from their encounters with CAM therapies or practitioners? We will consider the positive side of the coin, a favorable outcome from using dietary supplements, whenever grounds are available for such analysis.

Another major suspected basis for this shift may well be the mistrust bred by safety problems concerning prescription medicines. Reading and hearing of highly publicized withdrawals of drugs consequent to severe, often fatal adverse effects can be expected to instill fear in some portion of the population. Moreover, people are subject to being terrorized by reading the package inserts for their prescriptions, which list an array of potential adverse effects ranging from those as simple as headache to those as extreme as "sudden and unexplained death."[1] An array of Rx drug withdrawals is shown in Table 4.2.

Among recent examples of the former were the highly publicized withdrawals in 1997 of weight-reducing agents dexfenfluramine (Redux) and fenfluramine (Pondimin) used in fen-phen, in 1999 of the diabetes drug troglitazone (Rezulin), and in 2000 of the just-marketed alosetron (Lotronex) for treatment of irritable bowel symptoms, which after undergoing a reconsideration was returned to the market under a more restricted mode of usage.

Surpassing these, if only for its causing "single-handedly" a significant fall in the New York Stock Exchange, was the announcement of a voluntary worldwide withdrawal of Vioxx on September 30, 2004, after 84 million prescriptions had been dispensed. The decision by Merck was effective immediately. It was based on results of a new three-year prospective, randomized, placebo-controlled clinical trial called APPROVe (for the Adenomatous Polyp Prevention on Vioxx trial). Thus, a trial aiming to validate a new use for the drug instead revealed the facts that made it no longer acceptable for its former pain-relieving indications.

Of considerable interest is the response of the FDA. Acting commissioner Dr. Lester M. Crawford (2005) said the following:

> Merck did the right thing by promptly reporting these findings to FDA and voluntarily withdrawing the product from the market.
>
> Although the risk that an individual patient would have a heart attack or stroke related to Vioxx is very small, the study that was halted suggests that, overall, patients taking the drug chronically face twice the risk of a heart attack compared to patients receiving a placebo.

Dr. Crawford further stated that FDA would closely monitor other drugs in this class for similar adverse effects, saying, "All of the NSAID drugs have risks when taken chronically, especially of gastrointestinal bleeding, but

TABLE 4.2. Noteworthy withdrawals of prescription drugs in the United States.

Year	Generic name	Trade name	Producer	Basis for market withdrawal
2005	Valdecoxib	Bextra	Pfizer	Risk of serious cardiac malfunction
2004	Rofecoxib	Vioxx	Merck	Doubling rate of heart attack, stroke risk; returned with black-box labeling
2001	Cerivastatin	Baycol	Bayer	Cases of fatal skeletal muscle injury
	Rapacuronium	Raplon	Organon	Cases of life-threatening bronchospasm
2000	Alosetron	Lotronex	Glaxo Wellcome	Cases of fatal ischemic colitis
	Cisapride	Propulsid	Janssen	Risk for cardiac arrhythmias
	Troglitazone	Rezulin	Parke Davis	Cases of fatal liver toxicity
	Phenylpropanolamine	(PPA)	(various)	Increased risk of hemorrhagic stroke
1999	Astemizole	Hismanal	Janssen	Risk for cardiac arrhythmias
	Grepafloxacin	Raxar	Glaxo Wellcome	Risk for cardiac toxicity
1997	Dexfenfluramine	Redux	Wyeth-Ayerst	Valvular heart disease in women
	Fenfluramine	Pondimin	Wyeth-Ayerst	As dexfenfluramine + pulmonary hypertension
1992	Temafloxacin	Omniflox	Abbott	Withdrawn four months after entry to market caused by fifty serious adverse events, including three deaths; injury to blood, kidneys, liver; and low blood sugar
1982	Benoxaprofen	Oraflex	Lilly	Withdrawn after one month, five fatalities from liver injury. FDA accused Lilly of suppressing unfavorable research data. The company pleaded guilty to 25 criminal counts, paid a $25,000 fine

also liver and kidney toxicity. They should only be used continuously under the supervision of a physician."

However, this statement seems to overlook the three NSAIDs that are and have been for years available OTC, as nonprescription medicines. How is this consistent with the previous warning about all NSAIDs having risks for injuring the stomach/intestine, liver, and kidneys? If hazards in using Rx drugs and OTC medicines exist, how much more is it so for much less regulated botanical dietary supplements? If you rest securely in the thought that the FDA is looking after you, you are sadly and badly misinformed! Persons outside the FDA have been known to opine that the FDA pursues its "purpose in life" to ensure the major drug companies' ability to make major profits. When this author heard the same opinion in 2004 from a longtime scientist employee of the FDA, it was indeed rather disconcerting.

ANOTHER VIEWPOINT: AFTERNOON OF ALTERNATIVE MEDICINE

In a frank letter to the *British Medical Journal,* after listening to lecturer on CAM, Dr. Kevin Barraclough (2001), an English general practitioner, was driven to ask himself, "How do we know that they're not charlatans?" He anticipated the answer: "Ah!" say the cognoscenti, "you have to keep an open mind: even Van Gogh wasn't recognized in his own time." To which Barraclough replies:

> But if keeping an open mind means suspending scepticism, on the basis that it is tainted with prejudice, then surely we are all lost! We are at the mercy of every opportunist who flicks paint at a canvas, every shaman who claims to cure cancer. If we suspend systematic doubt in medicine, an area fraught with emotive self interest, then we risk plunging into an abyss of humbuggery. And the trouble is when it comes to humbuggery, the history of medicine is not squeaky clean.

DIETARY SUPPLEMENT REGULATION

The Dietary Supplement Health and Education Act of 1994 (DSHEA)

Aggressive lobbying by the dietary supplement industry, by physicians of nutritional or "natural" bent, and by the public toward the U.S. Congress resulted in this legislation that largely exempted supplements from before-marketing oversight by FDA for safety or efficacy. The Pure Food and Drug Act of 1906 similarly did not require that drug manufacturers prove a drug product to be safe before marketing it. Rather it permitted the government to remove it after showing it to be unsafe. That is what Congress gave as a gift to the supplement industry. However, the FDA received a new strengthened standing relative to regulation of the pharmaceuticals after the death of several hundred people in 1938 from an outbreak of fatal poisonings among users of a "sulfanilamide elixir," a name that implied a solution in alcohol (ethanol). Instead this product was a solution in diethylene glycol, what proved to be a toxic solvent that was untested for safety in human use. Seemingly, for the FDA to gain more oversight authority over the dietary supplements a "large enough" number of people dying from a comparable disaster will need to exist before Congress acts to grant such powers; e.g., an herbal must be recognized as a major source of fatalities. But this is not very different from regular occurrences about FDA-approved Rx drugs and vaccines. It is to be expected that at least a few of those products will disable or kill a certain fraction of the postmarketing exposed population. When the number becomes too conspicuous, the product usually is "voluntarily withdrawn" under FDA pressure.

Because the FDA has limited resources for laboratory analysis of the composition of drugs, foods, and related products, including dietary supplements, it does not routinely analyze drug or supplement products before they are sold to consumers. Consequently, a manufacturer alone is responsible for ensuring that all items on the ingredient list are present as per the labeled quantities, that those ingredients are safe, and that no other unlisted active materials are present. In Chapter 10 we will consider evidence that some unknown fraction, perhaps a large one, of supplement manufacturers have been failing to fulfill this responsibility to the consumer. Reasons for this may include both ignorance and incompetence, but greed also is a major suspect.

Efficacy is not at issue, as the required labeling on dietary supplements may not include any therapeutic claims and indeed must disavow any therapeutic intent. This is the standard disclaimer: "These statements have not been evaluated by the Food and Drug Administration. This product is not intended to diagnose, treat, cure, or prevent any disease."

FDA requirements further state that "The label of a dietary supplement must contain enough information about the composition of the product so that consumers can make informed choices." However, if the buyer is persuaded by extravagant promotional material (read elsewhere than on the package) saying that the item is indeed useful to "treat, cure, or prevent disease," that decision is the person's prerogative and responsibility. The manufacturer is instructed by the FDA to make sure the label information is truthful and not misleading. In fact, no basis exists for assurance that these requirements are followed, and many observations suggest that they frequently are not. Enforcement of this "truth in advertising" feature falls to the responsibility not of the FDA but rather to the Federal Trade Commission (FTC), which does periodically take action against supplement producers for false or misleading claims. A recent action of this in June 2003 was the FTC taking aggressive action to halt the deceptive advertising of coral calcium by its originator, Bob Barefoot, and associates.

Independent laboratory analyses demonstrated that some supplement products may not in fact contain the amounts claimed for the substances listed on the label. Furthermore, at times they contain added materials not shown on the label. These label "facts" need not to have been subjected to any external certification process. Label truthfulness is required by the FDA, but the FDA does not perform "unprovoked" testing to certify the accuracy of labeling, leaving it to the integrity of the producer. FDA is not empowered to automatically halt the sale of a product if an outside analysis should reveal that it doesn't contain what the label states, unless the product is found to contain a substance whose presence has been banned already because of known human toxicity, which makes it "adulterated." Aristolochic acid is an example of a natural product that will be considered in Chapter 29.

For another example, analyses of ginseng-labeled and ephedra-labeled products found that the amounts of the active ingredient in each dose unit ("serving") varied by as much as ten times among brands labeled as providing equal doses, whereas some products contained none at all (see Chapter 10). Such findings by an independent analysis may not provoke a change, because it is the responsibility (read: *option*) of the manufacturer to do so. Moreover, although the use of ephedra products had reasonably been alleged to have been a factor in a large number of severe and even fatal incidents, the FDA was for years unsuccessful in its efforts to implement restrictions designed to reduce the risk for more such incidents (see Chapter 8), much less to ban the marketing of ephedra.

Congress was apparently of a mind to say, "Well, so what if DSHEA legislation leads to [no, *demands*] a policy of 'let the buyer beware'? These materials are vitamins and other natural nutritive substances with little or no capacity for harm, are they not?" *Not!* This is a false argument, as vitamins are only a small fraction of all the dietary supplement agents. This book work will provide uninformed readers with abundant evidence to demonstrate that this view is mythology, or as some would say, "bunk."

THE CONSEQUENCES OF DSHEA

By enacting this legislation the U.S. Congress "freed" Americans to pursue better health or relief from illness by self-medication with often unstandardized botanical and nutritional or biochemical products that are nearly unregulated by governmental agencies. The act in essence dictates that regulation of dietary supplements by the FDA is limited to superficial labeling features. Premarketing data showing effectiveness or safety may be required. Indeed, the burden of proof is placed upon the FDA rather than upon the manufacturer in case a suspicion develops about the safety of a supplement product (see Chapters 7 and 8). In this respect DSHEA put supplements back to where pharmaceuticals were in 1906 under the initial federal regulation of drugs.

The FDA may not question efficacy, in return for which supplement producers are prohibited from making explicit claims on their product labels of usefulness for specific disease therapy. Indeed, the label must bear disclaimers with respect to the product being useful for diagnosis or treatment of disease, and that the FDA has not reviewed (or approved) the product. However, the claim's limitation may be readily circumvented by the producer claiming benefits in the contents of advertising separated from the product package.

The clearest contrast between conventional and alternative therapies is that the recent progress of the former has involved the requirement that new conventional therapies be scientifically tested to obtain rigorous validation of their safety and efficacy. This is done to satisfy regulations of the FDA. Such scientific testing must include gathering of extensive laboratory and clinical data before the FDA will consider approval of a new drug. This is followed by publication of such research in well-respected, peer-reviewed medical journals. The concept implicit in the phrase "evidence-based medicine" is now applied to all new prescription agents.

In contrast, alternative remedies or procedures generally have not undergone such scientific evaluation. Moreover, their advocates largely deny a need for such testing of alternative therapies, in many cases claiming a history of traditional usage as adequate validation. Admittedly, some older therapies used by conventional medicine also have not been rigorously tested. However, for the field of nonprescription, OTC medicines in the United States, in the 1970s a broad review process weeded out those OTC remedies judged to be of uncertain safety and/or efficacy.

Many persons who advocate alternative remedies tend to affirm that the scientific method is simply not applicable to their favorite therapies. They rely heavily on theories and anecdotal testimonials of benefit. Such anecdotal support for alternative remedies frequently is published as pamphlets or small books and likely do not undergo peer review as do papers in medical journals or in consumer-directed, health-related magazines. Some of the latter appear to be "simulated journals" directed to the public, especially to older Americans, to inspire more confidence than is warranted. These typically provide no substantial documentation nor any semblance of scientific evidence (as defined in Chapter 3). Such sources are presented to the public with photographs and names of endorsing physicians or sometimes the supposedly originating/discovering doctors—an age-old practice tarnished by its past association with quackery. That endorsement is presented as sufficient support for therapeutic claims. Printed materials that are not directly attached to the product, but which convey the claims made for its alleged benefits, are a means of avoiding the FDA's prohibition for such therapeutic claims in product labeling of dietary supplements, the main class of alternative remedies.

Several possible perspectives on the vast number of unconventional remedies are the following:

1. They are dangerous because they have serious toxic potential.
2. They may be safe alone, but they are susceptible to showing adverse interactions with ordinary pharmaceuticals.
3. They waste buyers' money and important time—potentially causing delay in a patient's receiving an effective conventional therapy.
4. They can't hurt and may even help people to feel better, if only by acting as a placebo.
5. They may actually constitute safe and effective therapy.
6. They may be equally or more effective than standard, conventional medicines, and they are likely to be less costly and less toxic as well.

Mildly skeptical persons may take position number four—whether or not they do good, they can't really do harm. However, many practitioners of medicine are highly convinced of the correctness of the first three viewpoints, which together comprise a strong case for the likelihood that dietary supplements may do more harm than good. Instead, emphasis should be shifted to the idea that we must in each individual case allow for any one of the six positions to be correct, and we should consider the question, "What are the odds for perspectives one through six to be true in this particular case?" Most of the promotional materials for supplements ask the reader to believe that only belief five or six could be true. In the promotion of botanicals and new nutrients, there never shall be heard a discouraging word.

THE FREEDOM TO PURSUE BETTER HEALTH: AT WHAT COST?

Among the latter day additions to basic freedoms, it would seem that one is an inalienable right to pursue health "freely," i.e., in whatever mode one may choose to self-medicate. This mind-set has resulted in many Americans following paths that comprise an *alternative* to conventional paths of health, hygiene, nutrition, and medicine that have prevailed over several generations. Another view is that many unconventional approaches can be profitably applied in addition to the conventional systems standard in medicine, public health, and nutrition. What should be the role of the FDA as many quasi-drugs are passed off as "foods"? Should it be certifying the safety and efficacy of these remedies? The U.S. Congress decided that manufacturers and distributors do not even need to be registered with the FDA or obtain FDA approval before producing or selling dietary supplements, unless they consist of a never-before-marketed substance. A level of purview over supplements that was already minimal was further reduced in 1994 by action of the U.S. Congress. Clearly, the manufacturer alone is responsible for ensuring that all items on the ingredient list are present as per the labeled quantities and that the ingredients are safe.

Subsequent to the 1994 DSHEA legislation, the floodgates have been opened (if not entirely swept away) by new botanical and nutritional products reaching the market without review and regulation by the FDA. In subsequent chapters evidence that such products may or may not contain the substances listed on the label and that the amounts claimed are not subject to certification will be shown. No one is empowered to immediately stop the sale if the product doesn't contain what the label states.

Does people having lost their liver function through toxicity of several different botanical products matter? Is the adulteration of imported traditional remedies with poisonous heavy metals important? Does loss of life from the misguided use of Eastern potions as aphrodisiacs count? How much concern is appropriate when one Chinese herbal used for weight loss causes more than 100 cases of kidney failure (to say nothing of its inducing cancer)? What should we think about the fraudulent addition of modern synthetic drugs to boost the effectiveness of products supposedly consisting of "efficacious" and "harmless" plants extracts? What can we foresee of future problems for long-term use of sex hormone precursor molecules by adolescent youths? What sympathy should we feel for the several hundred persons killed or left with long-term, serious illnesses because the amino acid they took had a toxic contaminant that for months went undetected because no agency was responsible for checking on the producer for good manufacturing practices? Should the U.S. population be free to expose themselves to these "costs," the potential illnesses or even death from unvalidated, unregulated alternative products? If such questions implying negative answers concern the reader, as they should, continue through the following chapters to learn more on misadventures with materials qualifying as dietary supplements.

Closing with a Positive View

One physician-patient (Baron, 2001) expressed eloquently her belief that individuals should have the freedom of access to complementary medicine because of the important factor of hope that it may sustain. CAM was endorsed by that physician who herself had experienced the hard struggle of cancer chemotherapy. Doctor Susannah Baron, who experienced B-cell, non-Hodgkin's lymphoma while still in training as specialist in dermatology, expressed:

> Why shouldn't alternative therapies that make you feel better boost your immune system? Complementary medicine does exactly what it says: complements conventional medicine which we know has so many limitations. It can give you that edge and sometimes that's what you need to survive. (Baron, 2001, p. 291)

Chapter 5

Historical Natural Remedies

HOW DID WE GET TO WHERE WE ARE NOW?

> The desire to take medicine is perhaps the greatest feature which distinguishes man from animals.
>
> Sir William Osler
> Professor of Medicine

The beginning of humankind's usage of natural remedies predates our best historical records. All that can be said about those earliest origins consists of speculation based on archeological and paleontological researches, extrapolations from the earliest written records and many educated guesses. In other words, the initial use of natural materials as remedies is hidden from accurate view in the proverbial mists of times past.

BOTANICAL MARVELS: "MIRACLE DRUGS" FROM LONG AGO

A "miracle drug" is a drug, usually one newly discovered, that evokes a dramatic positive response, i.e., it proves extraordinarily effective in improving a patient's condition (also often called a "wonder drug"). Although the phrase *miracle drug* may not have come into its highest popularity until the mid-twentieth century, in many prior instances the phrase might properly have been applied. Indeed, at least in the nineteenth century, it was used for various natural remedies as a part of the florid sales practices of that era. Such overblown claims of past centuries were not always well founded, as also in recent times. For example, tobacco was first hailed as a major new medicinal plant discovery, being described in 1571 as a remedy for 36 maladies over a wide range, from migraine headache to toothache, falling fingernails, worms, halitosis, lockjaw, and cancer. However, its medicinal image

doi:10.1300/5698_05

was not long sustained. Early on its major application became what in more recent times would be called a "recreational drug." The recognition of what later would be called addictiveness of tobacco became evident early to the Scottish novelist and poet Sir Walter Scott (1771-1832) who at the turn of the nineteenth century spoke of the use of tobacco as being "hard to quit." It took centuries more for the full scope of the damaging effects of tobacco smoking, especially its foremost adverse effects on the cardiovascular system and lungs, to be fully recognized.

This chapter will describe some botanical preparations that may in ages past have been household remedies and that by today's standards could be viewed as dietary supplements. However, they instead became mainstays of the physician for giving of comfort. They were among the first to provide an effective therapy for medical conditions, and consequently they played a major role in the development of modern Western pharmacotherapy.

Opium (Papaver somniferum): *"God's Own Medicine" for Relief of Pain*

Without doubt the availability of opium as a pain reliever was a tremendous advance over all previous attempts at finding solace from severe suffering from conditions such as serious traumatic injury (as in battlefield wounds), organic malfunctions (e.g., gallstones), or advanced cancer. For those so afflicted, the benefits of opium must indeed have been miraculous. Previously available plant preparations mainly were dissolved in alcohol, with their effects coming largely from the alcohol (ethanol). Alcohol is not a true analgesic, although it does serve as a sedative and sleep-promoting agent, especially when used as a vehicle for certain herbs that have minor pain-suppressing actions.

The initial discovery and ancient origins of the medical usefulness of the opium poppy are unrecorded by historical sources. Some authorities believe that from about 3400 BC opium poppies were being cultivated in lower Mesopotamia by the Sumerians, who called it the "joy plant" for its capacity to induce euphoria. They were followed in its use by the Assyrians and Egyptians. Its medicinal value was known in Greece by Hippocrates, "the father of medicine," in about 460 BC. Its medical use was recorded by the Greek physician Dioscorides in his catalogue of drugs written in about AD 60 or 70. A surgeon with the Roman army, Dioscorides had occasion to travel throughout much of the Roman Empire—Italy, Gaul, Spain, and North Africa. He used that opportunity to collect and record the existence and medicinal value of hundreds of plants. He compiled an extensive list of medicinal herbs and their alleged virtues. This work, which in its Latin translation became well known by its title, "De Materia Medica," served as the cornerstone compendium of Western pharmaceutical and herbal knowledge for the next 15 centuries. Moreover, it was also translated into Syrian, Arabic, and Persian languages, thus exerting a strong and widespread influence on the development of medieval medicine from Europe to the Near East. Dioscorides's recipe for an opium preparation called for the maceration of heads of the poppy flowers for extraction over two days in rainwater, combining the water with honey, and boiling the mixture until it thickened to the desired consistency.

In early centuries, the noted physician-philosopher Galen (AD 129-199), was not very enthusiastic about opium, saving it for very urgent cases. Moreover, use of opium was discouraged if not forbidden by the Roman Catholic Church from about 1300 until it was reintroduced by a renowned Renaissance physician, Paracelsus, who lived from 1493 to 1541. A native of Switzerland, his actual name was Phillippus Aureolus Theophrastus Bombas von Hohenheim (no wonder he chose a simple pseudonym). He was in his own time called by some a "Luther of medicine," e.g., a bold reformer of therapeutics. It is said that he owed much of his success to a liberal, bold application of opium in the form of pills at a time when his contemporaries were still adverse to its use. By 1600 one of his Dutch followers declared that the practice of medicine would be impossible without opium. A renowned English physician, Thomas Sydenham, is responsible for the phrase describing opium as being "God's own medicine." The actual quotation from which the phrase derives was, "Among the remedies which it has pleased Almighty God to give to man to relieve his sufferings, none is so universal and so efficacious as opium." He also recommended it for sleeplessness and diarrhea, for which it also is quite effective.

Paracelsus was first to give the name "laudanum" to medicinal opium, but "Sydenham's Laudanum" was a liquid preparation of opium made with sherry wine and herbs that dated from 1670 or 1680. Versions of this form of opium were perpetuated well into the twentieth century under the name of "tincture of opium" in the United States Pharmacopoeia (USP). The term *laudanum* derives from a root meaning worthy of praise. However, its misuse could cause a state of dependence that induced the addicted person instead to curse it as a source of veritable bondage (Anonymous, 1889).

A more renowned writing was Thomas De Quincey's autobiographical *Confessions of an English Opium-Eater,* although "opium eaters" were actually drinkers of laudanum, which supplied ethanol as well as morphine and other opium alkaloids. Besides Thomas De Quincey, other Victorian-era English writers of highest fame who are said to have become habitual users of opium in the form of laudanum included Charles Dickens and Elizabeth Barrett Browning (circa 1837).

The isolation from opium of its active ingredient, the alkaloid morphine, by the German chemist Friedrich Serturner in1803 made available a much more powerful drug. It was readily embraced by physicians, the more so after Dr. Alexander Wood of Edinburgh in 1843 introduced a new manner of administering morphine by hypodermic injection via a syringe and needle. He found that morphine's effects on patients were of much faster onset and were much more potent than those following an oral dose. It was a fateful discovery when in 1874 an English researcher named C.R. Wright converted morphine into diacetylmorphine, better known as heroin. This compound was then and continues to be accepted for medical use in Britain despite its being banned in the United States because of the great liking and preference held for it by addicts. Ironically, heroin (similar to cocaine in the 1890s) was advocated in the early 1900s in the United States as an aid to recovery from opium addiction!

For the remarkable history of opium poppy cultivation and the commercializing of opium distribution for nonmedical use, along with its strong sociopolitical aspects, see www.pbs.org/wgbh/pages/frontline/shows/heroin/etc/history.html, www.opioids.com/timeline/, or http://narcotichx.homestead.com/OpiateHistory1.html.

*Peruvian Bark (***Cinchona** *species): Conqueror of Malarial Fevers*

The area of South America that we now know as Peru was first explored by Europeans in 1513, and it came under the control of Spain about the middle of that century. Whether the bark of the cinchona tree actually was used by the indigenous people as a medicine is uncertain, but they clearly utilized it as a dye. However, they are said to have used the bitter bark of the "fever tree," which grew in the montane rain forests along the eastern slopes of the northern Andes, as a native remedy. Its recorded value as a febrifuge—an agent to oppose fever—is traced to 1638 when it was used to cure an "intermittent fever" for the Countess of Chinchon, wife of the Spanish Viceroy of Peru. This incident gave the tree, source of the bark, both a name and the beginnings of fame as a remedy. It is said that after her cure the Countess became quite a strong advocate for the new medicine. Accounts differ over who brought this remedy to be used for the Countess's therapy, but it is commonly attributed to the Jesuit missionaries who had been in the country for more than 50 years and were likely to know about native remedies. On the basis of this story, true or not, the renowned biologist and father of taxonomy, Carl Linnaeus, described and named the plant source but altered the spelling to be *Cinchona officinalis.*

When the Count and Countess returned to their home in Spain in 1640, Juan del Vego, their physician in Peru, also returned, bringing with him a considerable quantity of the cinchona or "Peruvian bark." His reports on the value of the material and his spread of it provoked a lively interest. Soon controversy existed over its acceptance as a cure for intermittent fever (this was a common phrase for malaria) between two schools of physicians. Those favorable were followers of Paracelsus, while those against were adherents of Galen. Perhaps of greater significance was the advocacy of cinchona by Jesuits, who imported a large supply to Rome from whence it was widely distributed over Europe among the members of their order. They were said to have supplied it as a powder without fee to the poor, while charging "its weight in gold" to the rich. In 1679 the head of the Jesuit order visited Paris, where he found the son of King Louis XIV ill with intermittent fever. The bark was recommended and supplied, and the patient soon became well. Such events made the "powder of the Jesuits" to be increasingly in demand over the next century, except among Protestants. The English Protestants' leader, Oliver Cromwell, rejected it. Supposedly, he died of malaria after refusing what he called instead the powder of the devil.

With the escalation of both demand and the price that many persons were willing to pay for a curative against the all-too-common fevers of the mid-seventeenth century, fraudulent substitutes began to appear. Spanish merchants were said to have replaced the difficult-to-obtain Peruvian import with botanical material from much more readily available sources. It must be acknowledged that the motivation of greed and dishonesty is no less evident in the early twenty-first century than in the seventeenth century. The possibility for similar fraudulent substitutions exists in the present-day botanical marketplace, just as counterfeits of prescription drug products in circulation also exist today.

In about 1671 an Englishman named Robert Talbor began a medical practice focused on treating fevers with cinchona. Talbor changed cinchona therapy by devising a liquid decoction rather than employing the traditional powdered form. Red wine saw major use as a solvent for the active components of the bark. This was the first step toward the eventual isolation of the active ingredient, the alkaloid quinine, from the bark. However, a major step toward widespread therapeutic use of cinchona depended on its being cultivated. Efforts in that direction failed in the 1700s, but around the mid-1800s both Dutch and British governments achieved success. The Netherlands established cinchona cultivation in their East Indies possession, Java, while the British did so in India. This had no small role in subsequent geopolitics of southeast Asia and tropical Africa.

The isolation of quinine, the active ingredient of cinchona bark, was accomplished in 1820. Subsequently, the use of quinine facilitated European colonization of the tropics and the operation of plantations and mines in their colonies. It was critically important in enabling the United States to construct the Panama Canal. In 1856 a chemist seeking to make synthetic quinine produced instead the first artificial aniline coal tar dye, derivatives of which much later became the basis for synthetic anti-infective drugs. When World War II threatened to deprive the Allies of critical access to cinchona plantations as source for the much-needed quinine, the search for a synthetic alternative was intensified. With the discovery of primaquine and other synthetic compounds, the dependence of antimalarial therapy upon quinine fell sharply, and its usage began to fade. This decline was accelerated by the malarial organism, *Plasmodium falciparum,* evolving to gain considerable resistance (lessened susceptibility) to quinine. Indeed, the story of quinine could be seen as an inspiration and pattern for further battles to be pursued in finding chemotherapies for many other infectious disease.

Purple Foxglove (Digitalis purpurea): *Restorer of Power to a Failing Heart Muscle*

The ancient history of foxglove is associated with its use by herbalists as an external preparation for complaints such as scrofula (tuberculosis of the lymph nodes in the neck). A few British physicians writing in the sixteenth and seventeenth centuries endorsed its internal use for the "falling sickness" (epilepsy), for which it has never been shown effective. It was also applied externally in a salve for all sorts of sores. However, in 1785 a physician and botanical scientist of Birmingham, England, William Withering, published "An Account of the Foxglove and Some of Its Medical Uses." He related that he became aware of the secret family recipe of an old woman in Shropshire for a remedy that had cured persons from "dropsy," which we now know as congestive heart failure with its familiar excess of fluid in the feet and legs and/or the lungs. He indicated that the recipe included about twenty herbs, but that he readily perceived foxglove to be the source of its benefit. Withering detailed his successful application of foxglove in hundreds of cases, concluding that it acted to benefit the heart but also provoked diuresis—increased kidney output—to remove the accumulated body fluid (edema) characteristic of dropsy. Foxglove for medical use in the form of the ground leaf became known as "digitalis," and it soon was recognized by an important drug compendium, the Edinburgh Pharmacopoeia.

Withering was concerned about physicians' using excessive doses of his marvelous new drug. Indeed, even now a considerable potential exists for adverse response with overdosage of digitalis such that a high-tech, antibody-based antidotal product has been developed to treat overdose toxicity.

Analogous problems in knowing the correct or optimal dose for botanical remedies persist to the present, more than two centuries later. To a large extent this arises from lack of knowledge about which component(s) among the variable mixture of chemicals in a plant may be responsible for the benefits associated with its use. To achieve chemically standardized preparations of a botanical one must know which chemical to use as basis for such a standardization. Research chemists are wrestling with this problem at many institutions, including the Thad Cochran National Center for Natural Products Research of the School of Pharmacy at the University of Mississippi.

Meadow Saffron (Colchicum autumnale): *The Herb That Puts Gout to Rout*

Meadow saffron or autumn crocus is a plant that had a reputation in early centuries of the Christian era as a poison. However, Dioscorides, a Greek surgeon in the Roman army during the rule of Nero (AD 54-68), described the meadow saffron in his influential pharmacopeia, "De Materia Medica," as also being a useful medicine. Despite the accurate characterization of it as a poison—a fatal overdose in medicinal application is possible—the crocus was used to treat joint pain as early as the sixth century. An early recognition of its selective benefit for gout is traced to 1763, and soon thereafter it was reportedly introduced into North American for this use by Benjamin Franklin. Its active component, the alkaloid colchicine, was isolated in 1820 by French chemists Pierre Joseph Pelletier and Joseph Bienaime Caventou.

Colchicine has continued in such use from then until now, but not so often as formerly because of the availability of less dangerous therapies. However a Mayo Clinic study described 22 patients having idiopathic pulmonary fibrosis, a quite threatening condition. When treated with colchicine they fared as well as they did on the standard therapy with a corticosteroid, but with far fewer side effects.

Not until 1951, when a synthetic anti-inflammatory agent indomethacin was discovered, could a patient suffering from acute gout receive comparable help via a safer drug. Newer synthetic drugs are now available for preventing acute attacks of gout: probenecid, sulfinpyrazone, and allopurinol. Although the suffering from the intense burning pain of gout does warrant a strongly favorable reputation for its remedy, gout is too rare for meadow saffron to gain a glory comparable to that of the opium poppy, Peruvian bark, or purple foxglove.

Coca Leaf/Cocaine: Nineteenth-Century Miracle Drug; Twentieth-Century Scourge

Cocaine is an alkaloid derived from the leaves of a South American shrub known as coca. It was first extracted from coca in the nineteenth century and was initially hailed as a miracle drug. It came into medical use most often in surgical applications that took advantage of its production of a strong anesthetic effect locally and also its ability to constrict small arteries, which reduced the tendency for bleeding. Indeed, it was the first true local anesthetic. However, it also has strong stimulatory effects on various functions throughout the central nervous system. By the 1880s in the United States it was freely prescribed by physicians for such conditions as exhaustion, depression, and morphine addiction, and was available in many patent medicines. In excess, cocaine causes a sudden increase in heart rate, blood pressure, and body temperature, which can threaten the health and life of a user.

Moreover, cocaine proved to provoke a dependency every bit as serious as the opium or morphine addiction, for therapy of which it was promoted by such a notable as Dr. Sigmund Freud, who is said to have experimented with its actions personally. Cocaine initially evokes a profound feeling of well-being, self-confidence, and alertness along with a lack of hunger. These euphoric effect last for 10 to 30 minutes, and they may seduce the person into frequent usage until his or her whole existence becomes oriented to usage of the drug. After a recognition of its dangers and social detriments grew, restrictive regulations were enacted. Its use decreased, and by the 1920s the epidemic had abated.

The discovery of alternative molecules to serve as effective local anesthetics, which were safer for their lacking the brain and behavioral effects of cocaine, led to its downfall as a therapeutic agent by mid-twentieth century. However, the nonmedical use of cocaine grew ever more prominent as the second half of the 1900s advanced. An epidemic began in the United States in the 1970s and peaked in 1988. Hundreds of young adults were caught up in the craze for use of "crack" cocaine. One of the most prominent tragedies of this era was the overdose fatality in 1986 of Len Bias, a prominent basketball star at the University of Maryland. He was the second overall NBA draft pick in 1986 and was signed by the Boston Celtics. Less than 48 hours after signing a million-dollar contract he was dead of a cocaine overdose (Smith, 1992).

After returning from a trip to Boston, Bias was with some friends in his dormitory suite. One of his friends made an emergency call for assistance because Bias had collapsed and experienced a seizure. After unsuccessful resuscitation efforts at a hospital, he was pronounced dead of cardiac arrest, which was later attributed to cocaine toxicity by a medical examiner. Bias had seemed destined in a few months to begin leading the team into a successful "post–Larry Bird" era. One friend of Bias was indicted and tried on charges of possessing and distributing cocaine and obstructing justice, but he was acquitted of the drug charges and the other charge was dropped. However, in 1993 he was sentenced by a federal court to ten years and one month in prison for further distributing of cocaine in years after Bias' death. A lack of understanding of the potential for serious toxicity with the "recreational" cocaine abuse cost 22-year-old Len Bias his promising career and his life.

The severe sociopolitical disruption in the South American coca-growing countries as well as the heavy adverse consequences of its North American abuse combined to make cocaine neither a magical nor miracle remedy. Instead it became a serious candidate, along with the stimulant methamphetamine, for being "the scourge of the century" with respect to drug abuse.

Galantamine: A Twenty-First Century Marvel

Galantamine (Reminyl) is a new Rx drug approved by the FDA in early 2001 that was derived from European daffodil (*Galanthus nivalis* L.), which bears lovely white flowers. The often lengthy process of detecting and validating a medical application for an active component from a plant material is well illustrated by this instance. The medicinal source reportedly was discovered among a field of wild flowers, Caucasian snowdrops, in Bulgaria. According to media sources, research on the plant was started in the early 1950s by a Bulgarian pharmacologist after one of his students said that the people in her village rubbed snowdrops on their forehead to ease nerve pain. This lack of correspondence between the folk application of this plant and the action later found of value to modern medicine is a fairly common occurrence. The upshot is that many useful medicinal agents derived from natural products do not prove to have the useful application attributed to them according to "folk wisdom" but may turn out to have some unrelated benefit.

DEVELOPMENT OF SCIENTIFIC MEDICINE

If one looks back to the Middle Ages it appears that the early representations of science were not far removed from the practices of traditional healers, shamans, or witch doctors. Witness to this can be found in a prescription by a professor of chemistry:[1] "For epilepsy in adults I recommend spirit [an alcoholic extract] of human brain or a powder to be compounded only in the months of May, June and July from the livers of live green frogs" (Cerf and Navasky, 1998, p. 34).

Despite such pessimism and negativity, the nineteenth century witnessed the launching of a scientific revolution in medicine by virtue of great advances in underlying biomedical sciences. Laboratory researches upon various natural products, especially toxic botanical ingredients, was fundamental to the development of the sciences of physiology and pharmacology, and they began to blossom abundantly at the outset of the twentieth century.

Indeed, in the late 1890s, aspirin became available as a new pain reliever and barbital became the first sedative of the barbiturate family, which subsequently grew to provide central nervous system depressants for various medical objectives. However, despite Holmes's negativity, the mid-nineteenth century already had witnessed a very major advance with the introduction in the 1840s of general anesthetics—nitrous oxide, ether, chloroform—to enable pain to be eliminated from both major and minor surgery.

New and improved anesthetics were developed throughout the twentieth century (However, those now available still are imperfect, too often associated with adverse after-effects on the brain [POCD, postOperative cognitive disfunction]). Risks are higher in more severely ill or injured patients and for those at older ages). The skills of surgeons improved and the technological aids to their efforts multiplied greatly as well. Local anesthetics and several other new classes of drugs greatly facilitated surgeons' often-marvelous procedures for removing malignant growths and restoring bodies from the devastation of trauma, the ravages of disease, or the defects of prenatal development failures.

In the mid-twentieth century the practice of medicine was revolutionized by the advances in treatments for infections—first the sulfonamide antibacterials and then successive classes and generations of antibiotics, beginning with penicillin. Following this came tremendous advances in psychopharmacology—the antipsychotic, antidepressant, and antimanic drugs that restore a semblance of normal life to persons afflicted by schizophrenia, major depression, or the mania of bipolar disorder. Cancer chemotherapy came into existence with progressively increasing help for surviving the dreaded diseases of leukemias, lymphomas, and even some carcinomas. Even such a daunting scourge as AIDS began to be brought under control. However, despite all of these major advances in the practice of medicine, a populace whose expectations had been raised to the point of seeking a chemical solution for *every* complaint has looked farther afield than merely the therapies offered by conventional medicine. A remarkable proportion of the people in Western nations during the late twentieth century embraced the hope offered by the natural remedies of CAM. Indeed, many natural wonder drugs of the far past are still important to modern medicine.

The prevalent approach to drug discovery research during the twentieth century was to study the chemistry of bacteria, fungi, and higher plants as sources of "lead compounds," which suggest new related chemicals having better chances of success as a medicine than the compound itself, and it has a better chance of being patentable. Many researchers employ the information derived from various systems of traditional medicine (ethnomedicine) for valuable guidelines to drug discovery objectives. Fabricant and Farnsworth (2001) identified 122 compounds of defined structure, which were obtained from merely 94 species of plants, that are used globally as remedies. They demonstrated that 80 percent of these had found an ethnomedical use that was identical to or related to the current medical application for the active constituent(s) of the plant. However, we must add that in many instances a modern medical application was discovered that cannot be related closely if at all to supposed beneficial actions in traditional ethnic lore.

An extra bright side of natural products research in the early twentieth century was its being a boon to the development of the biomedical sciences, first physiology and then pharmacology, and surely of toxicology. Investigating the active principles of important plant drugs, such as have been previously described, greatly aided in the formation of the basic constructs of these sciences, especially involving neurotransmitters both in the autonomic nervous system and in the peripheral neuromuscular control pathways. Those in turn paved the way for understanding of neurotransmission in the brain and the important areas of neuropharmacology and psychopharmacology.

PART II: Major Myths and Misconceptions

Be careful about reading health books. You may die of a misprint.

Mark Twain

Chapter 6

Botanical Supplements As Foods

One of the foremost myths fundamental to the dietary supplement trade is the mode of advertising for their products that might be called "organ-targeted nutritional supplementation." This concept is expressed by phrases of the following sort: "Compound X provides nutritional support for the [bladder/kidney/prostate/uterus/liver/eyes, etc.] so as to restore/maintain its healthful activity."

Statements such as these typically claim that a particular botanical (or a combination of several botanicals perhaps even with nutrients) has a special affinity for the organ in question and is able to benefit its healthy function by serving a role in vital "nutritional support." Never mind that decades of nutritional science research have established little if any scientific foundation for the "organ-targeted nutrition" concept expressed by those statements. Such unscientific (and at times nonsensical) statements constitute a solution to DSHEA legislation that restricts direct claim of a benefit for a particular disorder of a particular organ.

PAIN RELIEVERS AS FOODS?

However, as time progresses less and less lip-service is given to this principle and products are increasingly being described in terms of pharmacological actions. A prime example is the recent advent of products described as "a freedom formula," meaning freedom from pain. Relief of pain is quite certainly a fundamental aspect of pharmacotherapy. The foundation for these developments started with a new approach by the pharmaceutical industry several years ago which saw the introduction of selective COX-2 inhibitors, mainly for treating arthritic pain.

The first two of these were celecoxib (Celebrex) and rofecoxib (Vioxx), which were hailed as superceding the class of NSAIDs (nonsteroidal anti-inflammatory drugs), which act less selectively to inhibit both COX-1 and COX-2 enzymes. The desired pain relief is associated with COX-2 inhibi-

Consumer's Guide to Dietary Supplements and Alternative Medicines

doi:10.1300/5698_06

tion, while gastric irritation (and potential stomach ulceration) or injury to kidney function are associated with COX-1 inhibition. Although it is unclear that the superiority of COX-2 inhibitors is as great as was anticipated, it is remarkable that 2002 saw the launching of "natural alternatives"—botanicals acting as selective COX-2 inhibitors; this clearly is not a case for "nutritional support."

The truth is that these did not really comprise a new and distinct pharmacological class as the promotion sought to convince physicians and patients. Rather, they still were and are NSAIDs, and among that class some prior agents had considerable COX-2 selectivity, but they were not among the most prescribed NSAIDs, to which the new agents were compared. When those older, fairly selective inhibitors were developed, the discrimination between the two enzymes had not yet been uncovered.

One herbal COX-2 inhibitor formula contains curcumin from turmeric as the provider of a selective COX-2 inhibitory action. The other employs a new "patent-pending extract from the phellodendron tree" (Nexrutine). It should be emphasized that to whatever extent adverse effects accompany selective COX-2 inhibition, those risks logically would extend to natural inhibitors that share a common mechanism with the synthetic ones.[1]

Users of any member of the NSAID family, but mainly the "granddaddy," aspirin, are found to show a significantly reduced risk for the development of Alzheimer's disease (Etminan et al., 2003). The relative risk was 0.72 among NSAID use by people over the age of 55 years for all durations. However, the greatest benefit was for patients who used NSAIDs for more than 24 months, who had a lower relative risk for showing Alzheimer's disease of 0.27, only one-fourth as high as for those not using NSAIDs.

5-LOX stands for 5-lipoxygenase, one of a family of enzymes that acts to add oxygen atoms to the polyunsaturated fatty acids. This one acts on arachidonic acid to produce leukotrienes that act as mediators of inflammatory changes. Table 6.1 demonstrates these and other examples of the pharmacologic, not nutritional, character of many supplement ingredients.

WHAT DOES NUTRITIONAL SCIENCE SAY?

A brief review of basic nutritional science should help put these matters in proper perspective. Any textbook of nutrition will reveal that only the members of a limited group of chemicals are considered to truly provide nutrition, and thus nutritional support. They consist of the following:

1. *Carbohydrates:* consisting of simple sugars, complex sugars (or starches), and the "glyco" components of glycoproteins and glycosamino-

TABLE 6.1. Some supplements said to act by drug- or hormone-like actions.

Supplement and general descriptive phrase for the therapeutic effect	Mechanistic description of the product's claimed mode of action
Starch neutralizer to oppose uptake of calories ingested in the form of starches	Inhibition of the digestive enzyme amylase so that starch is not digested into absorbable sugars
Natural alternatives to NSAIDs for treating musculoskeletal pain	Selective inhibition of the COX-2 enzyme
Viagra substitutes for treating erectile dysfunction	Dilation of blood vessels to penis by raising level of cGMP[a] by inhibiting phosphodiesterase 5; same mechanism as sildenafil (Viagra), and others.
Fish protein powder or fish peptide extract	Inhibits ACE (angiotensin converting) enzyme, the antihypertensive mechanism of some Rx drugs
Niacin (vitamin B3) used in large, supra-nutrient doses	Vasodilation (flushing) and lowering of the blood level of cholesterol

glycans, which are complex molecules associated with connective tissue collagen.

2. *Fats:* Saturated and unsaturated, these are found as essential building blocks in all cells, being the fundamental component of the cell membrane. The fat found in what we call fat cells is not an active, functioning form, but rather comprises a storage depot for this class of molecules. From the broad biological viewpoint across a diversity of vertebrate species, storage of fat occurs for physiological purposes in only a few situations: (1) preparation of the female for reproduction, (2) preparation of either sex for surviving a winter period of limited food availability, and (3) preparation of both sexes, among the migratory species, for the metabolic stress of migration. Unfortunately, among the population of Western industrialized nations, excess storage of fat prevails in spite of most persons affected facing none of these three biological needs to warrant it. Many people are nutritionally well prepared for a really long migration, but would consider a walk around the block to be excessive.

3. *Proteins, peptides, and amino acids:* Among the 21 amino acids, eight or nine are classified as "essential," needing to be supplied by the human diet because we must have them for our biochemistry but cannot synthesize sufficient quantities of them for our needs. Thus, they must be included in

our food intake. These essential amino acids are isoleucine, leucine, lysine, methionine, phenylalanine, threonine, tryptophan, valine, and histidine (for children only). In addition both cysteine and tyrosine formerly were classified as nonessential amino acids but are now considered "quasi-essential." This is so because if the diet contains them, the body can use them to produce two essential amino acids, methionine and phenylalanine, respectively.

Nonessential amino acids are alanine, arginine, asparagine, aspartic acid (aspartate), glutamic acid (glutamate), glutamine, glycine, proline, serine, and taurine. Collectively, the amino acids are the building blocks from which our cells synthesize peptides, which are chains of connected amino acid units. In addition, we must have amino acids to build proteins, which consist of long and more structurally complex chains of hundreds of amino acids. The composition and sequence of amino acids are very critical to the functional biological properties of all proteins.

The synthesis of peptides and proteins is dictated by our genetic material, which is contained in long chains of nucleotides that comprise spiral, ladderlike biochemical macromolecules that are known as DNA (for deoxyribonucleic acid). Note that these nucleic acids are quite distinct from the amino acids. Despite their highly critical metabolic importance, nucleic acids are not required to be obtained as such from our diets but can be fully synthesized by the action of those highly crucial metabolic proteins that we know as enzymes.

4. *Vitamins:* These are relatively small molecules not fitting any of the previous classes, which cannot be synthesized by our tissues. In many cases vitamins act cooperatively with enzymes, which causes them to be called coenzymes. It is needful that we absorb enough of them *with* our diet. Several of the earlier-discovered class members were "amines" chemically, and they also were vital, thus, the name *vitamines* was coined, and subsequently the *e* was dropped. Note the use of the term *with* rather than *from* our diet. The former is used because in the case of vitamin K we can absorb the natural molecule from our intestinal tract even though it did not enter the alimentary canal as part of the food we eat. The reason for this paradox is that the normal bacterial residents of our intestine can and do synthesize vitamin K, a process of which we are benefactors. If all is well with our usual intestinal bacterial cohabitants, they will supply our normal need for vitamin K without a dietary source.

5. *Minerals:* All of the members of the previous classes are in chemical nature organic molecules, which means that they are compounds based on the element carbon. Minerals are inorganic (noncarbon) elements the atoms of which ordinarily occur in combination with atoms of another inorganic element in a compound known as a salt, for example potassium chloride. Or at times they are combined with an organic "carrier" molecule such as sele-

nium with the amino acid methionine. Familiar essential mineral elements include: calcium, phosphorous, sodium, chloride, and sulfur, plus the metals, iron, zinc, magnesium, manganese, copper, and a few other so-called "trace elements" that are less familiar—e.g., cobalt, selenium, vanadium, and chromium. Animal or human tissues may contain some other common elements, which enter our bodies via food, water or air, but that have no nutritional role, e.g., aluminum and silicon. Even as an excess of some of the required elements may cause injury—such as copper, iron and selenium—so also, other elements that have no biological role may accumulate to become poisonous if we are overexposed, especially to those known as heavy metals, such as lead, arsenic, and mercury. Even the light metal, aluminum, in a sufficient excess may cause neurotoxicity (causing "dialysis dementia"), which has supported the proposition that it may act as a factor in the brain injury of Alzheimer's dementia.

The amounts of material from classes 1, 2, and 3 that are required for adequate nutrition are large enough that they are called the macronutrients, whereas the much smaller required amounts of the vitamins and minerals cause them to be labeled the micronutrients.

Here is a very important point of information: plant and animal foods that we eat, and some beverages that we drink, contain multitudes of molecules of many different classes besides those outlined in classes 1 through 5. However, none among those thousands of chemicals in plants, besides those in classes 1 to 5, are actually considered true nutrients according to nutritional science. Instead, by the terminology of the science of pharmacology, such chemicals are called *xenobiotics,* defined as molecules that are not foods (nutrients) and are (with occasional exceptions) unnatural to the human body, that is, they are not produced by mammalian cells, nor are they involved in the essential, normal biochemical reactions. Thus, they are instead foreign (xeno-) to the body and its biochemistry. Indeed, these molecules have been the traditional research focus of the sciences of pharmacology, toxicology, and/or pharmacognosy rather than nutrition.

However, recent decades have witnessed nutritional scientists undertaking laboratory studies of xenobiotics for their exerting incidentally beneficial effects on normal life functions of animal species and human beings. Many xenobiotics have become known and used as diagnostic or therapeutic agents, or drugs, whereas others have made a reputation for themselves as poisons. A fairly common mode of action for such materials is by means of their inhibiting enzyme activities. In limbo or "a never-never land" are many food components that have become recognized as exerting favorable but nonnutritional effects. Among these are a great many that have been marketed as dietary supplements.

Some supplement sellers are deviating from the usual line and clearly acknowledging the nonnutrient basis for their products' supposed beneficial effects. An example besides those in Table 6.1 is as follows: "Studies show that it ["natural fruit extract"] is very safe. HCA [the active component, hydroxycitrate] helps inhibit fat production by temporarily inhibiting the enzyme ATP-citrate lyase, which converts carbohydrates to fats in the liver." This mechanism is supposed to be one that mobilizes fat, even when it cannot be regarded as excess fat, which is what makes it appealing to bodybuilders' fight against the last ounce of unsightly fat. The compulsive motivation of many bodybuilders to enhance their musculature to a maximum is accompanied by a drive to eliminate all of their subcutaneous fat that may hinder the best display of those muscles.

If we were to follow the lead of the current mythological concept, what should we say about caffeine? What if we should find caffeine-containing beverages—tea, coffee, or colas—being promoted by statements that "caffeine provides nutritional support for your brain activity"? I prefer to believe that most persons reading this page will find some humor in such a proposition. Caffeine is well known to be a stimulant, i.e., a drug, not a food that provides "nutritional support for brain activity." (However, the original version of what became Coca-Cola *was* called a "Brain Tonic and Intellectual Beverage.") Caffeine has an action that is pharmacological, not nutritional. In short, caffeine surely is a drug as defined by the science of pharmacology, whether it is being ingested as a component of a familiar age-old beverage or is being injected as a medicinal solution. Indeed, it formerly (more than currently) had medical application as a respiratory stimulant for persons whose brain center that controls breathing was impaired.

The antioxidant molecules in green tea have been subject to considerable scientific study in Japan and elsewhere in the 1990s. Laboratory animal data tends to support the conclusion from epidemiological studies that habitual users of green tea as a beverage are protected against malignant neoplastic diseases (cancerous growths). These findings make it possible to believe that green tea can serve as a preventive for certain cancers. Even that is a *drug* action. Drugs were long ago defined as foreign, nonfood molecules useful for the diagnosis, prevention, and/or alleviation of disease manifestations. To say that green tea serves as a "nutritional agent" when it is used for a possible protective action against cancer, or any other disease that it may benefit, is to distort long-established scientific and medical definitions for economic reasons. It is unreasonable for that to be happening, but it is happening in the United States. That view was expressed succinctly in a special issue of *JAMA* concerning dietary supplements by the title for an editorial (DeAngelis and Fontanarosa, 2003)—"Drugs Alias Dietary Supplements."

Because of the fundamental facts just stated on the xenobiotic components of plants, little or no scientific basis exists for the idea that the botanical supplements (herbals) are chemicals that provide special "nourishment" or "nutritional support" for persons' organs, whether it be the prostate, uterus, kidneys, or other. This is a fallacious concept that is foisted upon the U.S. public by the vendors of such products in order to sell the products while complying with the letter of the law—DSHEA. Admittedly, a few rare cases could have a valid argument that a botanical is a food component, such as when dealing with the food additives used as flavoring agents, spices (e.g., garlic and turmeric). Thus, in the promotion of dietary supplements, a molehill of evidence is frequently transformed into a mountain of promotional claims through endorsements by physicians whose level of sincerity and truthfulness we cannot measure. Scientific truth is not the issue; selling the product is the only issue. DSHEA used few facts and more fancy in declaring nonnutrient botanical products to be foods. The result was an oversimplifying of the issues and a failure to find the best answers for the regulation of botanicals and a few animal-source substances used as therapeutic remedies.

For fairness let it be noted that informational failings also exist concerning the promotional materials for Rx products that are directed to consumers. Those materials often project an arguably inaccurate, warm and fuzzy image for the product with an aim of getting consumers to insist that their physician prescribe the product. Also in this case, scientific truth seems not to be the issue; selling the product seems to be the overpowering issue.

Chapter 7

Natural Botanical Supplements

Herbal remedies are not inherently safe.

S. Bent and A.L. Avins (1999)

The toxicology of synthetic and natural toxins is similar.

Bruce N. Ames et al. (1990)

When we exercise the option to take a medicine, we generally believe that doing so will not lead to any harm. However, people in contemporary society have been made aware of altogether too many unsafe examples among conventional medicines. Many persons have become concerned, if not terrorized, by the lists of potential adverse responses to the prescription medicines they take. Some have become persuaded that their being synthetic is the key reason for the adverse effects of modern pharmaceuticals.

After 1994 the passage of the federal DSHEA legislation opened the way for a veritable flood of new botanicals and nutrients into the supplement marketplace. This torrent was accompanied by unprecedented promotional efforts by all available modes. A major theme of one basic sales pitch, which many of the American public seem to accept, is the false concept that says natural equals safe, whereas synthetic has been equated with being toxic. This fallacy was aptly described by University of Arizona pharmacologist-toxicologist, Ryan Huxtable, PhD (1992) in an article titled "The Myth of Beneficent Nature." His research on the chemicals of the group known as pyrrolizidine alkaloids showed that "Mother Nature" is not nearly so prone to avoid natural chemicals being poisonous as this myth would have us believe. Neither has the traditional usage of natural agents always successfully discriminated seriously toxic plants from safer ones.

Vendors of herbals and other supplements are highly motivated to promote the idea that natural equals safe to their potential customers. For a sub-

Consumer's Guide to Dietary Supplements and Alternative Medicines

doi:10.1300/5698_07

stantial number of people who use botanicals this may be a prime reason: they welcome and embrace the "myth of the natural." They are assisted in falling into this embrace by many promotional writings that clearly *promise* that natural remedies are somehow endowed with intrinsic safety, made available by kindly and caring suppliers. In contrast, synthetic medicines are much portrayed as dangerous products peddled by huge, greedy pharmaceutical companies that are insensitive to the benefit of consumers. Innumerable advertisements equate being natural with being safe, i.e., nontoxic. This is a major theme of many "natural" MDs who solicit subscribers for their newsletters promoting their favorite natural remedies. This chapter will debunk the myth of "natural safety" by showing that many natural products also are quite poisonous.

The division between "safe foods" and "unsafe medicines" is not at all what people generally think it to be. Good cooks know that raw vegetable materials are not always by any means safe, a feature not mentioned by advocates of ingesting high quantities of raw vegetables by "juicing." Some common and familiar vegetables need to be cooked to become edible rather than poisonous. A fine example would be insufficiently cooked red kidney beans, which in one report were described as causing of eight separate outbreaks of gastroenteritis (Noah et al., 1980).

Numerous natural products, mostly from higher plants, have been known since ancient times as the basis for potions used by professional poisoners because they contained powerful toxic constituents. Some turned into medicinals, especially when their active ingredients became available as purified active compounds permitting their chemical analysis that could ensure their safe use by assuring that the intended, proper dose of the powerful agent is used. Without chemical standardization a mixture that contains an uncertain amount of high-potency compounds cannot be assumed to be safe for human consumption. Examples of highly toxic active ingredients from plant materials that became medically useful are included in Table 7.1.

Any of the pre–twentieth century botanicals that contained these compounds could rightly be called poisonous. All of this group, if accidentally taken in an excess amount, could be fatal. At least two of those agents, digitalis and opium/morphine, were among those recently cited for their use by some physicians, and several nurses to end their patients lives' (Kinnell, 2001). However, each of them has shown medical value of great importance. Morphine and some others have been complemented but only partially superceded by newer agents, and they still have important usage in the twenty-first century. Their useful actions were able to be discovered because they are not subtle.

An herbal practitioner could easily recognize the response and receive patients' reports that a dose of opium (containing morphine as its active in-

TABLE 7.1. Examples of useful medicines derived from toxic plants.

Agent (Plant source)	Application	Overdosage toxic potential
Atropine (belladonna, or deadly nightshade)	gastrointestinal muscle relaxant; nerve gas antidote	delirium, coma, convulsions, possible death
Cocaine (coca)	local anesthetic	cardiac/respiratory failure, death
Codeine (opium)	suppress cough or pain	delirium, convulsions, respiratory failure and death
Colchicine (meadow saffron)	specific for pain of gout	confusion, delirium, neuropathy, renal failure, bone marrow aplasia
Digitoxin (digitalis)	enhance cardiac muscle action in congestive failure	color vision change, vomiting, heart slowing, fibrillation and death
Morphine (opium)	strong pain reliever	coma, respiratory failure, death
Physostigmine (ordeal Bean)	glaucoma therapy	many widespread symptoms leading to respiratory depression or death
Pilocarpine (jaborandi plant)	glaucoma therapy	similar to physostigmine
Quinine (cinchona bark)	antimalarial	dizziness, headache, nausea and emesis, circulatory collapse, death
Tubocurarine (curare)	muscle relaxant for better surgical anesthesia	paralysis, respiratory stoppage, and death

gredient) had relieved severe to excruciating pain, as from a kidney stone entering the ureter. A fever-lowering action of quinine in a malarial patient could also easily be detected, even lacking a thermometer, when a preparation of cinchona bark providing the benefits of quinine was administered. Colchicine was isolated from the meadow saffron *(Colchicum autumnale)*, which had long been observed to be useful for treating gout, another example of excruciating pain in affected joints being relieved in a short time. It is not difficult to see how a plant potion that was able to alleviate such pain would be clearly so recognized.

Indeed, researchers over the past century or more have been led to investigate plants known to be poisonous because, as will be noted, these are often sources of useful therapeutic actions when taken at low enough doses. Paracelsus, a founding father of the sciences of pharmacology and toxicology coined a truism often quoted as "the dose makes the poison." In other words, almost any useful chemical may become a poison if taken in an excessive quantity. Moreover, the old saying "one man's meat is another man's poison" can aptly be revised and reversed to "one man's poison may be another man's medicine!"

The action of a crude plant material known to the Yanomama tribe of Amazonian natives as "curare" could be recognized because it paralyzes the skeletal muscles, including those for breathing. The unfortunate person accidentally so affected would occasionally die in the course of their using the curare on the darts propelled from their blowguns to capture a monkey or other quarry sought for food. The French biomedical research pioneer, Claude Bernard, tested samples of those exotic materials and gained insight as to how it produced paralysis. This paved the way for its active component, d-tubocurarine, to eventually become a valuable drug for relaxing muscles of the abdomen or chest and greatly aiding the surgeon's task of operating in those areas.

Similarly, a native food-gathering procedure utilized the tropical American shrub, *Pilocarpus jaborundi,* which later yielded the active component pilocarpine for medical use. The presence in the plant's berries of a highly potent factor was evident from the plant being useful to catch fish for eating. When its berries were thrown into a small pond they produced such disability of the fish that they would float to the surface and be easily captured for food. Because of the much smaller dose needed to incapacitate the fish than to affect the eaters, they could dine with impunity. A solution of the purified pilocarpine has been useful in ophthalmology for treating glaucoma, but this use was incredibly unforeseeable from its application by the native food gatherers.

The dried seed of a woody vine from tropical West Africa was long called Calabar bean, or ordeal bean. It was obtained from *Physostigma venenosum,* and it proved to be the source for a potent and toxic alkaloid known to pharmacology and medicine as physostigmine or eserine. Tradition says that the Calabar bean was the "truth serum" of its place and time. When a person was accused of a serious offense, they might be required to swallow some ordeal beans to test whether their profession of innocence could be judged true or not. If they survived eating the required number of dried seeds, they were judged truthful; if they died after a dose, they were adjudged to have been guilty liars. Thus, trial, conviction and execution were sometimes combined in a single, efficient process! Again, the later medicinal applications of its constituents could hardly have been foreseen from this primitive forensic utilization.

Atropine is a major pharmacologically active alkaloidal constituent of the European plant, *Atropa belladonna,* commonly known as deadly nightshade. The presence of very toxic materials in this plant was not difficult to recognize, as the common name indicates. Perhaps an herbalist who made an aqueous solution of the plant ingredients by chance got a small drop in the eye and noted that it caused a profound and lengthy action to paralyze the internal ocular muscles. This produced not only a loss of capacity for focusing, but also a dilation of the pupils (mydriasis), which some women apparently perceived as having a cosmetic value. Medieval Italian ladies are said to have become so enamored of this application of the plant that the Latin name for the species became *belladonna,* meaning "beautiful lady," providing a lasting memorial to its cosmetic usage. What did it matter that the ladies so using belladonna could not focus well on the men who might look admiringly at them? However, this application gave no hint of its medical potential for relief of bronchial constriction in asthmatic persons. Might this usefulness have been was first noted by a Roman lady who happened to be asthmatic?

Excitatory properties of the strychnine alkaloid from *Strychnos nux-vomica* would not require a modern EEG (electroencephalograph) machine (brain wave recording apparatus) to be detected. It was long known for provoking convulsive seizures, which are easily observable. The idea that it could provide a benefit as a tonic persisted to the mid–twentieth century, when safer synthetic stimulants replaced it, except for its usage in homeopathic preparations, which are so greatly diluted as to be nontoxic. Similarly, the discovery of the sedative effects of various herbs, e.g., kava kava, likewise may be assumed to have required only one astute and careful observer. The same is true of others among the plant materials listed in Table 7.1.

However, credulity is stretched by many claims of herbalists for the benefits of using many traditional plant remedies, whether from North America, Europe, Asia, or Africa. It is difficult to believe that with unsophisticated conditions of observation even an astute observer could have made the necessary observations to detect subtle or slowly developing changes having therapeutic value or reflecting toxic injury. Persons who are acquainted with the process of establishing that a new candidate molecule has a valid use in drug therapy know that this involves extensive animal testing followed by complex human trials. Why are people so inclined to credit ancient herbal healers with great enlightenment or extraordinary perceptiveness, which they likely would deny to modern researchers? Do we subconsciously suppose that their supposed knowledge had some supernatural source? Perhaps this acceptance of the value of "traditional knowledge" harkens to an ancient respect for shamans—magicians or medicine men—who bring together religion and healing. Does a deeply rooted, unconscious hope exist in some or all of us that the traditional remedies, more than a contemporary drug product, will have some magical properties to heal the one who hopes, nay, believes that it will?

Detection of acute (immediate) or subacute (slightly delayed, but early) toxicity, which can occur within minutes to hours or at most a few days after exposure to the herb, could perhaps be readily possible. But how can we suppose that slow-onset or delayed toxic actions (weeks, months, or even years later) would be detectable by the shamans or traditional healers? The rigorous examinations and observations needed would seem to require a level of training and scientific sophistication that existed in very limited degrees prior to the nineteenth and twentieth centuries. The advent of human cancers after physical (e.g., x-irradiation) or chemical exposures that are capable of provoking it requires several years at a minimum, and more often several decades. Thus, how can we assume that herbals are safe and do not have a risk for provoking cancer? Indeed, it has become known in the past 10 to 50 years that several familiar, traditional botanical remedies contain cancer-promoting components—for example sassafras root, formerly used in making sassafras tea and flavoring candy and in herbal comfrey (Chapter 12).

Some plants provoke serious liver toxicity, including members of the *Amanita* family of mushrooms (see Chapter 12). Herbal healers' detecting such hepatotoxicity or the induction of cancer—delayed toxicities that manifest only weeks, months, or years after exposure—seems inconceivable. A cause-and-effect relationship in such situations could not reasonably have been discovered by primitive healers, yet these are the subtle sort of toxicity problems for which great concern must exist with respect to synthetic medicinals marketed after meeting the stringent requirements of the FDA for animal and human testing. Those safety requirements are being called "too excessive" for botanical remedies to meet because too small a profit margin exists in their marketing, but without them it will remain unknown whether a potential for serious organ toxicity or cancer lies undiscovered among hundreds of "nontoxic herbs."

TOXICITY PROBLEMS OF MODERN PHARMACEUTICALS

In recent years, the U.S. drug scene has been marked by the withdrawal of several widely used and highly valued medicines. A recent example is the oral antidiabetic therapy, troglitazone (Rezulin), which was recalled from the market because of rare cases of severe liver injury (that have also occurred with some closely related agents). These were regarded to be idiosyncratic reactions, which means that they cannot be foreseen from animal research, and that the risk seems not to be proportional to the dose but rather is determined by special, atypical traits (idiosyncrasies) of a small minority of users. Only rarely were cases of reversible jaundice, an indicator of possible liver toxicity, noted during the controlled clinical studies of Rezulin that supported the approval for its marketing.

After its introduction in early 1997, approximately 650,000 patients had been treated with Rezulin by the time of the first warning. Yet, additional millions of patient years of use were needed before evidence became conclusive enough for the FDA to on March 21, 2000, require the manufacturer to withdraw Rezulin from the market in the United States. Should it be any surprise that certain botanical materials cannot be demonstrated "conclusively" to be hazardous to the liver? Yet this is the standard that the FDA must meet to order withdrawal of a dietary supplement that seems to have caused a number of cases of liver injury. Does this indicate that the public can be assured of safety for their use of botanicals that are apparently toxic to the liver (e.g., chaparral, germander, and perhaps kava), merely because they are not forbidden in the American market?

The FDA in spring 2002 sent a "Dear Doctor" letter to physicians across the United States to be on the lookout for cases of hepatic dysfunction that might have been a consequence of kava preparations. This was triggered by an accumulation of dozens of case reports, mostly from European countries, of severe kava-associated liver disease.

Some authorities suspect that the kava preparations that might indeed have caused toxicity were concentrated extracts that supply a higher-than-usual amount of a toxic component. This may have amplified the likelihood of a rare toxic response. However, such an explanation does not deny the problem of uncertainty of what is an "effective and safe" level of exposure to a kava product.

It is impossible in general to supply numerical data on levels of danger in using some dietary supplements. Such hazard estimates, which are somewhat available for many prescription medicines, are derived from analyses of statistically validated results of the human trials required for a proposed new drug to reach the market. Only very recently are a few large-scale efficacy trials being conducted under federal support on a relatively small number of dietary supplements.

Surely no apology should be needed for raising safety questions based on single-case published reports in medical journals since the majority of "evidence" for the beneficial effects of botanicals or nutraceuticals consists of "information" that is comparably unsubstantial.

IGNORANCE IS DANGEROUS—NOT BLISSFUL!

"Traditional use" is often invoked for herbals, e.g., traditional Chinese medicine, which supposedly has much knowledge but little data available for evaluation based on the scientific standards of modern medicine of the Western world.

Some of the remedies being presented as newly discovered biochemicals or herbals are supported only by unpublished clinical observations, anecdotes, testimonials, or supposed tradition-based claims from some distant, exotic region of the world. Generally lacking is needed support of scientific evidence from well-designed, statistically sound human testing for efficacy and safety that has been published in recognized medical journals. Happily, exceptions to this rule are beginning to occur as federal support has funded more than fifty studies through the Office of Dietary and Herbal Supplements and NCCAM (National Center for Complementary and Alternative Medicine) of the NIH. However, the minimal assurance for which one would wish—that one can trust the label to be true concerning what a dietary supplement package is supposed to contain—is far from being fulfilled.

TRADITIONAL "HERBAL REMEDY" MAY CONTAIN ANIMAL SURPRISES

The column Minerva in the *British Medical Journal* (August 4, 2000) commented as follows regarding a warning letter to the *New England Journal of Medicine:*

> Vegetarians and others who would rather not eat bulls' testicles should look carefully at the ingredient list of any herbal dietary supplements before buying. Any product listing "Orchis" should be left on the shelf—that term does not allude to the familiar flower, "orchid," but rather to a male's testis! (Norton, 2000)

The letter by S.A. Norton, MD, that provoked Minerva's response related the list of 17 bovine organs in a "nationally distributed product" as: brain, spleen, lung, liver, pancreas, pituitary, pineal, adrenal, lymph node, placenta, prostate, heart, kidney, intestine, thymus, thyroid, and testicle. Dr. Norton raised the issue of a weaker regulation of imported cow parts when intended for use in dietary supplements than for those intended for use in food, medicines, or medical devices. His concern was with respect to the possible risk of such materials carrying the prions causative of the degenerative brain disease, vCJD (variant Cruetzfeldt-Jakob disease) (human equivalent of "mad cow disease").

The incorporation of nonmuscle components (especially brain and spinal cord) of cattle into the human diet in the United Kingdom via "processed foods," such as patés and sausages, is held most likely responsible for the human cases of the brain disease vCJD. This new disease of the early 1990s both followed and has been blamed upon the epidemic of mad cow disease (bovine spongiform encephalopathy or BSE) in Britain. The pituitary and pineal are highly suspect for possible risk because of their actually being extensions of the brain. Mechanical devices that are used to remove every scrap of flesh associated with the spinal column may cause the inclusion of nerve roots that have an intimate anatomical association with the spinal cord. Some scientists fear any cattle-derived material may have a yet-unrecognized hazard of contamination by the aberrant prion protein responsible for causing the human spinoff of BSE known as vCJD. Gelatin capsules, chondroitin, and various other supplement components have been identified as cattle-derived materials.

For some skeptics the question remains open as to whether the importation door is securely barred, as federal agencies claim, to entry of any overseas cattle-derived products having possible BSE contamination. That issue gained added importance in June 2003 when a case of BSE was discovered in a herd of Canadian cattle, from which some members had indeed already been exported to the United States. Importation of beef from Canada was halted, even for beef fat (suet) to be used as a songbird food! Then, at the end of December 2003, the diagnosis of BSE in a cow imported several years before from Alberta, Canada, showed that U.S. impunity was overrated.

However, a Stanford biologist in July 2004 emphasized that a geographically widespread contemporary human practice of eating animal brain—sheep, cattle, pigs, primates (in Africa and South America), and squirrels—exists for its flavorsome, high-fat nature. He suggests that this practice may have made unrecognized diseases caused by prions a feature of human pathology for millennia, long before the recent advent of disease acquired via BSE in cattle (Sekercioglu, 2004).

FAMILIARITY SHOULD NOT BREED CONTEMPT

Some botanicals sound so familiar that to suspect them of being risky may seem to be paranoid and unwarranted suspicion. However, the truth may not be comforting but rather disquieting, as will be seen in the following example.

European Mistletoe (Viscum album)

In the language of the Celtic tribes, the source of the word mistletoe is said to have meant "all heal." Currently it has attracted medical researchers' interest as a possible anticancer agent because of experiments that have shown that extracts of the plant are able to kill cancer cells in vitro as well as in vivo for certain types of cancer. Mistletoe extracts, or teas made from mistletoe leaves, long were regarded as a traditional remedy for diabetes. However, the various species called "mistletoe" complicate the picture, as do the multiple different bioactive components present in the plants. Moreover, the bioactive components may vary with the plant part and with the season of harvesting. North American mistletoes (*Phoradendron* species) are more toxic and should not be consumed.

The African mistletoe, *Loranthus bengwensis,* which was widely used in Nigerian folk medicine to treat diabetes, has indeed been shown to reduce blood glucose levels in rats, both those having and not having experimental diabetes. The active component(s) and the mechanism by which African mistletoe may exert a favorable effect on the symptoms of diabetes remain unknown. Nevertheless, usage of this or other plant materials for self-treatment of so serious a problem as diabetes would be very misguided.

European mistletoe also has shown an ability to stimulate the immune system. Thus, prospects of potentially significant therapeutic developments may be based on components of mistletoe, although activation of immune mechanisms can also be detrimental at times. Much careful investigation is required to find whether a safe and effective therapeutic response can be obtained from mistletoe. Concerning this plant material, the truism may apply that says if it is powerful enough to do good, it is also powerful enough to do harm.

Ingestion of North American mistletoe leaves or berries can have potentially fatal consequences, especially in children. Deaths have occurred after eating as few as two berries, with convulsions being followed by coma and death; the heart rate first may be excessively rapid and then becomes slow. A potential for adverse interaction of mistletoe with pharmaceuticals can arise from its content of a chemical known as tyramine. In a person who is taking Nardil, a drug used for treating depression that acts as an inhibitor of the crucial brain enzyme monoamine oxidase, tyramine elevates blood pressure excessively, acting similar to an overdose of adrenaline (epinephrine) with initially a racing pulse and later a slowed and/or erratic one. A fatal outcome is possible. Other responses may include headache, nausea and vomiting, or diarrhea.

CONCLUSION

In discussing pharmaceuticals, René Dubos (1901-1982), experimental pathologist, microbiologist, environmentalist, humanist, and Pulitzer Prize–winning author, stated: "Absolute lack of toxicity is an impossibility because absolute selectivity is a chemical impossibility" (in Basara and Montagne, 1994, p. 44).

Thus, safety is not to be considered an absolute condition, but must be seen as relative. The magical thinking that leads some people to think that natural equals safe, while synthetic equals poisonous, is totally misguided, as Professor Varro Tyler declared (quoted in Chapter 2). Most immediate and obvious poisonous effects of natural products are now known. It is the delayed and subtle toxicities that are mainly grounds for concern because of the greater difficulty for their being correctly recognized.

Chapter 8

FDA Regulations

CAVEAT EMPTOR (LET THE BUYER BEWARE)!

The FDA is responsible not only for safety of foods, dietary supplements, and drugs (both Rx and OTC pharmaceuticals), but also for medical devices. This is a very large plateful. We may wish that the FDA also were indeed responsible for the before-the-fact (i.e., proactive) certification of the safety of dietary supplements, but little or no prospect of such a change exists. This is because the DSHEA legislation assumed that the various types of dietary supplements are all more similar to foods than to drugs; therefore, it required no prior approval by the FDA on safety grounds before marketing. However, it might be argued that to call most botanicals "foods" is not nearly so valid as it is for the nutritional supplements. We have already presented evidence that botanicals frequently are used not for nutrition but rather for their pharmacological action (Chapter 6). This chapter expands on aspects of Chapter 4 with respect to matters of protecting the consumer welfare.

In the summer 2003 the European Commission, executive body of the European Union (EU), became involved in a disagreement between the European Chemical Industry Council and the environmental commission of the EU. This was because of a difference about the basic approach for regulating chemicals. The EU charter embraces an approach known as the *precautionary principle,* which says that a government should establish its regulatory policy on whether "a significant possibility of risk" exists. By this concept action might at times be taken before all cogent experimental data become available. This would be a proactive philosophy, and would stand contrast to the regulatory process in the United States, which is reactive. U.S. regulations are not applied unless or until a clear and concrete basis in evidence exists for needful action. The proactive principle is viewed by industry as causing an undue and burdensome expense in money and time for introducing a new product into commerce. This applies to any and all sorts of chemicals to which citizens may be anticipated to be exposed.

Consumer's Guide to Dietary Supplements and Alternative Medicines

doi:10.1300/5698_08

The situation that no premarketing evidence for safety is required for supplement sales represents a unique regulatory feature setting apart supplements from all the other categories.

MA HUANG

Although many botanical remedies are currently available in the United States, relatively few instances of serious disagreements exist on whether a particular supplement item should be allowed to remain available. The major example of such a controversy is the plant known as ma huang or ephedra, which was the first Chinese herbal remedy to find acceptance in Western medicine. Traditionally, ma huang was used for a wide range of complaints, including colds and influenza, allergy, nasal congestion, coughing, wheezing, fever or chills, headache, joint and bone pain, and edema. However, Western medicine did not accept the therapeutic potential of this plant until the work of a distinguished Chinese-American pharmacologist, K. K. Chen, with C. F. Schmidt, was published early in the twentieth century. This was a classic series of pharmacological studies on the properties of its primary constituent, ephedrine. The research established not only that ephedrine was the primary pharmacologically-active agent found in various species of the genus *Ephedra,* but also that it had medicinal value for asthma therapy and as either a local or systemic vasoconstrictor.

The family to which *Ephedra* belongs (Ephedraceae) consists of small, evergreen shrubs (thus not herbs) that grow in many regions of the world. The plants characteristically have a thick woody base and many slim, jointed branches covered with tiny scalelike leaves. The flowers typically are long, and the fruits (cones) are globular and red or yellow. These plants release a distinct pinelike odor and have a very astringent taste. The green branches of *Ephedra* plants are the source for the active factors, alkaloids, since the woody basal stem, root, flowers, and fruit are nearly devoid of such components. The alkaloidal content of *Ephedra* plants varies among geographic groups. It is reported that the North American and Central American species do not contain useful ephedrine-like alkaloids, although they contain other constituents that are less well-known. Thus, a botanical product could conceivably be labeled "ephedra" and yet not contain ephedrine! An example of a species found in the United States is *Ephedra nevadensis,* which is employed to make Mormon tea, a non-ephedrine-containing beverage. This should illustrate that a layperson or even an amateur student of botany may soon be out of their depth when dealing with a species of plant that has many close relatives.

Besides ephedrine, the different *Ephedra* species may contain varying quantities of other very similar alkaloids possessing equivalent actions. They are methylephedrine, norephedrine (or phenylpropanolamine [PPA]), pseudoephedrine, and norpseudoephedrine. These may be collectively referred to as "ephedrines." These molecules activate the heart and constrict arterial blood vessels, leading to an increase in blood pressure. Such effects are unlikely to endanger the great majority of persons who might be exposed. They were long used medically, and were deemed suitable for limited use without a prescription in oral products to oppose nasal congestion. In any form, ephedrines present an element of cardiovascular risk, especially for older persons who may have known hypertension or a cardiac or vascular defect, or for younger persons who may have unrecognized cardiac or arterial risk factors. Commercially available OTC or prescription ephedrine-containing products long ago began to depend on ephedrines produced synthetically rather than their being isolated from ephedra extracts. One trend was to use pseudoephedrine because it supposedly showed a better human safety margin.

Despite their longtime usefulness as OTC medications, the ephedrines no longer are of importance as Rx drugs. Because of their content of ephedrine alkaloids, during the 1990s ephedra products came to be widely marketed as botanical supplement products sold not primarily to treat asthma but rather to aid in controlling appetite and losing weight, to evoke euphoria and boost energy, and to attempt to enhance sexual arousal and performance in the pre-Viagra era. The stimulant effects and enhancement of energy led to the ephedra products being classed as illicit performance enhancers or "ergogenic aids." This caused their being banned from use among competitive athletes by the IOC (International Olympic Committee), NCAA (National Collegiate Athletic Association), and NFL (National Football League).

By 1994 some authors reported at least 15 deaths possibly attributable to ephedra and 395 serious adverse effects, which included strokes, heart attacks, and seizures, all associated with products containing ephedra. Furthermore, more than 800 adverse reactions were reported to the FDA from 1993 to 1998. In essence, these preparations containing extracts of ephedra truly constitute active herbal stimulants that were easily obtainable, and they became widely used for recreational rather than for medicinal purposes. They were made available not mainly from pharmacies but rather from health food stores, truck stops, fitness clubs, and nightclubs. They comprised a significant aspect of the "club drug" problem because these preparations not only exert potent actions with dangerous adverse effects alone, but they also may contribute to dangerous interactions with Rx drugs or street drugs.

The FDA called a conference in 1998 to consider whether the situation justified action to restrict ephedra-containing products for the sake of public safety. Despite much testimony that pointed to a need for some sort of limits, none were imposed.

Although OTC products continued to be permitted by the FDA after 1998, several states by 2003 had attacked abuse problems via restrictive legislation. Oklahoma, Tennessee, Florida, and Louisiana all passed statutes making it unlawful to sell ephedrine products (and in some cases pseudoephedrine products) for the purpose of stimulation, mental alertness, weight loss, appetite control, energy, or other indications not approved by federal over-the-counter drug policies.

In March 2003 a meta-analysis on publications evaluating the efficacy and safety of ephedra products for weight loss was published in *JAMA* (Shekelle et al., 2003). The reports available proved inadequate to show conclusive weight loss benefits; however, ephedra (and ephedrine) appeared to promote modest short-term weight loss (about two pounds per month more than placebo) in clinical trials. No data was given regarding long-term weight loss. Use of ephedra or ephedrine with caffeine was associated with increased risk of psychiatric, autonomic, or gastrointestinal symptoms as well as heart palpitations.

On May 26, 2003, the governor of Illinois signed legislation comprising the nation's first statewide ban on ephedra. He was flanked by the parents of a 16-year-old football player who died of a heart attack after using an ephedra-containing product. Earlier in May 2003 a major supplement retailer, General Nutrition Center (GNC), said it would ban sales of ephedra-containing products in its stores. Moreover, CVS Pharmacy, a major drug store chain, reported on July 11, 2003, that it would no longer sell ephedra-based products in any of its stores. Anticipation of the GNC action may have operated to bring some manufacturers to whom GNC is a critical outlet to modify their products by eliminating the ephedra component.

Human Toxicology of Ephedra and the Ephedrines

Nonmedical use of ephedra products may produce at least additive effects with the similar actions of another so-called "club drug," methylenedioxymethamphetamine or MDMA (ecstasy), so that the resulting cardiovascular hazard would be amplified over that of either one alone. Although the maximum CNS stimulant effects of ephedra alkaloids are less than the level attainable with dextroamphetamine or methamphetamine, these alkaloids may carry somewhat the same risks as for the stronger amphetamine group of stimulants and appetite reducers. A long history shows that a small proportion of persons may become abusers even after employing ephedrine products medicinally. This may involve a habitual usage with a compulsive aspect that may even progress into a paranoid psychotic state equivalent to amphetamine psychosis. This condition was documented widely after its first appearance in the latter 1940s (Connell, 1958). In the era following World War II, stocks of the amphetamine used by the military for alertness-enhancing aids were diverted into the street trafficking in Europe and Japan where their excessive use led to many psychotic episodes among abusers.

Ephedrine toxicity may develop after doses that are merely two or three times larger than the safe therapeutic dose range (Enders et al., 2003). Pseudoephedrine tends to be less toxic, and patients may show no symptoms until reaching doses four to five times the therapeutic dose. Thus, usage in OTC pharmaceuticals has tended in the latter twentieth century toward a choice of pseudoephedrine over ephedrine. Because the precise alkaloid content is not required to be shown on the label for ephedra products, the amounts of the several ephedrines that are actually supplied is nearly always unknown. This makes the situation very ambiguous when a person displays adverse symptoms in association with use of such products, especially when they possibly have also abused street drugs concurrently.

Because absorption of ephedrine is rapid and complete, its onset of pharmacologic effects should be evident within an hour after ingestion. The clinical toxicity of ephedra is manifested primarily on the cardiovascular system and the brain, and it continues for several hours (Haller and Benowitz, 2000). When sustained-release pharmaceutical products containing ephedrine are taken, the duration of symptoms and recovery usually requires six hours or more.

The major cardiovascular toxicity seen with ephedra includes hypertension and rapid heart rate. One report of a chronic, congestive cardiomyopathy was described in a patient who had abused ephedra for approximately ten years. This could represent a chronic state of excess strain on the heart, perhaps with a deficient blood flow and oxygen supply to the heart muscle. Moreover, cases of intracranial hemorrhage have been reported in association with ephedra use by persons having abnormalities of their blood vessels that predisposed them to having a cerebrovascular accident (stroke). In two such cases, ephedra was the only drug detectable in the body fluids by sensitive analytical technics. It was concluded that ephedrine caused systemic hypertension, which in turn provoked the intracranial rupture of vessels weakened by their prior malformation leading to a hemorrhagic stroke. A case of suspected obstructive stroke has also been reported as ephedra-associated. It was hypothesized that chronic high levels of ephedrine exposure caused an inflammation and excess constriction of cerebral blood vessels provoking an obstructive stroke.

Adverse effects associated with CNS toxicity of ephedra are anxiety, insomnia, restlessness, seizures, and psychosis. These effects are especially common when multiple stimulants are being used. Additional signs of ephedrine toxicity may include nausea, vomiting, headache, flushing, abnormal sensations, difficulty in urinating, and chest pain (Pentel, 1984). Patients with high doses of this type of agent may develop severe injury to the voluntary muscles (rhabdomyolysis), which can in turn threaten to cause kidney failure (shutdown). Ephedrines and amphetamines are especially dangerous if a person has a preexisting condition of hyperthyroidism. They also are prone to precipitate a state of mania in a person having bipolar affective disorder (manic-depressive illness).

During the interval of December 1993 to September 1995 the Texas Department of Health received more than 500 reports of adverse effects associated with the consumption of dietary supplements containing ephedrine and several other alkaloids associated with ephedra—pseudoephedrine, norephedrine, and N-methylephedrine (CDC, 1996). Reported adverse events ranged in severity from tremor and headache to acute fatality in eight ephedra users. It included reports of myocardial infarction, chest pain, stroke, seizures, insomnia, nausea and vomiting, fatigue, and dizziness. Seven of the eight fatalities were attributed to heart attack or stroke. Some examples follow.

Case Report 1

In December 1993, a 44-year-old man died from acute coronary artery thrombosis about three weeks after beginning daily use of a dietary supplement that was based on ephedra and contained ephedrine. He was an active swimmer and tennis player who had no known cardiovascular risk factors. He was provided the supplement product by his family physician at a routine physical examination when he requested a substitute for his daily stimulant sources of coffee and cocoa. He used the product as directed and stopped using coffee and cocoa. After playing tennis and returning home one afternoon, he sustained a cardiorespiratory stoppage. An autopsy revealed an acute thrombus in the left anterior descending coronary artery. All other coronary vessels were open, although they were found to be locally narrowed about 50 percent by calcium deposits (CDC, 1996).

Case Report 2

In May 1995, a 35-year-old woman who was taking no other prescription or OTC medicines began using a dietary supplement that contained ephedra for its aid in weight loss. She followed the dosage recommended on the label for about one month, then discontinued use of the supplement while on a one-week vacation, at the end of which she resumed the former intake on June 24, 1995. On June 25, while sleeping, she had onset of symptoms including acute anterior chest pain that radiated to her left shoulder and arm, numbness of the left arm and hand, sweating, and shortness of breath. She was taken to the hospital, and her pain ceased after she was given nitroglycerin and morphine. Although an electrocardiogram and cardiac enzymes indicated she had experienced an acute myocardial infarction, a cardiac catheterization showed normal heart action and a normal condition of her coronary arteries. She had no history of cardiovascular risk factors. She was discharged with a diagnosis of acute myocardial infarction resulting from spasms of the arteries, and was advised to discontinue use of the product that contained ephedrine. After discontinuing it, she had no further cardiac-related symptoms (CDC, 1996).

Case Report 3

On August 17, 1995, a 38-year-old woman with no history of seizures experienced two petit mal (absence) seizures beginning at 11:00 p.m. This was followed by two more such seizures on the following morning. That afternoon she developed a generalized tonic-clonic (grand mal) seizure that lasted for about two minutes, during which she required respiratory assistance. On that day she had taken two tablets of a dietary supplement containing ephedra at 10:00 a.m. and two more at 3:00 p.m. as directed on the product label. She denied use of any drug except an oral contraceptive. During one week in August, she experienced five additional seizure episodes consisting of periods of unresponsiveness while sitting or standing. While waiting in the office of a neurologist, she experienced another generalized seizure witnessed by the neurologist and staff. She was hospitalized for monitoring, was treated with anticonvulsant medication, and was diagnosed with new onset of tonic-clonic seizures plus complex partial seizures. Other possible causes of seizures besides the ephedrine were excluded. At discharge she was advised to avoid any products that contained either ephedrine, pseudoephedrine, or related agents. After stopping use of the ephedra-containing product, she had no additional seizures (CDC, 1996).

Case Report 4

A 21-year-old male entered an emergency department showing an elevated blood pressure of 220 over 110 mmHg along with ventricular dysrhythmias. He had taken four capsules of what was represented to him as "herbal ecstasy" (Zahn et al., 1999). Blood pressure readings of 160/90 or higher are sufficient to be considered hypertensive. He was treated with lidocaine, a drug acting against cardiac dysrhythmia plus an emergency drug to lower blood pressure, sodium nitroprusside. His symptoms were reversed after nine hours and no subsequent adverse effects were reported (CDC, 1996).

These reactions were totally predictable before the ma huang craze began to develop because of the past track record of self-medication with, or nonmedical abuse of, OTC pharmaceutical products containing ephedrine or closely related molecules (pseudoephedrine, norephedrine). One of the earlier predictions of this was provided by an article that appeared in 1984. The author warned of increasing risks from OTC products being widely marketed as nasal decongestants or appetite suppressants but being diverted to use as "legal stimulants," i.e., as alternatives to amphetamine or cocaine.

Ma Huang and Ephedrine-Induced Kidney Stones

Case Report 5

An additional danger was added in 1998 to the list of concerns that the FDA was reviewing (Powell et al., 1998). Researchers at Washington University School of Medicine in St. Louis determined that a male patient had developed kidney stones after 11 months of taking an ephedrine-containing "energy supplement" to enhance his bodybuilding goals (Powell et al., 1998). The removed stones were found to be composed of nearly pure ephedrine. Earlier, by October of 1996 the 27-year-old had been hospitalized four times and had experienced six episodes of extremely painful renal colic, which often occurs when kidney stones enter the ureter and prevent urine from leaving the kidney. The patient's diet was high in salts and he drank little fluid, both of these being factors reducing the solubility of minerals or organic matter in the urine and increasing the likelihood of such deposits forming a stone in the urinary tract. The subject also was born with only one kidney, which normally would lower the risk of developing stones, because a single kidney has to accommodate a larger volume of fluid to serve the body's needs. Despite this, he had experienced surgical removal of two stones from his kidney seven months before the November 1998 admission, and had passed another stone the previous month. He tested negatively in a determination whether he was prone to stone forming because of a metabolic disorder.

Two of this man's stones were sent to a company in Orlando, Florida, that specializes in chemical analysis of kidney stones by means of X-ray crystallography and other techniques. They found that the stones contained 95 percent of ephedrine or its metabolites. Rather than being a unique event, the company reported also that they had analyzed more than 200 stones that they had suspected of containing ephedrine and related metabolites. An additional 250 kidney stones of this type have since been identified. When the analytical laboratory sent out a confidential questionnaire to some of the sources of these stones, 13 of 15 respondents admitted that they had taken products containing ephedra. Seven admitted to ingesting dozens of dosage units per day, one person professing to have taken more than 500 "minitablets" daily for several years. (Could he have tolerated the supposed quantities of ephedrines? It must be questioned whether he was really receiving the amounts that he was paying for.) For his part, the bodybuilder said he had taken 4 to 12 tablets per day of a ma huang supplement for more than a year. Analysis showed the supplement contained 6 percent ephedrine in addition to closely related compounds known to occur in ma huang. It is quite likely that other herbal products would show rather different amounts (Powell et al., 1998).

The Final Irony

In 2000 the FDA took action requiring the removal from the market of numerous synthetic OTC products containing the active constituent phenylpropanolamine (PPA), or norephedrine. These products were mainly used orally for nasal decongestion with an antihistaminic component, because of PPA having a significant vasoconstrictor effect. Synthetic PPA was ruled to be too dangerous for continued OTC use on account of the number of adverse cardiovascular events. Yet the parallel situation occurring with norephedrine-containing ephedra products did not lead to the same action by FDA. It appears that the political clout of the supplement industry in addition to the hindering restrictions of DSHEA made a difference in the actions in the two situations. Thirty-five years ago, a student's MS degree thesis research (Davis and Pinkerton, 1970) in the Department of Pharmacology at the University of Mississippi found that a stimulant action of norephedrine in rats could be amplified when combined with an anticholinergic (atropine-like) component. This project was provoked by reports that teenagers in south Mississippi were abusing the commercial nasal decongestants that combined PPA with an anticholinergic agent to obtain an amphetamine-like "rush."

THE BAN ON EPHEDRA PRODUCTS

At the outset of the preseason football practices in 2001 there was a much-publicized death of a Minnesota Viking NFL player, in which ephedra use was implicated. On September 5, 2001, the activist Public Citizen Health Research Group (PCHRG) petitioned the FDA to ban production and sales of supplements containing components of ephedra similar to those involved in these celebrated cases as well as in numerous reported adverse or even fatal occurrences with their use by ordinary citizens.

In July 2002 Department of Health and Human Services (HHS) Secretary Tommy Thompson announced an initiative to expand scientific research on the safety of ephedrine alkaloids and to pursue the illegal marketing of nonherbal synthetic ephedrine alkaloid products. HHS funded the RAND Corporation to conduct a comprehensive review of the existing science on ephedrine alkaloids, particularly those in dietary supplements. NIH would then use the information as a guide to an expanded research effort to clarify the safety status of ephedrine alkaloids.

Despite the temporary hullabaloo aroused by the deaths in the fall of 2001 no action was taken, and press coverage fell off. However, in the Major League Baseball preseason training camp period of early 2003 another fatal incident again seemed to highlight the dangerous potential of ephedra products. Steve Bechler, a Baltimore Orioles pitcher, died on February 17, 2003, a day after the 23-year-old was unable to finish a team workout and arrived at an intensive care unit in a state of heatstroke. He allegedly was using an ephedra-containing product, which was found in his locker, because of a need to reduce his weight. After a premature announcement that the death was related to use of the ephedra product, the medical examiner recanted and admitted that other factors must be considered. These included an enlarged heart, a state of borderline hypertension, abnormal liver functions, an overweight condition, dieting, and the use of the ephedra product, Xenadrine. Nonetheless, this event renewed calls, including one from the Orioles' owner, for banning ephedra products marketed for use in weight reduction.

One of the further results of the highly publicized concerns about the safety of ephedra was that the American Heart Association urged a ban on sales of ephedra. In addition, a major biomedical science organization, the American Society for Pharmacology and Experimental Therapeutics (ASPET), issued a statement in early 2003 expressing the concerns of its members regarding the use of dietary supplements and ephedrine and suggesting that the handling (nonregulation) of the class of dietary supplements as a whole should be reformed so that FDA would treat them more as they treat pharmaceuticals.

The FDA called a conference in 1998 to consider whether the situation justified action to restrict ephedra-containing products for the sake of public safety. Despite much testimony that pointed to a need for some sort of limits, the pressure that industry exerted through members of Congress to the contrary was unsurmountable, perhaps because of the risk of potential risks to the overall programs of FDA. The director of Public Citizen Health Research Group, Sidney E. Wolfe, MD, asked in an April 18, 2003, editorial:

> Does it make a difference, in terms of FDA regulation, that a drug is natural, having been around for thousands of years and is dispensed as "servings" rather than doses, if the drugs has been known for decades to cause increased blood pressure, increased pulse rate, and an increased risk of cardiac arrhythmias? For dietary supplements containing ephedra alkaloids, the answer is yes, it has made a difference. (Wolfe, 2003)

Finally, on December 31, 2003, it was announced that the Bush administration was taking action effective at the end of the first three months of 2004 to ban fully any continued production or distribution of ephedra in the United States. It seemed that the case against ephedra known for years to the FDA medical staff had finally reached "the highest levels" of the administration, where a decisive step was taken at long last. Of course, an immediate "run" on sales of the available stocks of those products still containing ephedra occurred. The FDA Commissioner Mark McClellan in an address at the University of Mississippi in January 2004 indicated that action against ephedra would serve as a model for increased attention to safety matters regarding other supplements. It was of interest to follow subsequent developments on the supplement regulation issue, seeing that a bill had been introduced in the Senate to bring about a broader restrictive action for the sake of public safety. Pro-supplement forces in latter 2003 were marshaling to oppose legislation to give greater responsibility to the FDA for supplement regulation, fearing that FDA would be acting in the best interests of the pharmaceutical industry to reduce the competition of the supplement industry more than in consumers' best interests.

Moreover, the move by manufacturers to alter their weight-reduction products so as to maintain sales without ephedra is noteworthy. The FDA immediately took an aggressive stance in the first week of 2004 as seen by a press interview given by FDA Commissioner Mark McClellan. He warned that the "ephedra substitutes" being trotted out comprise mostly materials concerning whose safety even less is known than was for ephedra.

One of these natural products, *Citrus aurantium,* or bitter orange, does contain a component known as synephrine, a molecule popular as a synthetic pharmaceutical ingredient during the second half of the twentieth century. It served as a vasoconstrictor to oppose ocular or nasal congestion. Although being of lesser potency, its pharmacological profile has more in common with rather than in contrast to the profiles of the several ephedrines, including PPA. Especially of concern is its tendency to raise blood pressure and heart rate, and probably body temperature if taken in excess quantities. Moreover, botanical material providing synephrine contains ingredients similar to those of grapefruit, which are prone to inhibit drug-metabolizing enzymes (especially a prominent one, CYP3A4). Thus, it would posses an ability to exaggerate (or inhibit) the actions of many Rx pharmaceuticals.

The situation of "ephedra substitutes" is reminiscent of the 1970s when "designer drugs" were spewed out by the underground chemists in response to the scheduling and thus banning of opioids or psychedelic/hallucinogenic agents by the Drug Enforcement Administration (DEA). The game was to produce, market, and accrue profits from a new chemical while it was not yet illegal because it had not yet been given a schedule number by DEA, and thus to avoid the stiffer legal liability incurred by distribution of a scheduled compound. Also to be expected would be prospects of an Internet black market for ephedra developing.

A LESS NOTORIOUS AGENT

Some botanicals sound so familiar that to accuse them of being risky may seem to be an excess of suspicion. However, the truth may not be comforting, as will be seen in the following example.

Comfrey

This homey-sounding herb has a long history of use as a traditional folk remedy in the United Kingdom and the United States. Taken internally, it has been thought useful to treat a number of conditions including arthritis/rheumatism, colitis, diarrhea, gallstones, gastritis and gastrointestinal ulcers, pleurisy, bronchitis, internal bleeding, and as an antidiarrheal. However, it has become recognized as a member of the group of plants that contain chemicals known to be hepatotoxic (liver-injuring by obstructing of its blood supply). These pyrrolizidine alkaloids not only may injure the liver so as to impair its function, but also may provoke cancer formation.

An expert advisory committee of the USP (United States Pharmacopeia) in 2000 determined that consumer use of comfrey as a dietary supplement can be harmful. That prompted the USP to issue a negative monograph, discouraging its use. Reports were given of liver damage in humans after oral comfrey use, occurring after long-term or short-term use (a few weeks to several months) from various amounts and forms (leaves, roots, pills, and teas). The USP particularly emphasized a danger for the use of comfrey by children, pregnant, or nursing women, and by people with liver disease, because these persons may be especially at risk for toxic effects of comfrey.

The FTC began at the same time (2001) to act against a manufacturer and marketer of a variety of products containing the herbal ingredient comfrey, for both external and internal uses. The FTC charged that the company, its president, and its vice president made unfounded claims regarding diseases and conditions and that they were safe via their Internet promotions and sale of the material. Despite this action, one who desired to do so could still obtain and ingest a comfrey tea if they should choose to tempt fate.

Chapter 9

Botanicals and Prescription Drugs

A major concern in modern medicine is avoiding adverse interactions between two or more different medications being taken. This commonly may occur when one of the agents causes a reduction or an increase in the rate of elimination of the other. In the first case, an exaggerated, prolonged response could occur that could lead to toxicity. In the second case, a reduced degree and duration of the intended response could occur, which may undermine the efficacy of the medication. The discovery that St. John's Wort lowers the available blood level of anti-HIV drugs and other medicines, jeopardizing their effectiveness, has been most revealing. Now we have on our hands the unanswered question of how many more botanicals have similar unrecognized detrimental effects on conventional pharmaceutical therapies.

ALTERED DRUG RESPONSES AND ST. JOHN'S WORT

Chemotherapy of HIV/AIDS

Interactions between botanical products and Rx or OTC drugs parallel better known drug-drug interactions. In February 2000 an important example of this principle was reported. The staff of the Clinical Center at the National Institutes of Health performed a study on eight healthy volunteers to determine whether a widely used herbal product, St. John's wort (SJW), could significantly alter the efficacy of the anti-HIV agent, indinavir, which belongs to the class of antiviral drugs known as protease inhibitors. These are among the most potent agents available for treating HIV disease, and they have proven able to slow the progress of the infection and thus prolong survival.

The researchers first measured the amount of indinavir in the volunteers' blood when a dose of it was taken alone. Next, participants in the study took

doi:10.1300/5698_09

only SJW for two weeks. Finally, indinavir and SJW were given together and the blood levels of indinavir were again measured. All the participants showed a marked drop in their blood levels of indinavir after taking SJW, ranging from 49 percent drop to 99 percent. These effects on indinavir levels are large enough to be clinically significant and to jeopardize the effectiveness of the antiviral therapy. However, an HIV patient would be unaware of this hindrance to his or her medication regimen. They simply would fail to receive the benefit available from their medication against the infection, and they might as a consequence experience a severe and life-threatening opportunistic infection—fungal, viral, or bacterial. Another potential detriment would be a greater tendency for the HIV to become resistant to the antiviral agent by exposure to a subeffective level, which might even carry over to decreasing the susceptibility of the virus to several other protease inhibitors.

The inference is that the persons' exposure to the herbal had provoked (referred to technically as "induced") a higher production of a drug-metabolizing liver enzyme that acts on indinavir. Knowing that indinavir is mainly metabolized by a particular liver enzyme (CYP3A4) allows the forecast that numerous other drugs also metabolized by CYP3A4 could be similarly rendered less effective by the use of St. John's wort. Without so much publicity, it was already anticipated in 1999 that a similar decrease in availability might occur for digoxin and theophylline because of SJW.

Antagonism of Immunosuppression in Transplant Patients

In 2000, cases of SJW interaction reducing the availability of transplant patient's needed dosage of cyclosporine, an important immunosuppressant, were reported (Barone et al., 2000; Breidenbach et al., 2000). Two more cases were reported by mid-2001 (Barone et al., 2001; Turton-Weeks et al., 2001).

Case Report 1

A 29-year-old white woman received a cadaver kidney and pancreas transplant in July 1994. After two early episodes of rejection she achieved stable kidney and pancreas functions, and was maintained on two immunosuppressants, cyclosporine (Sandimmune, Neoral) and prednisone. Unknown to her transplant physicians, in November 1998 she began to self-medicate with SJW, one or two tablets daily for improvement of mood. A month later, a periodic measure of cyclosporine in her blood showed that it had sharply dropped below the needed therapeutic range. When asked about a possible neglect of her medicine, she insisted that she had taken it is usual and had not begun taking any new prescription or OTC medications. Another reading was obtained in three weeks that was even lower, when a blood enzyme measure also was elevated, suggesting a pancreatic problem, along with pain over the site of her pancreas transplant.

These facts combined to indicate an acute rejection reaction despite her drug regimen designed to oppose it. A kidney biopsy showed evidence of acute rejection. During a two-week period of treatment with a therapeutic antibody, her use of SJW was discovered and stopped. Over the next two weeks she responded rapidly to a temporarily elevated dosage of cyclosporine by reaching and exceeding the therapeutic blood-level range. However, she subsequently displayed chronic transplant rejection. It was concluded as "probable" that the inadequate cyclosporine blood levels were the cause for the loss of therapeutic response, and that the tragic failure of her transplanted organs was a result of the patient's using St. John's wort without the approval of her transplant team (Barone et al., 2001).

St. John's Wort and Antagonism to a Cancer Chemotherapy Agent

Results of a randomized crossover clinical trial were presented in April 2002 to the American Association for Cancer Research meeting from the Rotterdam Cancer Institute in the Netherlands. Mathijssen and colleagues (2002) gave cancer patients a course of the anticancer drug irinotecan (Camptosar) alone, followed three weeks later by a second course that combined irinotecan and SJW. Another group first received a combination of SJW with irinotecan, followed three weeks later by only irinotecan. The patients who first received irinotecan alone showed more than a 50 percent decrease in the systemic level of its active metabolite when taken with SJW. Moreover, the reverse group also had a lesser response when receiving irinotecan alone, showing that they had not completely recovered from the effects of the prior SJW exposure that lowered its blood levels. "Our findings indicate that patients on chemotherapeutic treatment with irinotecan should refrain from taking St. Johns wort," the authors wrote. Their data did not permit saying how long a period of abstinence from SJW would be sufficient to regain the normal response. They further stated that "since about 50 percent of all drugs are metabolized by CYP3A4, the combination effect we found with St. John's wort and irinotecan might occur with many other anticancer agents."

SEROTONIN SYNDROME AND ST. JOHN'S WORT

St. John's wort indeed has an oft-demonstrated usefulness as a treatment for mild to moderate depression. Although the mechanism of the antidepressant action of SJW is still uncertain, it is likely to be the result of multiple simultaneous actions. One of these is that of monoamine oxidase (MAO) inhibition, which comprises the blocking of the enzyme, MAO, that is mainly responsible for inactivation of brain monoamines such as norepinephrine, dopamine, and serotonin. This is the mechanism for the earliest class of antidepressant drugs originated in the 1950s, the MAO inhibitors.

An excess accumulation of serotonin in the brain can cause unpleasant and at times dangerous changes known as the "serotonin syndrome" (Table 9.1); it may also occur with the newer antidepressants known as selective serotonin reuptake inhibitors (SSRIs), because they too act to enhance the availability of serotonin (Gordon, 1998). These drugs include sertraline (Zoloft), paroxetine (Paxil), fluoxetine (Prozac), trazodone (Desyrel), and citalopram (Celexa). However, whatever the circumstances allowing excess serotonin to exist it may result in the same sort of symptoms.

Case Report 2

An 88-year-old man was taking the antidepressant sertraline, 50 mg per day, having been diagnosed with major depression (Lantz et al., 1999). He had shown improvement in his mood disorder from this therapy. However, upon the advice of a family member, he began also taking SJW at a dose of 300 mg twice daily. After two days he began to show nausea and vomiting, and to feel anxious and confused. When he was brought to an emergency room, all diagnostic tests were negative. A computerized tomography (CT) image of his brain revealed only evidence of a prior stroke. He was advised to discontinue taking both sertraline and SJW because of the presumptive diagnosis of serotonin syndrome. He was directed to take three 4-mg doses daily of cyproheptadine, which is a blocking agent against serotonin at its receptors in the brain. After four to five days his symptoms were improved, and he was able to resume taking the sertraline without any further problem (Lantz et al., 1999).

TABLE 9.1. Symptoms of the serotonin syndrome from excess serotonin.

Motor effects	**Autonomic effects**	**Other brain-level effects**
Shivering, rigidity	Flushing, sweating	Poor concentration
Incoordination, ataxia	Fever, chills	Confusion
Muscle spasms, tremors	Nausea, vomiting	Agitation, anxiety
Hyperreflexia	Abdominal pain	Headache
Dysarthria (speech deficit)	Diarrhea (local effect?)	Excitement, restlessness
Muscle weakness, jerking	Tachycardia	Hypomania
Involuntary flinging motions	Fainting (hypotension)	Coma, death (rarely)

Case Report 3

A 78-year-old woman with a recent history of depression was being successfully treated with sertraline 50 mg per day (Lantz et al., 1999). She began taking SJW, 300 mg three times a day, upon the advice of a clerk in a natural food store. Four days later she developed nausea, vomiting, and headache. Evaluation at an emergency department revealed no reason for her symptoms. She was advised to stop all medicines. Thereafter her symptoms receded over two to three days. She later was able to resume sertraline without any problem. The authors suggest that elderly persons not only tend to have a high consumption of nutritional supplements, but also are more at risk for drug-herb interactions as exemplified by serotonin syndrome (Lantz et al., 1999).

Moreover, case reports link the use of only St. John's wort with a serotonin syndrome in "sensitive patients" despite the absence of another antidepressant agent (Nierenberg et al., 1999; Parker et al., 2001).

The task of obtaining information comparable to that for St. John's wort concerning the potential herb-drug interactions among the hundreds of botanical preparations that might be used is a mind-boggling prospect. A person who self-prescribes botanicals in addition to receiving conventional medicines is risking possible trouble with his or her ongoing therapy. Further specific cases will be illustrated in this chapter.

RISK OF BLEEDING FROM USE OF BOTANICALS BEFORE SURGERY

Persons anticipating elective surgery should stop using supplements that contain some commonly used herbal remedies to avoid problems of excessive bleeding that might result in serious complications. This warning was carried by U.S. media outlets such as ABC News, MSNBC, and others in the summer of 2001 based on a July report in the *Journal of the American Medical Association* (Ang-Lee et al., 2001) that recommended new precautions for patients scheduled for surgery who are users of several popular herbal remedies. Examples are described in the following cases.

Risky Outcomes with Use of Dong Quai and Danshen

The major oral Rx anticoagulant, warfarin, is a synthetic compound that was patterned after the natural chemical in the coumarin family, bishydroxycoumarin (or dicumarol). Before being replaced by warfarin, dicoumarol was the first and long the leading orally active anticoagulant drug. It was discovered by researchers seeking an explanation for bleeding in cattle that had eaten spoiled clover silage. Coumarin-type agents oppose the action of vitamin K in the liver to enable the production of proteins that act as clotting factors of the blood. Dong quai may also favor bleeding by inhibiting the aggregation of the blood platelets, which are vital to the clotting process. Thus, this patient taking dong quai may have shown a dual, synergistic action by being combined with the prescribed medication, warfarin. These facts show that it was foolhardy for a herbalist, or anyone, to recommend use of dong quai to a person already receiving warfarin therapy.

Case Report 4

A 62-year-old man underwent surgery to replace the mitral valve in his heart with a prosthesis at the Prince of Wales Hospital at the Chinese University of Hong Kong (Izzat et al., 1998). Following uneventful postoperative progress, he was discharged on day seven after surgery in good cardiovascular function. He was taking a heart medicine, digoxin, an antihypertensive agent, a diuretic, and 5 mg daily of the anticoagulant warfarin with his clotting status well stabilized. Upon review after two and four weeks, he was making quite satisfactory progress, and his warfarin dosage required no alteration.

However, at six weeks from discharge the patient came to the emergency department with complaints of a general, central chest pain, increasing difficulty in breathing, and a decreasing tolerance to exercise. Chest X-ray and echocardiography disclosed that he had a massive accumulation of fluid in his right lung cavity as well as a large accumulation in the pericardial sac around his heart. His blood showed a deficit of platelets and a low hemoglobin level. His clotting time was prolonged, indicating an excess anticoagulant response even though he had been taking the correct dose. A detailed history-taking revealed that over the prior two weeks he had begun taking daily a liquid preparation of the herb danshen *(Salvia miltiorrhiza* root*)*, upon recommendation of a Chinese herbalist, for the purpose of "mending his heart."

Both warfarin and danshen were halted, but the patient required seven units of packed red blood cells and six units of fresh frozen plasma over two days time, which brought his hemoglobin and clotting measures back to normal. A chest drain was inserted, and a 4.5-liter volume (more than one gallon) of unclotted blood was removed from the pleural cavity. Further fluid accumulation in the pericardium stopped. In the subsequent two weeks warfarin therapy was gradually resumed without problems. It seems likely that the bioavailability of warfarin was increased by an interference with its metabolism or its binding to plasma proteins to cause this interaction. A review by Heck et al. (2000) considered broadly the subject of known or potential supplement interactions with the anticoagulant warfarin. The results are tabulated in Table 9.2 (Izzat et al., 1998).

Discussion

A great many drug-drug interactions have become known for altering the response to warfarin or other oral anticoagulants. Thus, it is not surprising that the same should occur with a botanical preparation with more than 300 different coumarins having been identified from natural sources, especially green plants (Table 9.2). Thus, many more potential instances of this type of

TABLE 9.2. Supplement ingredients and interactions with warfarin.

Documented reports of interactions	May increase risk of bleeding or synergize warfarin
coenzyme Q10 danshen devil's claw dong quai ginseng green tea papain vitamin E	angelica root, arnica flower, anise, asafetida, bogbean, borage seed oil, bromelain, capsicum, celery, chamomile, clove, fenugreek, feverfew, garlic, ginger ginkgo, horse chestnut, licorice root, lovage root, meadowsweet, onion, parsley, passionflower herb, poplar, quassia, red clover, rue, sweet clover, turmeric, willow bark

Source: Adapted from Heck et al. (2000).

interaction could occur. Indeed, ginkgo, ginger, garlic, feverfew, cayenne, and bilberry are among other herbs besides dong quai and danshen that are reported (or suspected) to be able to provoke bleeding when taken with warfarin if its dosage is not adjusted to compensate for their interaction. *Ginkgo biloba* extract has by itself been noted in several cases to cause spontaneous bleeding, since it reduces clotting capacity. On the contrary, a popular herb Asian ginseng *(Panax ginseng)* is generally well tolerated, but has been implicated in *decreasing* the action of warfarin.

The results of an interaction with warfarin might be more injurious if there were to be only internal bleeding without visible skin bruising as a warning sign. The interactions of a combination can be particularly dangerous for people who have risk factors for stroke. If bleeding occurs within the skull, the outcome may be a fatal stroke. Inhibition by constituents of dong quai toward the metabolism of medicinal agents is in need of added research. Researchers on grapefruit chemistry discovered that a furocoumarin found in grapefruit may be responsible for its effect on the CYP (cytochrome P450) enzymes that metabolize many medications, an effect that has been well publicized in recent years. It seems that no one has yet studied dong quai to see if its furocoumarins may exert a similar effect.

Besides interactions involving blood clotting and drug metabolism, dong quai may have a serious tendency to sensitize the skin to sunlight by virtue of known properties of several coumarin compounds that it contains, especially psoralen and bergapten. This may result in a severe reddening of the skin, looking similar to a sunburn or a rash, even though sun exposure has been minimal—a photosensitivity reaction. These compounds are said to react upon light exposure to form new products that are carcinogenic. Experts in their chemistry recommend that people avoid ingesting coumarins if possible. Although no data show that people who take dong quai have experienced photosensitivity reactions, anyone taking it would be wise to minimize sun exposure and to avoid tanning lamps. A similar, apparently weak, photosensitizing action has also been noted for SJW.

OTHER INTERACTION EXAMPLES

A review of interactions of herbs and drugs was published in the distinguished British medical journal *Lancet* (Fugh-Berman, 2000). Some examples from the study are the following:

- *Panax ginseng* taken concurrently with certain prescription antidepressants has been found to induce mania. Ginseng also may cause headache, tremulousness, and manic episodes in patients treated with the antidepressant phenelzine sulfate. It should also not be used with estrogens or corticosteroids because of possible additive effects.
- An increased risk of hypertension exists if tricyclic antidepressants are taken with the alkaloid yohimbine or its herbal source *Pausinystalia yohimbe.*
- Licorice *(Glycyrrhiza glabra)* and oral contraceptives can interact to promote hypertension in women, and licorice could hinder the antihypertensive effects of drugs, especially spironolactone (Aldactone).
- Betel nuts *(Areca catechu)* taken with a psychosedative, flupenthixol (Depixol), or the anti-Parkinson's disease agent, procyclidine (Kemadrin), caused distressing jaw tremors and rigidity.
- Cathartics such as senna and cascara, as well as soluble-fiber laxatives such as guar gum and psyllium, would tend to decrease the absorption of and reduce the benefit from various important prescription drugs taken by mouth concurrently.
- Valerian should not be used concurrently with barbiturates, benzodiazepines, or alcohol, because excessive sedation might occur.
- Evening primrose oil and borage should not be used with antiepileptic agents because they may lower the seizure threshold and reduce the agents' efficacy.
- Shankapulshpi, an ayurvedic medication, may lower blood levels of the antiepilepsy therapy, phenytoin (Dilantin) and thus diminish its efficacy.

- Although considered to be a mild anxiolytic sedative, kava reportedly has resulted in a coma when used jointly with the benzodiazepine alprazolam.
- It would be illogical to use immunoenhancers such as echinacea and zinc at the same time as an immunosuppressant such as systemic corticosteroid or cyclosporine.
- Despite that numerous herbs (e.g., karela and ginseng) may alter blood glucose levels, none is known to be safe and effective for control of diabetes mellitus, and they should not be substituted for insulin or for oral antidiabetic drugs.
- Tannic acids present in many herbs (e.g., St. John's wort or saw palmetto) may inhibit the intestinal absorption of iron.
- Kelp as a supplemental dietary source of iodine may cause an oversupply that could interfere with ongoing thyroid replacement therapy.
- Kyushin, licorice, plantain, uzara root, hawthorn, and ginseng all are believed to oppose the therapeutic action of the vital cardiac drug, digoxin (Lanoxin).
- Additive interaction will occur between a source of phytoestrogen and a medicinal estrogenic product that might produce unfavorable consequences.

Chapter 10

Supplement Labels

UNRELIABLE LABEL DATA

Pharmaceuticals are subject to FDA inspection and review of their processes of manufacturing and the analytical integrity of their ingredients and products, but this is not true for dietary supplements. Several academic research groups have tested various dietary supplements, including botanical products, for the reliability of their stated amount of certain (possibly the active) ingredient(s). Results of such testing paint a picture of unreliability for supplements that generally makes it very difficult for a purchaser to trust what they propose to buy and use. A very deplorable deficiency of quality control has clearly occurred in the production of dietary supplements. It has begun to threaten the progress of the supplement industry as the public increasingly has become aware of the situation. Please note that sources on the following topic, and others throughout this book, were recent enough at the writing that one may not assume that situations have changed for the better.

Ephedra Analyses

A remarkable study was published by Bill J. Gurley, PhD, and his colleagues of the University of Arkansas College of Pharmacy (Gurley et al., 2000). They tested 20 products of ephedra (ma huang) for their content of ephedrine, one of four closely related active components that have been used either to aid weight loss or simply as a brain stimulant. Fully one-half of the products showed an actual alkaloid level that was more than 20 percent higher than the labeled quantity. For one product a significant lot-to-lot variation of the alkaloid content existed that ranged from 1.8 times to ten times for different constituents. The recognized hazards for high doses of this group of alkaloids (Haller and Benowitz, 2000) are amplified by such excesses beyond labeled quantities, even if the user takes only the suggested number of "servings." At the other extreme, one product contained abso-

doi:10.1300/5698_10

lutely no detectable amount of the ephedra alkaloids for which the product would be purchased. The buyers may not have been put in danger by the product, but they were defrauded of its cost.

A pharmacokinetic study by Gurley and co-workers (1998) concluded that excess variability in pharmacokinetics between individuals was not an evident factor in adverse responses to ephedra. They inferred that excessive dosage appeared to be the primary explanation.

Feverfew Analyses Are Disquieting

Two recent studies from the research program of Ikhlas A. Khan, PhD, at the Thad Cochran National Center for Natural Products Research at the University of Mississippi School of Pharmacy examined the active components in the traditional herbal feverfew (Abourashed and Khan, 2000; Abourashed et al., 2003). This botanical, which is touted as effective for preventing migraine attacks, is available in the United States in a variety of forms and compositions. The products analyzed (by different methods) showed a wide range (from zero to 0.36 percent) in content of the supposedly active component, parthenolide. Only three out of 13 products tested even showed on the label an exact amount of parthenolide that supposedly would be obtained from each "serving." None of the three actually came near to containing the indicated amount. Only four contained the minimum percentage recommended by a French Ministry of Health standard, and only two achieved the Health Canada minimum standard. Thus, most of the products could not be expected to produce the expected and anticipated benefit.

St. John's Wort Shows Problems

ConsumerLab.com reported in April 2004 that they had recently purchased and tested 14 St. John's wort supplement products. Three were described as being "contaminated." Another offered less than 25 percent of the standard dose. Two failed to disclose which part of the plant the products' ingredients were taken from, which violates the FDA labeling requirement (ConsumerLab.com, 2004).

Ginseng Analyses

Similar analytical studies (Huggett et al., 2000) on a widely used herbal tonic, ginseng, showed that quality control in herbals, as one researcher characterized it, "ranges from good to nonexistent." However, purchasers do not have such analytical data available and surely cannot discriminate by the labels of products between the good, the bad, and the ugly!

HELPING THE SUPPLEMENTS ALONG—ILLEGALLY

Fraudulent adulteration for the purpose of "fortifying" supposedly traditional remedies has been detected repeatedly over the past several decades, especially involving Chinese herbal products or their raw materials imported into the United States. This fraud involves adding to a ground botanical powder one or sometimes even several synthetic pharmaceuticals used in scientific medicine, which are not mentioned on the label. Presumably this is done to make certain that the herbal remedy will produce impressive therapeutic benefits. By this action users may be convinced that a "natural" herbal preparation has great value, when in fact it is acting by virtue of the presence of modern synthetic medicinals. This situation recently was reported also for a home-produced skin remedy marketed in the United Kingdom, rather than for an imported product. It was also noted for some therapies obtained by Americans crossing the border into Mexico. Such practices must be seen as a major fraud that can be a serious health hazard to users while also tarnishing the image of legitimate supplements.

Poisoning from a Chinese Proprietary Remedy for Epilepsy

Case Report 1

A 31-year-old female Chinese patient with an eight-year history of epilepsy was being well controlled with the use of carbamazepine (Tegretol), sodium valproate, and phenobarbital (Lau et al., 2000). On the day of hospital admission in Hong Kong, she had been found in a comatose state. When she was examined she was unable to follow any instructions, her impaired consciousness being the only sign of brain dysfunction except for some jerks. Her blood pressure and pulse were normal, as was an examination of her eyes. Serum analyzed on the second day showed the presence of a nonprescribed epilepsy drug, phenytoin (Dilantin), at a level that was 2.5 times higher than the upper limit of the normal therapeutic range—reaching the range that would predict a severe toxicity. Two days later her alertness improved but she still had impaired movement and nystagmus (strong involuntary eyeball movements). Fortunately, she showed no permanent residual motor deficit, which might have been possible after such a serious level of overdosage, but her toxic signs disappeared within ten days.

It was learned that one month before admission, the patient, at the suggestion of relatives, had begun taking a regimen of three different-colored capsules, a number of each daily in addition to her prescribed epilepsy medicines. These capsules were a proprietary antiepilepsy remedy from mainland China that was labeled as including only a combination of pure, "harmless traditional Chinese medicines." Analysis revealed that one capsule contained 41 mg of phenytoin, while the other two contained other epilepsy drugs, carbamazepine and valproate. Unregulated intake of these capsules resulted in a serious degree of phenytoin neurotoxicity, which is not always reversible.

The authors of this report concluded that such adulteration of Chinese proprietary medicines constitutes a major public health problem, and that long-term ingestion of the Chinese remedy by itself would be a hazard for overdose neurotoxicity. Although this case occurred outside of the United States, the present-day level of trans-Pacific commerce and travel can bring this problem to our shores (Lau et al., 2000).

Because of the evident unreliability of Chinese remedies contents seen here (and also in Chapters 12 and 20), it was unsettling to see a paper reporting positively on an ages-old TCM approach—a 20-ingredient therapy (Bensoussan et al., 1998). Such a medicine was evaluated with favorable results against irritable bowel syndrome by Australian researchers in a 1998 report in *JAMA*. The concern would be that reliability of even this same product might be lacking, and the same ingredients might not be provided by the same name elsewhere.

Recall with Warning to Stop Use of Prostate Support Supplements

In early February 2002 FDA's Safety Information and Adverse Event Reporting Program issued a notice warning consumers to stop using two herbal supplements, PC SPES and SPES capsules, because they contain undeclared prescription drug ingredients that could cause serious health effects if not taken under medical supervision. Analysis of the products by the California Department of Health Services found that PC SPES contained warfarin, and that SPES contained alprazolam, both of which are legally available only by prescription under their generic names or the trade names Coumadin and Xanax, respectively. The illegal presence of these agents is puzzling because neither is appropriate for the claimed purposes of the products—PC SPES and SPES are marketed for maintaining prostate health and strengthening the immune system. Botanic Lab, the manufacturer of the products, immediately issued a nationwide recall.

Chuifong Tokuwan for Pain Relief

In August 1988, the Texas Department of Health (TDH) investigated illegal sales in rural west Texas of products manufactured in Asia. These agents were identified by TDH and FDA agents as chuifong tokuwan, a remedy in pill form that had been manufactured in Hong Kong (FDA, 1991). The drug usually had been repackaged and relabeled. Analyses revealed that the chuifong tokuwan contained not merely a Chinese herb, but also a combination of modern drug components—hydrochlorothiazide, indomethacin, mefenamic acid, dexamethasone, and diazepam—as well as the metals lead and cadmium! The former five drugs are legitimate Rx pharmaceuticals, but were not approved by the FDA for use in this form, and thus were illegal for sale or importation into the United States. The two metal elements are clearly not legitimate for medical use. Sixty-six persons (71 percent of the sample) reported having taken the pills to relieve symptoms of painful medical conditions such as joint pain or other pains such as back pain, headache, and stiff neck.

The Texas Department of Health tested 93 persons who had ingested the pills for their exposure to lead and cadmium. Of these, 61 percent were female, more than 90 percent were non-Hispanic white persons, and the mean age was 55 years. Twenty-two (24 percent) persons had elevated urine levels of cadmium; none had elevated levels of lead. However, 42 percent had elevated urine values for a protein that signals kidney dysfunction. Cadmium is known for being toxic to the kidneys and for accumulating in the body. It essentially remains indefinitely, having a biological half-life of greater than ten years in humans, which means that only half of the original amount will be excreted after ten years, and merely three-fourths after 20 years.

Increasing the body stores of cadmium might be responsible for reduction of kidney function in some persons using this product. With continuing exposure, the level of cadmium builds, especially in the kidneys. However, not only the cadmium but also the two NSAID analgesics present, indomethacin and mefenamic acid, might injure the kidneys. For persons who might have been taking other prescribed pain medications for arthritis, the risk for analgesic-induced kidney injury would be amplified by concurrent exposure to the cadmium in chuifong tokuwan. Fortunately, neither indomethacin nor mefenamic acid, the NSAIDs present in all the pills analyzed, is among members of the class that are most likely to endanger kidney health.

Chuifong tokuwan first was noted in the United States in 1974. Although it was banned by the FDA in 1978 (FDA, 1991), the drug continues to be imported and distributed illegally in various parts of the United States, and is sometimes sold by mail. Whereas the primary users in this study were longtime residents of Texas, use of unapproved imported drug products is most common among recent immigrants to the United States, especially those immigrating from southeast Asia and from Latin America. Although these imported products are typically represented to be nonhazardous herbal folk remedies, they often contain components having the potential for serious adverse side effects. Other such adulterants have included corticosteroids or anabolic steroids, antibiotics (tetracycline and chloramphenicol), or controlled substances (opioid analgesics; diazepam, Valium). Indomethacin adulteration of chuifong tokuwan also was reported from Panama (Lasso de la Vefa, 1982).

Zhen Qi, Tongyi Tang, and Pearls for Diabetic Patients

In February 2000, the California Department of Health Services (CDHS) issued a warning to consumers about five herbal diabetes products. These products were claiming to contain only some traditional Chinese ingredients, but were actually found to contain one modern oral antidiabetic drug, glyburide, and an older one discontinued in the United States, phenformin (FDA, 2000). Oral antidiabetic agents are prescription-only medicines in the United States. The products in question bore label names of Diabetes Hypoglucose Capsules, Pearl Hypoglycemic Capsules, Tongyi Tang Diabetes Angel Pearl Hypoglycemic Capsules, Tongyi Tang Diabetes Angel Hypoglycemic Capsules, and Zhen Qi Capsules (California Department of Health Services, 2000).

The investigation by CDHS into the five herbal remedies was launched following the report that a diabetic patient in northern California experienced hypoglycemic episodes after consuming one of the products. For a diabetic sufferer to be taking a remedy containing these oral antidiabetic drugs without his or her physician's knowledge, authorization, and supervision is not only illegal but downright dangerous. A person who undergoes an attack of hypoglycemia when alone or in a place where no knowledgeable person is available to give assistance could experience a convulsive seizure leading to irreversible injury to the brain from insufficient oxygen, causing coma and death. Adjusting the dosage of an oral antidiabetic agent depends upon initial laboratory monitoring and later daily self-monitoring of the person's blood sugar. That would not occur for persons taking a fraudulent preparation such as one of these five, which would be unlikely to bear proper instructions about side effects or precautions for a self-medicating person. Scientific medicine has accomplished wonders in saving and easing the lives of diabetics. Those achievements cannot be equaled or replaced by a "simpler" unconventional approach using supposedly antidiabetic botanical remedies. Diabetic persons who attempt to do so are gambling dangerously with their health and life. Certainly, a parent should never endanger a diabetic child by following such practices; moreover, to do so would likely incur criminal legal liability in case of injury or death.

Herbal Weight-Loss Mixture Contains Banned Fenfluramine

Metcalf and colleagues (2002) reported concern arising from more adverse responses in young women undergoing an herbal regimen supplied by a particular Chinese herbalist for weight loss with "spectacular" results. Several women reported that they experienced significant cardiovascular symptoms but were reassured that Chinese medicines were natural and would cause no harm. Chemical investigation was directed at the combination that claimed as many as nine components (a normal approach for traditional Chinese medicine), examining the possibility that the preparations might contain ephedra alkaloids (ma huang). However, ephedrine was not detected, but instead a rather high concentration of the synthetic appetite suppressant fenfluramine, which was withdrawn from U.K. use in 1997 after it was incriminated in causing pulmonary hypertension and damage to heart valves. At the issuance of this report, it had not been established where in the chain of supply the adulteration with fenfluramine occurred. It appears clearly to have been a matter of intent rather than an unlikely accident, because the appetite suppressant nature of the adulterant coincided with the use for which the "herbal remedy" was sold. In Japan and Singapore four or more deaths were attributed to a similar product appearing under different names.

On August 8, 2002, the FDA issued an alert to the U.S. public about the two Chinese weight-loss products labeled Chaso (Jianfei) Diet Capsules and Chaso Genpi because they posed a potential public health risk if imported and sold (FDA, 2002a). Although the FDA has advised its personnel conducting import operations to be on the alert to intercept Chaso Diet Capsules or Chaso Genpi, it was possible that such materials might already have entered the country and might be offered for sale at small urban markets as alternatives to Western weight control medicines. The agency urged consumers not to take these diet pills and to notify the FDA if the products should be found in their area.

British Inquiry into Fraudulent Skin Treatments (not Dietary Supplements)

The January 8, 2000, issue of *British Medical Journal* contained a report of an official parliamentary investigative group concerning nonregulated skin products having dangerous side effects. It was revealed that some products sold as natural remedies had actually contained a potent synthetic steroid, and they were being widely marketed to patients with skin diseases (Yarney, 2000). The group was assisted by an advisory committee of skin specialists and patient representatives. They collected written and oral evidence of the fraudulent practices in therapy of skin disease. Besides the finding that some herbal products had excess "help," other cases involved products touted as cures for dermatologic problems that contained no active ingredients at all. Moreover, some "skin clinics" had been providing harmful dietary advice.

A mail-order product called "SkinCap," was marketed to patients with psoriasis at a cost of more than £30 (about $48) per week, yet the manufacturers claimed that it contained nothing more active than zinc pyrithione. Patients did indeed report dramatic resolution of their symptoms, and they were inclined to continue using it on a long-term basis. However, an independent analysis of the cream showed that it contained a potent topical corticosteroid, which would raise questions of safety for its continual use. This is in addition to it being an illegal, mislabeled product. One clinic in London charged £950 (about $1,500!) for a 50-gram (less than 2 ounces) pot of cream to treat vitiligo, a patchy loss of normal skin pigmentation. When analyzed this product contained a small amount of a corticosteroid, fluocinolone, in a white, soft-paraffin base. For such contents that price is surely exorbitant. Let the buyer everywhere beware!

Systemic Corticosteroids: "Mexican Asthma Cure"

A 1990 report indicated that asthmatic patients from western Canada and the United States who visited an asthma clinic in Mexicali, Mexico, returned with their symptoms substantially improved or even temporarily eliminated. They were told that the medicine was a new bronchodilator agent supposedly unavailable in the United States or Canada because of hindrances by "the big drug companies." However, analysis of the medicines revealed that instead they usually contained a synthetic cortisone substitute (triamcinolone) and a commonly used OTC antihistamine, chlorpheniramine (Rubin et al., 1990). Sometimes benzodiazepine-type sedatives were included in the mixes. However, the patients were told that medications they received were free of side effects, and were assured that corticosteroids were not being used.

Such fraudulent therapy is hazardous to patients who not only are ignorant of the composition of their south-of-the-border medications but also are unlikely to inform their doctor that they are taking it. In doing so, persons may risk drug interactions or side effects from unwittingly using duplicate medicines. A particularly serious danger is the likelihood of an unrecognized suppression of their adrenal cortex function, which is a predictable effect of sustained oral intake of any corticosteroids such as triamcinolone. As a result, a user may experience life-threatening adrenocortical insufficiency when they undergo a severe stress, or even at the mere withdrawal of the medication. A risk also exists that a person so misled will abandon a safer form of asthma therapy because of their encounter with "a miracle cure."

Sex-Enhancing Supplement Enhanced with Viagra

On April 4, 2003, the FDA announced that Ultra Health Laboratories, Inc. and Bionate International, Inc. were warning consumers not to purchase or consume a product known as Vinarol tablets. This item, which was being marketed as a dietary supplement, contained an unlabeled Rx drug ingredient, sildenafil (Viagra), that might pose a serious health risk to some users. This situation exemplifies illegal fortification of a supposed "natural" supplement formula, and makes one wonder how many other "effective" remedies for increasing sexual desire, confidence, and performance benefit from the same ingredient (NCCAM, 2003).

On November 2, 2004, the same scenario repeated with a warning from the FDA to consumers not to purchase or to consume Actra-Rx or Yilishen, two products offered for sale on Web sites as "dietary supplements" for treating erectile dysfunction and enhancing sexual performance for men. The two products did in fact contain an active prescription drug ingredient, sildenafil, which might comprise a hazard for excessive fall in blood pressure under certain circumstances. A research letter was published in *JAMA* describing the results of a chemical analysis of Actra-Rx, which found that each capsule analyzed contained prescription-strength quantities of sildenafil (FDA, 2005).

EPHEDRINE

From Alaska comes a case of legal action taken against a weight-reduction product alleging a deceptive practice leading to harm. An Anchorage jury decided in favor of a local women who at age 32 years began taking a product advertised as herbal and natural. After two years of use the woman experienced a stroke and permanent brain damage. She believed the product to be all natural as labeled. Instead it combined caffeine with diethylaminoethanol and ephedrine, the latter in particular being alleged at trial to be a synthetic material used for "spiking" the product. A Washington Post story of February 8, 2001, indicated that the jury found that the supplier was liable for her injuries and levied a judgment for $12 million in punitive damages and $1.3 million in compensatory damages. No prior action of this sort had occurred in the U.S. courts. The attorney for the plaintiff said that both the FDA and the Montana Department of Public Health and Human Services had notified the manufacturer repeatedly that their product was implicated in users suffering heart attacks and strokes (Gugliotta, 2001). Fortunately (in context) for the woman the ephedrine was synthetic, because when encountered in herbal form the potential adverse actions of ephedrine are protected by DSHEA. Only when an "extra" amount, of synthetic origin, is added to the product can the manufacturer be held at fault.

UNRELIABILITY OF SOME NUTRITIONALS' LABELS

Conjugated linoleic acid, commonly known as CLA, represents a concentrated 50:50 mixture of two special fatty acids. They began to be promoted in the latter 1990s as a means to reduce the proportion of the body weight consisting of fat (Raloff, 2001). Initially, studies in immature growing animals found that a higher intake of CLA promoted a more lean body composition (Larsen et al., 2003). However, a 2004 study from France found no such effect in adult rats, whether combined with exercise or not (Mirand et al., 2004). Validation of these findings has not been accomplished for the human body. A research report from the United Kingdom found divergent effects on blood lipids depending upon the nature of the fatty acids in a CLA mixture (Tricon et al., 2004). Moreover, neither an effective dose regimen nor its long-term safety has been established, although a 12-month human safety trial was reported in 2004 (Whigham et al., 2004). A review of a number of human studies suggest that CLA supplementation has no effect on either body weight or insulin sensitivity. In humans and pigs, the effects of CLA on fat deposition seem to be marginal and equivocal in contrast to the results observed in rodents. Another review suggests, moreover, that some persons may experience adverse responses to CLA products used for weight reduction.

However, once a concept of this sort is put forward by legitimate scientists, efforts at commercial exploitation become so rampant that one must wonder whether reliable product sources are available. One also must wonder whether test materials differ between different research projects. The grounds for such doubt are illustrated by this example. An analysis early in the wave of CLA marketing found the following results for a sample of 15 off-the-shelf samples of products claiming to supply CLA:

- One contained absolutely NONE of the purported CLA.
- Several contained about 90 percent of the claimed components.
- The great majority had various proportions less than the claimed level.
- All were qualitatively inconsistent in their composition.

Can a person always rely on the label when buying a dietary supplement consisting of a relatively simple constitution such as CLA? Evidently not. Again, the labels lack the one most appropriate phrase—caveat emptor!

Chapter 11

If a Little Is Good for You, a Lot Will Be Better!

The use of complementary and alternative therapies has become widespread, and many patients use alternative medicines or seek care from alternative medicine practitioners without the knowledge of their usual primary physician. However, persons need an awareness that many seemingly harmless self-treatments and dietary practices exist that can be carried too far for health or safety. We will consider examples of people getting into serious trouble by highly excess usage of agents that hardly anyone, including the FDA, would believe to deserve being tightly regulated or called unsafe, namely licorice, milk of magnesia, and large quantities of fruit juices!

LICORICE ROOT EXTRACT

Since 1950 it has been known that an extract of licorice exerts a significant hormonal activity in humans, similar to that of the first-known mineralocorticoid, desoxycorticosterone, which acts on the kidneys to conserve sodium and to excrete potassium to excess.

Case Report 1: Near Fatality from Licorice Abuse

One day in March 1997 a 44-year-old woman walked into the emergency department of a hospital in Sweden where she promptly experienced the first of a series of life-threatening attacks known as ventricular tachycardia (Eriksson et al., 1999). In this situation the main pumping portion of the heart muscle, the left ventricle, beats at a highly excessive rate. Such tachycardia is especially threatening because of the serious possibility of progressing into ventricular fibrillation, in which the heart's pumping action fails because its contractions are totally out of synchrony and coordination. The result is that no effective pumping of the blood occurs. Death will ensue if a reversal (defibrillation) is not rapidly achieved. Among the laboratory measures obtained on the woman's blood, it was found that her serum potassium was quite de-

doi:10.1300/5698_11

pleted (hypokalemia). After various investigations that included cardiac ultrasonic imaging and endoscopic imaging of esophagus, duodenum, and colon, the physicians remained bewildered about the cause for her condition. She finally admitted having eaten 1.5 to 3.5 ounces (40 to 70 grams) of licorice every day for the previous four months. This patient was far from the first to have an adverse encounter with licorice. Indeed, for a substance having so innocent a face, licorice has quite a record for unfavorable effects. The most clearly documented problem is for excessive licorice intake to promote hypertension because of its increasing the secretion of aldosterone, an important hormone of the adrenal cortex. It is an extension of the actions of aldosterone that provokes the deficit of potassium (Eriksson et al., 1999).

Despite its long use in candies and as a flavoring agent in medicinals, whole licorice has pharmacologic actions that may become significant when a person severely overdoes it. It causes sodium retention and potassium loss when taken in sufficiently large doses (Epstein et al., 1997). These indirect effects of high amounts of ordinary licorice on kidney function, are known since 1977 to be able to cause toxicity by severely reducing the body's supply of potassium ions, which are necessary for maintenance of normal heart action (Blachley and Knochel, 1980; Luchon et al., 1993). The present incident was by no means the first one published, but was said to be the first recorded case of an overindulgence in licorice resulting in an attack of the especially dangerous form of tachycardia (rapid heartbeat), torsades de pointes. Many cases of the type of heart condition (from different causes) that was experienced by this fortunate patient have seen a fatal outcome. Torsades de pointes has increasingly been recognized in recent years as a serious risk associated with many prescription medications.

Extracts of licorice root are widely used in many other countries (more than in the United States) as flavoring agent, breath freshener, or candy, and many people are exposed to its constituents. Moreover, some herbalists advocate use of licorice to cleanse the colon, relieve bronchitis (by increasing the fluidity of mucus secretions), oppose bacterial infections by *Staphylococcus* or *Streptococcus,* control fungal infections by *Candida,* relieve inflammatory disorders (rheumatism and arthritis), promote adrenal gland function, and stimulate the production of interferon. A form that has the component glycyrrhizin removed, known as deglycyrrhizinated licorice (DGL) (mostly as chewable tablets), is said to avoid the unwanted effects of ordinary licorice. It is advocated for suppressing acid reflux and to prevent ulcers by increasing the number of mucus secreting cells in the digestive tract.

Guidelines and Other Cautions

Acute poisoning has not been noted, but chronic (days to weeks) licorice poisoning is possible. It is rare in North America, but apparently more common in Europe. In short, high intake is ill-advised. It is advised that one should not take licorice for more than seven days in a row, and, of course, always follow package directions if using a product intended not as candy but as a dietary supplement. As for botanicals generally, women who are pregnant or nursing should not use licorice. Use of licorice is not recommended when any of the following conditions exists: hypertension, heart disease, kidney or liver disease, diabetes, glaucoma, menstrual problems, prior stroke, and for persons taking thiazide diuretics.

Moreover, a 1999 report described the results of a test on seven normal, healthy men ranging from 22 to 24 years of age (Armanini et al., 1999). The men were given for one week a seven-gram (one-quarter ounce) daily dose of a commercial preparation of licorice in the form of tablets. This amount of licorice is said to be eaten daily by many people in Italy. The researchers then evaluated the effect of licorice on gonadal function before, at four and seven days of licorice intake, and at four days after it was stopped. Their serum levels of testosterone, androstenedione, and 17-hydroxyprogesterone (17HP) were measured as indicators of hormone synthesis and secretion by the testes. During the period of licorice intake the men's serum testosterone levels decreased and their serum levels of the testosterone precursor, 17HP, were increased. The results showed that licorice inhibits both of the enzymes that are necessary to convert 17HP, first to androstenedione and then to testosterone.

The authors conclude that not only men with hypertension, but also those with decreased libido or other sexual dysfunction, should be questioned about their possible excess intake of licorice. Overall, a greatly excessive intake of licorice can cause a remarkable variety of symptoms, such as the following:

- Dark urine (muscle-injury-induced myoglobin appearing in the urine)
- Weakness (from hypokalemia and/or muscle injuries)
- Fatigue and muscle cramping
- Muscle spasms (tetany)
- Reduced reflex activity, muscle wasting and weakness, or flaccid paralysis
- Polyuria/nocturia (increased urination)
- Edema (swelling from increased extracellular fluid volume)
- Dyspnea (difficult breathing from pulmonary edema, excess fluid in the lungs)
- Headache (from hypertension)

- Paresthesias (abnormal feelings, e.g., burning sensations of the extremities)
- Impotence and/or diminished libido (from lowered testosterone action)
- Amenorrhea (from altered female hormone metabolism)
- Collapse and possible death from cardiac arrest or cardiac dysrhythmias (rare)

MAGNESIUM

Fatal Outcome from Excess Milk of Magnesia

Case Report 2

A 28-month-old boy arrived at an emergency department in a state of cardiopulmonary arrest—an absence of both heartbeat and spontaneous respiration (McGuire et al., 2000). He had a medical history of severe mental retardation, spastic paralysis of all limbs, and a seizure disorder. He required mechanical ventilation nightly via an intratracheal tube for lack of normal breathing, and he received nutrition and medicines via a gastric tube.

In the three weeks before being taken to the hospital his mother had been giving the boy high doses of vitamin and mineral supplements on recommendation of "a nutritional consultant" without the patient's physician being informed. The boy's regimen included multivitamins, essential fatty acids, lactobacillus, bifido bacterium, and two minerals, calcium carbonate and magnesium oxide, which the mother was told would help relax his muscles and relieve his constipation. She had been instructed to give a half-teaspoonful of magnesium oxide suspension ("milk of magnesia") four times per day (800 mg) and to watch for loose stools. Several days before admission she decided to triple the dose to a half-tablespoonful four times per day (2,400 mg) because of the continuing constipation. The mother reported that two days previously he appeared drowsy and less easily arousable. On the morning of admission, she found him unresponsive, unarousable, and with big pupils. Because of concern about his enlarged pupils, she disconnected him from his ventilator and rushed him to an emergency department, which required merely a five-minute trip.

On arrival, the boy showed no pulse, no breathing, and was unresponsive to stimulation. His pupils were wide and unreactive to light and his muscle tone was generally flaccid. His torso was warm but he had cool extremities. Cardiopulmonary resuscitation was initiated. Epinephrine (adrenalin) was administered, after which heart action and blood pressure returned to a normal rate. The pulse became detectable, but the heart rhythm remained abnormal. Early laboratory data obtained after the initial resuscitation showed a highly elevated serum level of magnesium, whereas most other results were within the normal range. His electrocardiogram showed abnormalities of rhythm and a low ventricular rate of 60 beats per minute and occasional premature beats. An echocardiogram test revealed a severe reduction from the normal strength of cardiac contraction. An external pacemaker was applied, which resulted in an adequate blood pressure. Dialysis was used to reduce the overload of magnesium.

Despite a prompt correction of the biochemical abnormalities and the aggressive provision of cardiopulmonary support, the patient died 20 hours after admission from uncorrectable cardiac dysrhythmias and consequent profound cardiac dysfunction. Postmortem examination showed tissue changes in the heart that reflected a deficient oxygenation, an acute interstitial pneumonia in the lungs, early necrosis of the small and large intestines, and a pronounced congestion of the kidneys. The stomach and small bowel contained a soft, chalklike material. This patient suffered from a rarely seen condition of severe hypermagnesemia—a great excess of magnesium in the blood despite his having normal kidney activity, which normally prevents such a condition. This clearly was a consequence of extreme overdosing with an ordinarily very safe compound, magnesium oxide, which has long been used in the laxative products titled milk of magnesia. Magnesium taken by mouth is poorly absorbed, and any excess absorbed beyond needs is readily eliminated in the urine by persons having adequate kidney function. A review of past medical records demonstrated that the child's previous kidney function testing showed normality by several measures (McGuire et al., 2000).

Magnesium has been rightly regarded as safe, except for very special circumstances under which it may prove to be distinctly unsafe, most commonly an elderly person with diminished kidney excretory capacity. However, in this instance excretion by the kidneys could not match the highly excessive intake, even despite that much of the material remained unabsorbed in the alimentary canal. The pediatricians who reported this case stated the problem correctly in saying that many patients do not view OTC "patent medicines" and dietary supplements as being drugs. This case demonstrates why people need to inform their child's pediatrician, and all other physicians, of *all* sorts of remedies being used, including alternative remedies. However, to be realistic, physicians in the main have not been trained to know or evaluate the possible significance of most such items, and many are disinclined to ask for such "nondrug" information. Moreover, they have only in recent times being urged in medical journal articles to become prepared to utilize patient information on nonprescription remedies.

FRUIT AND FRUIT JUICES: HELPFUL BUT NOT HARMLESS

Beginning in 1991, many evidences have accumulated to show that citrus juices, especially grapefruit juice, can be not only a desirable, healthful drink for its ascorbic acid and citrus bioflavonoids but also an unwanted modifier of therapeutic drug actions. It became well established that several citrus components have an appreciable capacity to interact by virtue of their inhibiting an enzyme (CYP3A4) found in the liver and in the wall of the small intestine that is responsible for the metabolism of many drugs and, generally, their inactivation. Such an action, especially prominent for grapefruit, would enhance the blood and tissue levels of various drugs and increase their effects. However, a minority of agents (those classed as "prodrugs") would be affected in the opposite direction because their activity requires their being metabolized to become activated. Thus, the effects of grapefruit can be complex.

Moreover, an even further effect of grapefruit complicates the picture. It also inhibits a mechanism in the intestine that opposes some drugs being absorbed, thus acting to decrease their blood levels and effects.

An example of an important agent affected is cyclosporine, an immunosuppressant medicine of importance to organ transplant patients. As with most drugs for that purpose, its therapeutic range must be carefully monitored and maintained. If levels are too low it may be ineffective and fail to prevent rejection, resulting in loss of a transplanted organ, and too high levels can be a risk for dangerous toxicity. St. John's wort is well known to have the former action by *increasing* levels of the enzyme CYP3A4 so much that blood levels of cyclosporine fall below a minimal effective level (see Chapter 9).

Dangerous Elevation of Blood Potassium from Too Much Fruit Juice

Case Reports 3 and 4

A patient with chronic renal deficiency began regularly self-treating with an alternative remedy, noni juice, a product obtained from the fruit of *Morinda citrifolia* (Mueller et al., 2000). This patient appeared at the clinic after becoming ill and was found to be in a serious state of hyperkalemia (elevated blood potassium level) despite his claiming to have followed the low-potassium diet required by his kidney disease. The authors reporting the case analyzed the noni juice and found the level of potassium to be 56.3 mEq per liter, similar to concentrations reported for orange juice and tomato juice. The noni plant, which originally was native to islands of the South Pacific, provides a juice that is now widely available and promoted for use against more than 20 health problems (including cancer) as an "adaptogen" (Mueller et al., 2000).

In another case, a diabetic man became hyperkalemic because of an excessive affection for drinking apple juice, which was reported to have a level of merely 28 to 32 mEq per liter (Jarmon et al., 2001). There recently has been a marketing push for foods or beverages that provide a high ratio of potassium to sodium—e.g., by orange juice companies, as one daily serving of a citrus juice is said to reduce the risk for acute ischemic stroke by 25 percent. The case above illustrates that the beneficial effects of fruit juices do not prevent their being a hazard when taken to excess by persons whose health problems put them at high risk for getting "too much of a good thing" by excessively increasing potassium intake (Jarmon et al., 2001).

ANOTHER HAZARD FROM GOOD JUICE TURNED BAD

Fatal Amplification of Anticoagulant Action Attributed to Excess Cranberry Juice

Case Report 5

After a chest infection that was successfully treated with antibiotic, a man in his seventies had a poor appetite and ate next to nothing for two weeks except for cranberry juice *(Vaccinum macrocarpon).* The Rx drugs he was taking were phenytoin, digoxin, and warfarin (Suvarna et al., 2003). He was admitted again to hospital with an elevated prothrombin time (blood not clotting as quickly as normal). Previously, his anticoagulation response had been stabilized at a desirable level. He died of a massive hemorrhage into the gastrointestinal tract and the pericardial sac. He had been not been taking OTC or herbal products, and had taken his Rx drugs (especially warfarin) correctly (Suvarna et al., 2003).

This is the eighth case reported to the U.K. Medicines and Healthcare products Regulatory Agency about a possible interaction between warfarin and cranberry juice leading to an unfavorable change in the blood clotting time reading or a bleeding incident. None was so dramatic or devastating as this one. Little information was provided on whether these patients were taking the warfarin correctly. Warfarin is metabolically inactivated primarily by the enzyme CYP2C9, but it is not known whether the flavonoids found in cranberry juice inhibit this enzyme. Such an interaction is known for other CYP enzymes and flavonoids, as in citrus fruits. Physicians prescribing warfarin need to warn their patients against excessive fruit juices as well as certain botanical supplements.

PART III: Questionable Supplement Marvels

How prone we are to come to the consideration of every question with heads and hearts pre-occupied! How prone to shrink from any opinion, however reasonable, if it be opposed to any, however unreasonable, of our own!

Frances Wright, Scottish author

There is no expedient to which a man will not go to avoid the labor of thinking.

Thomas Alva Edison, American inventor

Chapter 12

CAM: Hope, Help, or Hazard?

> These observations raise questions about the frequency and control of hepatotoxicity associated with ingestion of herbal medicines. The frequency of such hepatotoxicity has probably been underestimated.
>
> Larrey et al. (1992)

Various factors implicated in the onset of liver disease include injury from a bacterial endotoxin from an excess of endogenous tumor necrosis factor-alpha (TNF-alpha) or from oxidizing free radicals. Free radicals can become injurious by their activating a production (transcription) of TNF-alpha, a major proinflammatory cytokine (an immune cell secretion) that can initiate hepatitis. Thus, an action to halt the progression of such injury might logically be directed against endotoxins, TNF-alpha, or free radicals.

The adverse action of free radicals is referred to as oxidant (or oxidative) stress. This process appears to play a key role in pathogenesis of liver disease. Using animal models and cultured liver cells in vitro, researchers have established a firm link between actions that generate free radicals and the development of alcohol-induced liver injury. Thus, complementary and alternative treatments that diminish/oppose oxidant stress have a theoretical merit of protecting the liver from damage induced by free radicals. Research on animal models tends to support this hypothesis, but validation from human research is very much lacking. Antioxidant supplements now under study include NAC (N-acetylcysteine), vitamins C and E, phosphatidylcholine, and silymarin (milk thistle).

A NEW PLAGUE: HEPATITIS C VIRUS

Hepatitis C virus (HCV) is emerging worldwide as a serious problem, and it has already reached the point in the United States at which the mortality rate is predicted to triple in the next decade, rivaling the numbers of

doi:10.1300/5698_12

deaths from HIV/AIDS. The disease has an incubation period of 10 to 30 years before manifesting. A minority of people never do develop serious health effects from HCV, however many experience a progression of liver ailments until either cirrhosis or cancer destroys the liver. Symptoms or signs may not appear until the disease has reached the stage of severe injury called cirrhosis. HCV is an infection whose transmission is mainly body fluid/blood related, similar to HIV. Injected drug abuse is a major mode of exposure if sharing of syringes or needles between infected and uninfected persons occurs; the prevalence of hepatitis C doubled in the United Kingdom from 2000 to 2003 among persons who had recently started injecting abuse drugs. Former transmission via transfusions was interdicted by testing of donor blood. Tattoo parlors were another site of transmission besides the medical and addiction contexts.

Early diagnosis is a vital component of successful management of hepatitis. A large increase in the number of adults needing liver transplantation because of hepatitis C occurred in the 1990s, and the upward trend continues. Unfortunately, no reliable and effective therapy exists for chronic HCV infection. The current standard therapy uses interferons, highly expensive antiviral agents and biotech pharmaceuticals, but the cure rate is no greater than 30 percent. Moreover, an additional extremely costly step of liver transplantation is not a permanent answer because viral infection of the new liver is very likely without the prior eradication of the virus, which presently is seldom possible.

CAM Products for Treating Liver Diseases

However, a number of lower-tech alternative therapies are also being examined—glycyrrhizin, catechin, silymarin, phytosterols, and the antioxidants N-acetylcysteine and vitamin E, according to a recent review (Bass, 1999). The most prominent of these is a preparation known as silymarin, which consists of a standardized extract from the fruit of *Silybum marianum.* It is a mixture of four isomers in a flavonoid subclass flavonolignans, which are believed to exert such actions as free-radical scavenger and membrane stabilizer. In several experimental models of liver injury those actions have prevented the occurrence of lipid peroxidation and its associated damage to cell membranes. In laboratory animals not only the liver but also the kidneys, pancreas, red blood cells, and blood platelets are protected by silymarin against the effects of model hepatotoxic chemicals such as carbon tetrachloride, cyclosporine, and alcohol. It is interesting that the historical background on milk thistle use for liver problems is extensive from the early sixteenth to the eighteenth century.

A clinical review (Flora et al., 1998) concluded that

> most of the clinical trials designed to assess the effects of silymarin are difficult to interpret, as they are flawed by the small numbers of subjects, variability in etiologies, and severity of the liver disease studied, as well as inconsistency of alcohol usage by patients, heterogenous dosing, inconsistent use of control groups, and inadequately defined endpoints.

The most common uses of silymarin have been the acute liver toxicity of mushroom poisoning by the *Amanita phalloides* and the chronic injury from excessive exposure to beverage alcohol.

In 1999 B. M. Berkson, MD, PhD, of the Integrative Medical Center of New Mexico, reported on three hepatitis C patients to whom he provided an unconventional treatment regimen (Berkson, 1999). This consisted of a triple antioxidant combination that included silymarin, selenium, and alpha-lipoic acid (also known as thioctic acid). All three people responded favorably to the triple antioxidant program. Their clinical signs of illness were soon reversed, and their laboratory values improved to a remarkable degree without liver transplantation. The patients were said to be able to return to work and carry on normal activities while feeling healthy again. Their feeling better could be dismissed as a mere placebo effect, but the laboratory findings suggest that a real benefit could have existed.

About one-third of HIV-infected patients are also infected with HCV. In any person, HCV infection is prone to progress to liver failure, but it may do so more rapidly in HIV-infected patients. Because milk thistle is reported to decrease the risk of developing liver failure, it is not surprising that HIV-infected persons who are also infected with HCV are inclined to take milk thistle. Thus, it was important to test whether the supplement interacts to hinder the action of anti-HIV agents. One major anti-HIV drug, indinavir, was recently tested and found not to be subject to such an interference through fourteen days of concurrently administered silymarin despite the latter having two actions that might be expected to favor herb-drug interactions (Berkson, 1999).

Whether silymarin, or its major active component, silibinin, fulfill the hopes held for their benefit to persons with liver illnesses, other plant components in prospect have shown even better effects in animal studies. A success of the sort suggested by Dr. Berkson's report would indeed revolutionize hepatitis C therapy.

THE DRINKER'S DEADLY DESTINY: ALCOHOLIC CIRRHOSIS

A controlled trial on the use of silymarin in patients with alcoholic liver disease was reported in 1992 from Chile. Seventy-two patients admitted to the trial were randomly assigned to experimental or placebo control groups that did not differ in their initial laboratory assessment. They were monitored for an average of 15 months while taking either placebo or silymarin daily. Ten patients died during the follow-up—five in the placebo and five in the silymarin group—displaying no difference in mortality between the two. It was concluded in this small trial that silymarin did not alter the course or the risk of fatal outcome of alcoholic liver disease. As in hepatitis C, therapy of alcoholic liver injury is unlikely to succeed if it is begun only after reaching advanced stages. However, many alcoholic persons resist being brought into any therapy before their liver disease is advanced. Thus, a solution to this serious and costly pathology would be highly desirable (Bunout et al., 1992).

Persons who abuse alcohol are more likely to become infected with HCV and are more likely to experience persistent, long-term infection. Excessive alcohol intake also tends to increases the degree of viral burden and interferes with antiviral therapy. For such persons the liver disease is more likely to progress to cirrhosis and liver cancer. Thus, appropriate interest in the possible value of CAM agents to oppose this deadly progression has developed. In 2002 the National Institute for Alcoholism and Alcohol Abuse and the NCCAM issued a call for research proposals concerning the possible value of SAMe (S-adenosylmethionine) in treating alcoholic liver problems. SAMe is a donor of methyl groups that supports biochemical methylation reactions and thus it has a great many important roles. Another valuable metabolite for liver health is N-acetylcysteine, which serves as a precursor of glutathione, the main protective antioxidant present in liver cells. Ensuring the adequate availability of glutathione tends to bolster the body's chemical defenses, which are put to the test by an intake of various poisons, including drinking an excessive amount of alcoholic beverages on a continuing basis (NIAAA, 2005).

Human studies of SAMe include a randomized, placebo-controlled, double-blind, multicenter clinical trial that was conducted by prominent medical researchers in Spain. The study included 62 SAMe-treated and 61 placebo-group patients, all having the diagnosis of alcoholic hepatic cirrhosis. The daily treatment was three 400 mg tablets of SAMe or a placebo, and the trial lasted two years. Upon entry into the trial no significant difference existed between the two groups regarding sex, age, previous major complications, or the severity of cirrhosis by liver function tests. The two-year period of observation revealed that SAMe was safe and well-tolerated. Reasons for a few persons stopping therapy were nausea, diarrhea, and/or a form of heartburn (Mato et al., 1999).

The overall rate of death or liver failure requiring liver transplantation at the end of the trial was 30 percent in the placebo group, but only 16 percent in the SAMe group. The level of probability for this difference did not quite attain the standard for statistical significance. However, when eight patients in the most severe class of the disease were excluded from the analysis for both groups, the mortality rate (from any cause) or the rate of liver transplantation was significantly lower in the SAMe group than in the placebo group (12 percent versus 29 percent). The results suggest that long-term treatment of alcoholic cirrhosis patients with SAMe may improve their survival time or delay their need for a liver transplant, especially for those having less advanced cirrhosis. The usual dose for liver disorders is 1,600 mg/day. Maintenance of protective levels of glutathione by SAMe therapy is a major possible explanation for these effects.

Such favorable results deserve further confirmatory studies by other research groups. Moreover, they raise the question of whether a person who is a chronic heavy drinker of alcoholic beverages could gain more significant protection by the use of SAMe or NAC. Obviously, their better choice should be to abstain from continued detrimental exposure of their liver (and other organs) to the injurious effects of alcohol. However, a physician dealing with a patient who is determined not to change their drinking habit, despite warnings of potential liver cirrhosis or cancer, might be warranted in prescribing a potentially liver-protective measure such as the long-term intake of SAMe or NAC.

A RECURRING TRAGEDY: AMANITA *MUSHROOM POISONING*

Hepatic injury often results from a mistaken identity between safe, edible species of mushrooms and the highly poisonous death cap mushroom, *Amanita phalloides,* or other members of the toxic *Amanita* genus (Larrey and Pageaux, 1995). A large proportion of persons eating a poisonous mushroom will experience such a high degree of injury as to die from liver failure and its complications, although toxicity to the nervous system or heart may also be responsible. The value of finding an effective antidote for the toxic components of amanita is clear.

UNWISE SELF-PRESCRIBED "LIVER CLEANSING"

The application of an herbal such as milk thistle for a disease condition is one issue, but its prophylactic use by a person having no physician-diagnosed liver problem is quite another matter. When we take a substance as a medicine we expect not only that it will have a high probability of helping but also that it generally will not be likely to do harm. For an adverse consequence to arise from a material taken as a supposed *preventive* of illness would be unacceptable. Thus, it is necessary to mention a report of an adverse outcome in such use of milk thistle.

Case Report 1

A 57-year-old woman came to her physician with complaints of a two-month period during which she experienced intermittent episodes of illness consisting of sweating, nausea, colicky abdominal pain, watery diarrhea, vomiting, weakness, and collapse. Although these episodes lasted as much as 24 hours, she felt entirely well between attacks, which were not clearly related to food intake or other activity. Her drug intake consisted of an estrogen and a tricyclic antidepressant, neither of which could be blamed for such manifestations. An examination revealed no abnormalities, but she was admitted to the hospital for study one day after an attack. Test results tended to exclude several possible explanations.

Upon further questioning about any history of changes during the past two months, she acknowledged that she had indeed begun taking a certain brand of milk thistle capsules for headache and "liver cleansing" two months before. After cessation of this remedy she had no further episodes for several weeks. She took another capsule and experienced a strong reaction similar to the prior one that led to hospital admission. The association in time between the herbal use and an adverse response tends to support a causative role of the herbal capsule in her prior problems. The Australian Adverse Drug Reactions Advisory Committee, which reported this case in 1999, had received only two other adverse reports on milk thistle, one of which was similar in that it also included nausea and abdominal pain as well as listlessness and insomnia. The authors acknowledged the possibility that these reactions were idiosyncratic, or that they were attributable to factors unrelated to the supposed active ingredient(s). The committee's main emphasis was upon the urgency for patients to fully reveal to their physicians usage of all unconventional remedies, i.e., all agents classed in the United States as dietary supplements (Australian Adverse Drug Reactions Advisory Committee, 1999).

MORE ABOUT SAMe AND THE LIVER

S-Adenosylmethionine (SAMe) is a natural metabolite having a pivotal role as the most important methyl donor for reactions essential to a myriad of biological events via biochemical processes. SAMe is widely distributed throughout the body in every living cell, but it occurs at especially high concentrations in the brain and liver. About 85 percent of all methylation reactions occur in the liver. Besides serving as a methyl donor, SAMe is an activator of enzymes in many biochemical reactions, mostly in the liver. Recent data suggest that SAMe also acts as an intracellular control switch to regulate such essential liver functions as regeneration, differentiation and sensitivity to injury.

The essential amino acid methionine is metabolized by the enzyme SAMe-synthetase mainly in the liver to produce SAMe. For patients with liver disease, the production of SAMe may be among a multitude of liver functions that become impaired by a deficit of SAMe-synthetase activity. Because exogenous SAMe may be expected to overcome a loss of the SAMe-synthetase activity, liver problems have been a major focus for the therapeutic application of SAMe in Europe, where the compound was first developed.

Synthesis of SAMe is linked to the metabolism of both folic acid and vitamin B12. Deficiencies of B12 are associated with reduced levels of the SAMe in the central nervous system, which may be an explanation for the neurologic and psychiatric disorders associated with pernicious anemia or other states of B12 deficit. SAMe seems also to enhance the synthesis of a vital component, the proteoglycans, of chondrocytes (cartilage cells) when they are grown in vitro after being obtained from the joint cartilage of patients with osteoarthritis. Such data support the use of SAMe for that widespread, age-related, and painful joint disease.

However, the most impressive human responses were after injections of SAMe, which left open the question of whether equal responses could be achieved by oral dosing that is necessary for its use in the United States as a dietary supplement. An obstacle to its medical acceptance is that most clinical trials were conducted in Europe, and, of course, that a major North American pharmaceutical company is not promoting it as an Rx product. SAMe is relatively free of adverse effects, which consist mainly of mild gastrointestinal distress with large doses. It appears to have no supplement-drug interactions except for synergism (rarely) with concurrently used antidepressants of two major classes, monoamine oxidase inhibitors (MAOIs) and selective serotonin reuptake inhibitors (SSRIs) to cause the toxic response known as the serotonin syndrome.

SAMe administration was tested by Chinese researchers for an ability to oppose experimental liver injury. Their results reported in 2001 supported earlier evidence for an important hepatoprotective effect by SAMe. From Spain comes a 1999 study that compared SAMe to the "standard" antidote, N-acetylcysteine (NAC), for a protective action against liver poisons. The two agents were tested in mice for their ability to oppose a toxic dose to the liver of the common analgesic acetaminophen (Tylenol, and other equivalents). SAMe was found to show equal efficacy as that of NAC. The data indicate that SAMe at doses of 1.0 g/kg was equally effective in preventing liver injury and death from the acetaminophen overdose in mice as was 1.0 g/kg of NAC. The levels of SAMe are enhanced by NAC administration, which is a less expensive product. The authors suggested that SAMe may be a useful alternative to NAC for the treatment of acetaminophen poisoning in human beings.

In summary, SAMe is a hepatoprotective drug commonly prescribed by physicians in many European nations. It seems likely that SAMe constitutes an underutilized medicine by U.S. doctors for several wrong reasons. That it was not licensed by a major pharmaceutical company for similar uses, as in Europe, and lacked the consequent promotion to physicians, left the door open for SAMe being marketed here as a dietary supplement. It evidently it was not seen as offering enough profit to justify the cost of licensing in addition to the clinical research necessary to obtain FDA approval for its marketing. Along with its not being promoted by pharmaceutical sales representatives, its classification as a supplement automatically causes SAMe to be ignored by many U.S. physicians. This is aggravated by clinical studies by U.S. researchers not being funded by a pharmaceutical company, so such trials are unlikely to happen here except as federal funding occurs. Thus, it will tend to remain essentially true that "all the human data are from overseas," which is an all-too-strong, prejudicial argument against any medicine, and hardly a scientifically valid one.

BOTANICALS CONTAINING HEPATOTOXIC CONSTITUENTS

According to a review on hepatotoxicity associated with botanical remedies (Stickel et al., 2000), "Severe liver injury, including acute and chronic abnormalities and even cirrhotic transformation and liver failure, has been described after ingestion of a wide range of herbal products and other botanical ingredients" (p. 113). This is a reasonable inference when one considers that diagnosing the cause of a case of hepatitis is a difficult process.

One source suggests that eight different types of causation for liver injury may exist, of which three are relevant to this topic: (1) cholestatic, (2) autoimmune, and (3) hepatotoxic. Among these, several pharmaceuticals have been known for causing a cholestatic problem, i.e., one in which the bile is blocked from draining out of the liver normally (*chole-*, bile; *-stasis,* stand still). Other drugs have been implicated in causing an immune-mediated response; this requires passage of time after a first exposure. This may be quite difficult to differentiate from other hepatic problems, which may also have systemic signs such as fever or rash.

Many potential drugs have never reached the market because of their hepatotoxicity that was detected by chronic toxicology testing in animals. It is believed that about 2 percent of all cases of jaundice result from drug-induced hepatotoxicity (Stickel et al., 2000). However, some drugs that do reach the market are associated with the rather rare cases of idiosyncratic liver dysfunction, which cannot be duplicated in animal tests and is not necessarily related to dosage. Instead, it is more determined by one or another special characters (idiosyncrasies) of a patient suffering the reaction—age, sex, prior disease, other chemical exposures, and particularly genetic traits.

In view of the extent to which the liver enters into problems for pharmaceuticals, it is not surprising that examples of botanical-induced liver injury have existed for a long time, with new ones surfacing during the 1990s to the present. It follows that an association between liver injury and botanicals is as complicated a problem as it is for pharmaceuticals. Some cases may indeed be a manifestation of intrinsic ("classical") hepatotoxicity, whereas others may derive from an immune-mediated response, and some could occur as an idiosyncrasy. The association of liver injury and the taking of a botanical remedy can present a difficult puzzle because of such remedies often containing many herbs, according to labels (if such information is even available), as well as the uncertainty about whether labeling is accurate. When MacGregor and colleagues (1989) reported on four women showing evidences of hepatotoxicity plus recent use of botanical remedies, they were able only to speculate that skullcap (*Scutellaria* species) might have been a common ingredient previously suspected to be hepatotoxic.

Estes et al. (2003) reporting from the Division of Liver and Pancreas Transplantation of the Oregon Health & Science University emphasized the extent to which their transplant patients seemingly owe their problem to the use of botanical remedies. Their analysis considered all 20 patients referred for liver transplantation service for fulminating hepatic failure (FHF) (fulminating indicates rapid progression into encephalopathy) from January 2001 through October 2002. All patients underwent investigation for possible causes of their liver injury. Potentially hepatotoxic supplements were defined as those with previously published reports of hepatic injury related to their use. Ten patients (50 percent) were recent or current users of potentially hepatotoxic supplements; the ten others had no history of supplement use. Of the supplement group, seven (35 percent) had no other identified cause for hepatic failure. Six patients in the supplement group and two in the nonsupplement group underwent liver transplantation. Five patients in each group died. No significant differences in transplantation rate or survival existed between groups; however, the different proportions requiring transplantation would have reached significance with a slightly larger group size. Supplement use alone accounted for the most cases of FHF during this survey period, exceeding rates for acetaminophen toxicity and viral hepatitis. The authors closed with the statement: "Enhanced public awareness of the potential hepatotoxicity of these commonly used agents and increased regulatory oversight of their use is strongly urged" (Estes et al., 2003, p. 852).

The plants most clearly identified with a classical hepatotoxic hazard are those that contain members of a chemical group known as the pyrrolizidine alkaloids. These plants may be the cause for poisoning when consumed by livestock or by people as food, when ingested by people for medicinal purposes, or as accidental contaminants of agricultural crops. Pyrrolizidine-producing weeds sometimes contaminate cereal grain crops and forage crops so that alkaloidal chemicals can be introduced into flour or other foods, or into milk through cows consuming such plants, and even into honey collected by bees foraging on toxic plants. The plants involved include members of three major families—Boraginaceae, Compositae, and Leguminosae—and they supply more than 100 different hepatotoxic alkaloids.

From 1990 through 1995 at least six reports were published of hepatotoxicity from the United States, Canada, and Australia that were associated with the botanical chaparral, which comes from leaves of a shrub native to the southwestern United States, *Larrea tridentata.*

Case Report 2

In April a previously healthy 33-year-old woman was found to have a benign breast lump (Katz and Saibil, 1990). On the advice of a concerned friend she began to take a botanical product, chaparral leaf tablets, 15 per day. She was well until July when she developed loss of appetite, nausea, and burning epigastric pain. In early August she noticed a darkening of her urine, which caused her to decrease her intake of tablets from 15 to merely one. She became markedly better with a return of her appetite and cessation of the pain and darkness of urine. However, later that month she increased her intake to seven chaparral tablets per day. The pain and nausea returned along with new symptoms of fatigue, yellowness in the whites of her eyes (icterus or jaundice), edema of her feet, and a swelling of her abdomen.

In early September she ceased taking the tablets, and her appetite returned within a few days. However, the discoloration of the sclera, fatigue, and increased abdominal girth persisted and were joined by a paleness of her stools. At this time she was admitted to hospital. She had no known risk factors for hepatitis, including no history of tattoos, acupuncture, use of blood products, or needle sticks. She had no personal or family history of liver or biliary tract diseases, and she did not smoke or drink alcohol. Physical examination revealed jaundice, abdominal fluid (ascites), and edema of the feet. Tests for hepatitis A and B, cytomegalovirus, or Epstein-Barr virus were negative. Her bleeding time was markedly prolonged, indicating a deficit of circulating clotting factors. Upon use of a diuretic agent and supportive care she responded and was able to leave the hospital after three weeks. A liver biopsy revealed a 60 percent loss of liver cells without significant inflammation. On follow-up her biochemical measures had normalized, but a CT scan of the liver showed focal scarring that did not progress upon further imaging (Katz and Saibil, 1990).

Evidence for human toxicity may appear in a few days or, more commonly, it may not be evident until weeks after the alkaloid is first ingested. The acute onset of illness has been compared to a known disease that is characterized by thrombosis (clotting) in the hepatic veins, which causes liver enlargement and hypertension in those vessels, which in turn leads to ascites—fluid exuding into and accumulating in the peritoneal cavity. Clinical signs are jaundice, nausea, fever, acute upper gastric pain, and acute abdominal distension with prominently dilated veins on the external abdominal wall. Biochemical tests reflect liver dysfunction. The lungs also may be affected by fluid accumulation (pulmonary edema) from pleural effusion (seepage from lung capillaries). Injury to the lungs may be prominent and has been fatal. Chronic illness from ingestion of small amounts of the alkaloids over long intervals may give warning merely by a loss of appetite and undue fatigue. Yet it still can cause fibrosis of the liver, which may progress to cirrhosis that is indistinguishable from cirrhosis of other causes.

Relatively few reports of human poisonings exist in the United States, but in worldwide terms a great many more cases have been documented. Such incidents in the United States have been growing over the past 20 years and likely will continue to increase in view of the popularity of botanical remedies. Most hepatotoxic incidents in the United States have involved the consumption of either an herbal tea or a supplement in an oral dosage form (Huxtable, 1989). The first patient ever diagnosed in the United States was a woman who had used a medicinal tea for six months while visiting in Ecuador. She developed typical hepatic veno-occlusive disease (closing down of veins in the liver), with copious accumulation of ascites in the abdominal cavity, congestion of the central lobe of the liver, and increased hepatic portal vein pressure. The patient completely recovered within one year after ceasing to consume the tea.

From Los Angeles came a report (Woolf et al., 1994) of seven persons who developed acute hepatitis after a mean of 20 weeks (range 7 to 52) of using tablets of Jin Bu Huan *(Lycopodium serratum)*. This is a pain relief remedy that is said to have been used in China for 1,000 years (obviously not in the modern tablet form), but became available in the United States only in 1984. However, all seven patients were Caucasian, and none had a history of prior liver problems. All denied a history of excessive alcohol usage or contact with known hepatotoxic chemicals. Their symptoms were characteristic of acute liver injury—fever, fatigue, nausea, itching, and abdominal pain, as well as signs of jaundice and liver enlargement. One patient had a liver biopsy that showed signs "consistent with a drug reaction." Reduction of dosage in one person led to improvement of blood tests of liver function. Resumption of taking Jin Bu Huan by two other patients led to an abrupt return and flaring up of hepatitis.

The authors further reported that the tablets were not typical for Chinese medicines in that they contained a single active ingredient, levotetrahydropalmatine, rather that a botanical mixture, and declared that the compound is also found in two additional genera of plants. The single-component nature, if true, would be a remarkable deviation from usual practice in TCM of mingling a dozen herbs, which is a confounding claim that obviates the validity of safety proven by "millennia of prior usage." Wolf and colleagues (1994) also state that the chemical structure of the levo-tetrahydropalmatine is such as to suggest a toxic mechanism similar to the mechanism of the pyrrolizidine alkaloids.

Another herbal poisoning arose from a toxic species of *Senecio* being mistaken for a harmless plant and used to make an herbal cough medicine. Two infants were given this preparation for several days. One, a two-month-old, was ill for two weeks before being admitted to a hospital, where he died six days later. The second child (a six-month-old) also developed acute liver disease with ascites, portal hypertension, and a pleural effusion. She improved with treatment, but after six months a liver biopsy showed extensive hepatic fibrosis that progressed to cirrhosis over the next six months.

Another case of hepatic veno-occlusive disease was in a 47-year-old nonalcoholic woman who had consumed large quantities of comfrey (a species of *Symphytum*) tea and pills for more than one year. Liver damage was still present at 20 months after the intake of comfrey consumption stopped. This herb has long before been banned by Germany and Canada. Similarly, germander has been banned also in France, where more than 30 cases of liver toxicity associated with germander have been seen (Larrey et al., 1992).

Other plants that can injure the liver are listed in Table 12.1., including some containing pyrrolizidines and others without such constituents. Another not listed by the sources of Table 12.1 is usnic acid, an antibacterial chemical that occurs in lichens of the genus *Usnea.* In a November 2001 Talk Paper from the FDA it was stated the agency had received at least six reports of persons between 20 and 32 years of age developing liver injury or failure after the use of a dietary supplement weight-reduction formula known as LipoKinetix marketed by Syntrax Innovations Inc. (FDA, 2001).

The product contained not only sodium usneate, a salt of usnic acid,[1] but also four other components: norephedrine or phenylpropanolamine (PPA), caffeine, yohimbine, and diiodothyronine. The Talk Paper was a warning to consumers not to use LipoKinetix, which claimed to cause an increased rate

TABLE 12.1. Botanical materials known or suspected of having hepatotoxic action or possible carcinogenicity to the liver.

Containing pyrrolizidine alkaloids	Not containing pyrrolizidine alkaloids
Borage *(Borago officinalis)*	Deathcap mushroom (*Amanita phalloides* and related spp.)
Paraguay tea (maté) *(Ilex paraguayensis)*	Locoweed (*Astragalus* spp.)
Heliotrope *(Heliotropium europium)*	Indian tobacco/cardinal flower (*Lobelia* spp.)
Rattlebox[a] *(Crotalaria ssp)*	Fo-Ti *(Polygonum multiflorum)*
Chaparral (or creosote bush) *(Larrea tridenta)*	Jin Bu Huan[a] *(Lycopodium serratum)*
Life root, ragwort *(Senecio spp.)*	Paeonia spp.[a] (*P. suffructicosa, P. lactiflora* [others?])
Comfrey *(Symphytum spp.)*	Ma huang[a] (*Ephedra* spp.)
Germander *(Teucrium chamaedrys)*	Oak tree (*Quercus* spp.)
Colt's foot *(Tussalaga farfara)*	Rue *(Ruta graveolens)*
	Periwinkle (*Vinca rosea* [now *Catharanthus roseus*])
	Cockleburr *(Xanthium strumarium)*
	Mistletoe[a] *(Viscum album)*
	Pennyroyal[a] (*Mentha pulegium* [and *Hedeoma pulegoides*])
	Sassafras[a] *(Sassafras albidum)*
	Skullcap or Scullcap[a] *(Scutellaria spp.)*
	Valerian *(Valeriana officinalis)*

Source: Fetrow and Avila (1999), pp. 838-843.

[a]From Stickel et al. (2000).

of metabolism to burn off excess fat. This followed an April 2001 seven-patient case series (Favreau et al., 2002) published from a Los Angeles hospital affiliated with UCLA and from the FDA on severe hepatotoxicity seen in users of LipoKinetix.

None of the persons had been taking Rx or OTC medicines, but four were taking other dietary supplements. All were negative for hepatitis viruses A,

B, and C, as well as two other significant viruses, and for autoimmune disease. Symptoms in all cases appeared within four weeks of beginning to take LipoKinetix.

Case Report 3: Kava Comes Under Suspicion

A 50-year-old man presented to his Swiss physician having noticed jaundice appearing over the prior month along with fatigue and dark urine. He had no remarkable medical history except for a slight anxiety. He had not consumed alcohol or taken any drugs, but he had been taking three to four capsules of kava for the anxiety daily for two months. The maximum recommended dose was three capsules. A liver function test showed a 60-fold and 70-fold increase in plasma levels of two liver enzymes, aspartate and alanine transaminases, respectively, which reflected serious liver injury. Other clinical chemistry values also were elevated, but only slight enlargement of the liver was detected and no accumulation of ascites fluid in the abdominal cavity. Blood tests were negative for hepatitis A, B, C, and E plus HIV, EB virus, and cytomegalovirus. The patient's clinical condition deteriorated over the next 48 hours, with an advanced-stage encephalopathy. His test for blood clotting was very impaired. Fortunately, he was able to receive a liver transplant two days later, and he recovered uneventfully. Microscopic characterization of the liver pathology was consistent with a hepatotoxic action of the kava (Escher et al., 2001; Humberston et al., 2003).

The FDA responded (with snail-like speed) to this January 2001 report, among several from Europe that associated liver failure with use of kava, by sending in spring 2002 a "Dear Doctor" to U.S. physicians alerting them to possible events of this sort in users of kava. It also called for any such events to be reported directly to the FDA. Also, on March 25, 2002, the FDA issued a consumer advisory titled "Kava-Containing Dietary Supplements May Be Associated with Severe Liver Injury" was posted on the FDA Web site (FDA, 2002). The site displayed 21 alternate names by which kava might be seen on supplement labels as well as a statement saying that the "FDA will continue to investigate the relationship, if any, between the use of dietary supplements containing kava and liver injury."

The relative "promptness" of this action may have reflected some impact of the extremely poor, *decade-long* failure to take note of the Chinese herbal nephropathy disaster in Europe (Chapter 29). France followed Switzerland in banning kava products. Germany planned to do the same, and a voluntary recall had just been completed in Britain. A European Union–wide ban was being considered by the EU's pharmaceutical regulatory committee. At least thirty European cases of hepatitis, with four of them requiring liver transplantations and one death attributed to kava products, were insufficient grounds for FDA action. In January 2002 Health Canada issued an advisory, followed by a ban in August 2002, on the sale of herbal kava. At one month after the advisory 67 percent of 33 Canadian health food stores visited were still selling kava. Two months after the ban, 57 percent of 30 stores continued to sell kava (Mills et al., 2003). These data indicate that health food stores may not be well-informed about the sale of restricted natural products.

Case Report 4: Fatal Use of Pennyroyal in a Futile Abortion Attempt

An 18-year-old young woman came to a hospital emergency department with abdominal pain, nausea, vomiting, and a state of consciousness varying between agitation and lethargy. She admitted having taken two half-ounce bottles of oil of pennyroyal two hours before with intent to terminate a suspected pregnancy (Sullivan et al., 1979). Her state of depression suggested that she may have intended suicide. She had previously on many occasions drunk tea made from pennyroyal leaves to induce menstruation. At admission her vital signs were: blood pressure, 120/60; pulse rate, 80 beats per minute; respiratory rate, 24 breaths per minute; and body temperature, 37°. Physical signs were normal except for abdominal tenderness and a generalized rash that receded while she remained in the emergency room. Vomited material was strongly positive for blood, and her pregnancy test was negative. She was admitted to intensive care for monitoring and supportive care. Admission laboratory studies showed no remarkable findings except for metabolic acidosis.

During the next 24 hours she had continued abdominal pain and blood-tinged vomit. At about 40 hours she began to show signs of disseminated vascular coagulation resulting in a prolonged clotting time from depletion of her prothrombin clotting factor. This led to excessive bleeding at venipuncture sites, nosebleed, vaginal bleeding, and ocular hemorrhages. Her liver was tender to abdominal palpation and enlarged. Laboratory values showed deterioration of hepatic and renal function, and bleeding despite repeated administration of plasma and platelets. At 64 hours on the third day after the ingestion plasma levels of enzymes indicated severe liver injury, while clotting time and platelet level were distinctly abnormal. That evening she became unresponsive and required intubation for assisted ventilation for failing respiration while showing bilateral lung infiltration on chest X-ray. At 80 hours post-ingestion the liver measures began to improve, but renal function continued to deteriorate. On the fifth day she experienced cardiopulmonary arrest with a successful resuscitation. She died after a second arrest 48 hours later on the seventh day. Postmortem findings included widespread petechial hemorrhages in multiple organs, pale and enlarged kidneys, 4.5 liters of blood in the peritoneal cavity, plus massive necrosis and a small laceration of the liver (Sullivan et al., 1979).

CONCLUSION

Consumers need to remember that the liver is just as much a vital organ as the heart; the difference is that a person dies more quickly when the heart fails than when the liver fails. Lifestyle factors can aid in keeping both organs in good health. Sources of hepatitis must be avoided if possible. Unfortunately, the danger can be lurking nearby while being unrecognizable.

Witness to this is the fall 2003 outbreak of about 600 cases of viral hepatitis A in Pennsylvania (later also Georgia, Tennessee, and North Carolina) that were traced to eating meals at a particular restaurant. Public health sleuthing by the CDC (Centers for Disease Control) followed a trail that led to a conclusion that green onions (scallions), apparently imported from Mexico, were the source of the viral infection. This type of hepatitis arises through oral ingestion of food or water subject to fecal contamination. The chopped green onions were incorporated into salsa and a variety of dishes on the menu.

Not only did four people die, but the business also expired, a victim of food contamination that likely occurred long before the onions entered its doors. The FDA banned imports from four scallion growers after identifying them as a possible source for the hepatitis A outbreak. Mexico has 22 other producers of green onions whose exports are not affected. On November 25, 2003, Mexico announced its closure of those four growers along with a plan to conduct more intensive inspections intended to restore consumer confidence in the country's produce. Strawberries are another crop that has been associated with a hepatitis A problem.

Hepatitis does not always kill rapidly, nor is it caused only by viral infection. In the case of alcoholic liver toxicity, the process is slow and insidious, but also capable of leading to irreversible loss of liver function and death. Just as what we eat can affect our state of heart health, so also through diet or dietary supplements we can ensure that we attain a lower risk for liver problems. Avoiding toxic levels of beverage alcohol is an especially obvious step in a healthful direction. Avoiding exposure to natural poisons is another, e.g., toxic mushrooms and the potentially hepatotoxic herbals/botanicals described in this chapter. In either an occupational or a household context we should avoid frequent or continual exposure to possibly hepatotoxic chemicals—e.g., inhaled vapor of volatile hydrocarbons used as cleaning fluids or degreasing agents, exemplified by hexane, toluene, or xylene. Sometimes these occur in the laundry room as household products. If one is unable to avoid or is unwilling to abstain from contact with a potentially hepatotoxic agent, such as alcohol, it might be justifiable to use the dietary supplements described in this chapter for their possible protective actions. Sometime in the future adequate clinical data may be available to confirm their clinical value, but most of us cannot wait until then. Nutrient supplements, SAMe, NAC, and alpha-lipoic acid have much to commend their use in this fashion, with seemingly their cost as the sole negative factor if the buyer really receives what he or she intends to purchase.

Chapter 13

Hormonal Supplements: Fountain of Youth Formulas?

BASIC CONCEPTS

Despite the failure of scientific and medical research in the United States yet to provide a clear answer to the problem of senescence (aging), it is said that

> the retention of youth, the preservation of beauty, and the defiance of death are a billion-dollar industry. Their bases are a curious mixture of science and nostrums, the latter no more effective than those peddled for centuries off the backs of carts in village squares . . . The triumphs and the promise of biomedical research have raised huge expectations about the ultimate goal: longer, healthful human lives. (Bunk, 2002)

Clearly, dietary supplements are prominent among the methods of youth-pursuit alluded to in Bunk's quote. They are not the only product in which people put hope for achieving such goals, but they are indeed a major aspect. Antiaging goals are pursued also by mainline medicine via the practice of cosmetic surgery and by clinics existing to supply prescription drugs for weight reduction or to provide liposuction to remove the infamous love handles or cellulite deposits. More recently we see cosmetic medics providing injections of the muscle paralyzant drug Botox, based on the botulinus bacterial toxin, in order to hide signs of aging by smoothing forehead wrinkles and crow's-feet at the eye corners. Most recently a "cosmetic medicine" has become available that employs drugs injected under the skin to mobilize and drive out subcutaneous depots of excess fat!

Even before the New World explorer Ponce de Leon allegedly searched for the fountain of youth,[1] hoping to find it in Florida, humans have desired and sought a longer life and a better health for old age. The Hebrew Bible

Consumer's Guide to Dietary Supplements and Alternative Medicines

doi:10.1300/5698_13

recounts how in ages past a much greater longevity and, apparently, better health and quality of life in old age existed. It is recorded that Moses was taken up to his God Jehovah being "a hundred and twenty years old when he died, yet his eyes were not weak nor his strength gone" (Deuteronomy 34:7, New International version). Many today would wish for that condition at merely 70 years! Life expectancy in the United States as of 2001 had risen to 77.2 years (74.4 for men and 79.8 years for women) for all races, an increase of about 26 years since 1900. Declines in mortality were apparent among most racial, ethnic, and gender groups. Although life span has risen in the Western world across the twentieth century, the quality of life and the level of health enjoyed by persons in advanced age brackets have left much room for improvement.

What Is Normal About "Normal Aging"?

What is widely described as "normal aging" is a concept about which researchers do not agree especially as to whether it should be seen as a pathological or physiological process. Aging often results in diminished cognitive ability; decreased muscle mass, bone mineral content, lung capacity, and sexual function; and a reduction of the ability for the immune system to resist infection or cancer. A growing tendency is to think of aging as a biologically programmed fact of life that cannot be avoided, and thus should not be regarded as pathological. However, other evidences on the nature of aging focus on the existence of slowly progressive, accumulative injuries at the cellular and subcellular levels, which comprise the basis for most changes that characterize aging. Even the concept of a programmed, clocklike determination of a "normal" life span (e.g., that any higher organism has a certain inherent "quota of heartbeats") does not necessarily imply an occurrence of the multiple physical deficits that are commonly encountered in old age.

However, enough rather healthy centenarians are alive today to justify a view that "normal" for an aged person could—perhaps should—be for one to retain both mental and physical functions with minimal impairment into their eighties and nineties, or even past 100 years for some. It is tempting to view this as a luck-of-the-draw situation, that some people have genes inherited at conception that make them well suited both to longevity and to good health into old age. In contrast, others may receive an unfortunate array of genetic traits that are inconsistent with longevity. A concept of this sort has inspired contemporary efforts to locate and identify a "controller gene" serving as a physiological programmer to determine such outcomes.

Many time-related diseases become more likely to occur as age increases that can and must and be differentiated from the aging process. A rather popular idea is that an accumulation of "genetic injuries" causes misreading of the person's genetic information. This leads to the biochemical changes that eventually become incompatible with health and life. A more recent view is that the DNA that matters most in this regard is not the DNA residing in the nucleus of the cell but rather those DNA molecules that exist in the cellular energy organelles, the mitochondria. Because our mitochondrial DNA is inherited only from our mother, her longevity factors may determine our status.

Insight from an Unnatural Aging Disease

As for many aspects of physiology, we can gain some insight from research on the abnormal condition, in this case, Werner syndrome (WS). Pathology sources tell us that WS is an uncommon, autosomal recessive human genetic disease that mimics premature aging. In other words, a child who inherits the genetic deviation associated with WS is doomed to show very premature changes that we associate with "normal" aging. The person with WS appears to age rapidly after puberty, and has a greatly increased risk of developing cancer and cardiovascular disease. The characteristic signs of WS include premature graying and loss of hair, muscular atrophy, cataracts, osteoporosis, wrinkled skin, a tendency to have atherosclerosis and diabetes, and hardening (scleroderma-like) changes of the skin. The pathological process that begins in adolescence or early adulthood results in the victim having the appearance of old age when they reach 30 or 40 years of age, and their life span is abbreviated. An aberrant gene (named WRN after the syndrome) has been identified as the origin of WS, and a protein that is normally produced in response to the gene also is known. However, the normal function of the protein is uncertain. Thus, the molecular role of WRN in WS remains to be proven, as does the probable role it may have in the normal aging process. Clearly, this a crucial and difficult research area.

ENDOCRINOLOGY AND AGING

A major experimental approach to aging has focused on the endocrine system because of its broad physiological regulatory roles and because of a clear pattern of age-related reduction in its functions. Aging is paralleled by a long-familiar decrease in the production of the gonadal hormones in both women and men. More recently it was recognized that decreases occur in the secretion of various other, less familiar but also vital factors, e.g., an adrenal gland hormone, dehydroepiandrosterone (DHEA), human growth hormone (HGH), and growth factor-1. The principle of hormone replacement therapy to deal with such reductions is an important but uncertain issue facing medicine and the aging population today. Replacement of the gonadal hormones in either sex seems to entail significant risk of adverse consequences (see Chapter 3).

Human Growth Hormone

HGH is produced by the pituitary gland and is necessary in early life for a person to grow to a normal body size. The consequence of a serious early deficit of secretion is known as pituitary dwarfism, whereas an abnormal, excessive release leads to rare cases of giantism. Within the normal range, the period of linear skeletal growth (in height) caused by HGH is normally terminated by an opposing action of the gonadal hormones beginning at puberty. HGH levels begin to decrease gradually after the age of about 30 years.

In the mid-twentieth century growth hormone was extracted from human cadaver pituitary glands by a federal laboratory, and a limited amount was available for physicians in the United States to treat children showing seriously deficient growth. However, this was halted by the discovery that some patients had developed a very rare, fatal, and incurable degenerative brain disorder, Creutzfeld-Jakob disease (CJD). It was realized that one or a few pituitaries had entered the HGH supply from donor(s) unrecognized as having CJD, and thus the causative agent for CJD had been transmitted to recipients of HGH. Fortunately, it was only a short time later that recombinant-HGH became available from production by a genetic engineering technology—in vitro microbial biosynthesis of the hormone by recombinant-DNA methods. Since then a sufficient supply of the recombinant hormone has been available, but it is quite expensive.

Because HGH is a protein, it is available only as a sterile solution to be injected as prescribed by a physician for an FDA-approved purpose—treating serious hormonal deficiencies in adults as well as in children. It is certain that some physicians are also treating wealthy persons who are able to pay dearly to obtain regularly repeated injections of HGH to oppose its normal age-related reduction. This would be a legal off-label (non-FDA-approved) application, but the monthly cost for injections would be more than $1,500 and would not be reimbursed by medical insurance because no legitimate pathologic diagnosis could be truthfully be supplied. Moreover, illicit usage of HGH as a performance enhancer by athletes has occurred, tantamount to blood doping—the administration of whole blood to provide a better oxygen-carrying capacity. This is forbidden by Olympic and other national and international athletics bodies, and efforts to detect and punish such practices continue to grow, often amid controversy, as in the March 2005 Major League Baseball hullabaloo with involvement of the U.S. Congress.

Evidence exists that HGH secretion is reduced in normal elderly persons as well as patients with Alzheimer's disease (AD). Research findings have tended to confirm that the potential benefits of HGH supplementation in older adults are as follows:

- Help retain muscle mass and strength at normal levels
- Reduce the proportion of body fat
- Restore or maintain the sex drive
- Decrease blood cholesterol
- Thicken hair
- Lower blood pressure
- Sharpen vision
- Provide a heightened sense of well-being and vitality

However, adverse effects reported with relatively short-term HGH supplementation include joint pains and carpal tunnel syndrome. From the well-known properties of HGH it may be assumed that its use would carry a increased risk for developing type 2 diabetes. A possible heightened risk of cancer is currently under investigation. Anyone taking HGH needs to do so under the care of a physician for hormonal blood levels to be properly monitored. The long-term effects of any hormone may be more risky than any short-term ones. (To which many elders might respond, "I don't need to worry about long-term effects!") The American Association of Clinical Endocrinologists has issued a warning and recommendation against using growth hormone as an antiaging treatment or to oppose ordinary obesity. However, the doctors who gravitate to "antiaging medicine" in their practices have not endorsed such a cautious statement, which is not surprising.

Alternative Routes to HGH

The expense of HGH, plus its need for injection, opened the door for promoters of "cheaper and easier, but equally effective" oral alternative remedies that sometimes claim even "super-HGH" capacities. The usual supposed source of their activity is a mixture of several amino acids, perhaps with a vitamin such as niacin. Such products are claimed to provide a secretagogue action, which is the scientific term for any agent having the capacity to stimulate greater glandular secretion, in this case of a hormone.

Indeed, research in the past decade has shown that receptors exist in the anterior pituitary gland, the source of human growth hormone, which are called secretagogue receptors. Those receptors have been found to respond to two or more endogenous (naturally occurring) polypeptides, the larger of which consists of a chain of 28 amino acids. A smaller molecule having secretagogue activity seems to be a mere hexapeptide—composed of only six amino acids. One synthetic peptide that serves as an effective secretagogue was found to be only a tetrapeptide, consisting of a precise sequence of merely four amino acids. However, even the activity of this short a peptide would probably be largely destroyed by peptide-digesting enzymes if it were administered by mouth. Be assured that pharmaceutical research is ongoing to find a small, synthetic, nonpeptide molecule that would be orally effective as a secretagogue. A pharmaceutical alternative of this sort would be advantageous for the currently approved uses in place of taking injections of recombinant HGH. One must believe that off-label use of such an agent would soar.

However, although major pharmaceutical industry research teams have yet to find a small nonpeptide secretagogue, various supplement sellers some years ago began to put forth audacious claims they had solved the problem. They declared that a mixture of several individual amino acids, if combined in an oral dosage form with a vitamin or two, can act as a nonpeptide HGH secretagogue. A simple example of this includes only four amino acids: arginine, glycine, lysine, and glutamine. A newer, more elaborate example contains eleven: arginine, glycine, glutamine, ornithine, methionine, valine, tyrosine, taurine, leucine, cysteine, and gamma-aminobutyric acid. This proposition is unvalidated by scientific data published in medical or scientific journals.

Although promotional literature suggests that evidence for HGH secretagogue action is "out there somewhere," no citations of where or whether they were published are given, or if such supposed findings are from merely animal or also human research. Lacking any substantiation of the claims for their activity, these oral remedies cannot be taken very seriously. Products based on this premise appear likely to be a total waste of the serious amount of money ($100 per month) that they cost for continuous therapy. In such circumstances, one might rightly say, "I wish that it were true, but wishing won't make it so!" Despite actions by the FTC and the Department of Consumer Affairs of New York City against some companies marketing products with misleading or false claims as releasers of HGH, no slowing of the promotion of such products is evident.

GONADAL HORMONE REPLACEMENT THERAPIES FOR WOMEN

Therapeutic use of ovarian hormone replacement therapy (HRT) during and for months or years after menopause has been practiced in the United States for decades despite the lack of a complete consensus among medical authorities that it is safe and desirable. Besides the physical benefits attributed to estrogen supplementation, in recent times researchers began to report evidence that women might be at lower risk for age-related benign memory impairment or even Alzheimer's disease because of estrogenic action. However, after nearly a half-century of this practice, it was not uniformly agreed that HRT had a sufficient benefit-to-risk ratio. Furthermore, advocacy by some medical authorities of lifelong postmenopausal estrogen supplementation was even more controversial. However, the revelations concerning estrogenic hormone replacement in 2002 must have stopped the tongues of all such advocates. For many years HRT was nearly synonymous with the prescribing of Premarin, despite other applicable products being available. Environmental and animal abuse concerns have arisen against this industry that requires large herds of horses to be kept in western Canada solely to obtain the pregnant mare urine from which the equine estrogens of Premarin are extracted.

The recognition of a heightened risk for uterine cancer with chronic postmenopausal estrogen HRT, when not counterbalanced by cyclic progesterone secretion, led to a modified approach. Except for women whose uterus had already been surgically removed, the standard treatment became the newer product, Prempro, consisting of Premarin combined with a synthetic derivative of progesterone. However, these products were hard-hit by the results from several large randomized controlled trials of such therapies announced in mid-2002, as was discussed in Chapter 3.

"Natural medicine" practice has turned away from the natural but *equine* hormones to support a bioidentical hormone mix. The phrase *bioidentical hormones* refers to use of the normal *human* steroids estradiol, estriol, estrone, progesterone, and testosterone rather than Premarin or Prempro-based HRT or plant-derived hormones (phytoestrogens). A contention exists that the bioidentical therapy is better tolerated and safer than equine or synthetic gonadal steroids and without a risk for favoring breast cancer. However, the limited relevant clinical findings are equivocal and insufficient to clearly support the argument that bioidentical is better. Validation of the concept would require a very large and expensive research project, which seems unlikely to occur. Such preparations must be obtained from compounding pharmacies or through dispensing clinics and physicians who deal with such outlets.

Another hormonal replacement approach of recent times is for supplementing the endogenous secretion from the adrenal cortex of a compound that can be converted to both androgenic and estrogenic products, serving as a precursor. This compound, DHEA, has been reported to have favorable effects for older women (Yaroch, 2001) as well as for men.

A widespread view that using a natural phytoestrogen (plant-derived) is somehow preferable and advantageous over estrogens prescribed in pharmaceutical form exists. A review paper (Whitten and Patisaul, 2001) evaluated the status of both in vitro and in vivo (animal and human) research concerning the phytoestrogens. Receptor binding studies show that the soy isoflavonoids react with a high affinity for estrogen receptors, especially ERB (estrogen receptor beta). However, they have less potency in whole-cell assays and also in the whole animal situation, presumably because of their interactions with other proteins. In vivo results show that phytoestrogens exert a broad range of biologic actions at doses and plasma levels that can result from normal human diets containing phytoestrogens.

Significant in vivo responses have been found in animal and human tests showing that phytoestrogens affect bone, breast, ovary, pituitary, blood-vessels, prostate, and serum lipids. Whitten and Patisaul (2001) tentatively concluded that phytoestrogens exert a significant inhibitory effects on steroid hormone production and on brain functions, specifically on the inhibitory feedback system known as the hypothalamus-pituitary-ovary axis. Inferences of the reviewers were tentative because of the inadequate knowledge regarding the dose-response relationships for many physiological end points. The multiplicity and degree of uncertainties were seen to make the phytoestrogens an unsuitable alternative to HRT-employing pharmaceutical estrogens, because the latter have a track record of nearly half a century of medical use and study. Moreover, that there is so high a level of concern about safety and benefits of pharmaceutical HRT should indicate that a favorable majority consensus on the desirability and safety of sustained usage of phytoestrogens hardly exists. Surely a dearth of sound data from clinical trials is apparent for phytoestrogens in comparison to pharmaceutical HRT trials.

ANDROGEN REPLACEMENT FOR MEN

The latter twentieth century saw an increasing but hardly universal acceptance of the idea that men experience an analogue to women's menopause—an androgen deficit state called "andropause." This is different from a state of testicular malfunction developing earlier than andropause (in a person's fifties or sixties) known as hypogonadism. For hypogonadism the FDA has approved topically applied testosterone in the form of a patch or gel. To the surprise of only terminally naive persons, physicians have come under pressure from their aging male patients to prescribe such testosterone products for "andropausal complaints."

In November 2003 a committee of the Institute of Medicine of the National Academies (United States) concluded a one-year review of existing research on testosterone replacement therapy (TRT). Their report described finding only 31 trials that focused on older men, and most involved less than 50 subjects, with durations of all but one being less than one year. Moreover, many were not done on a placebo-controlled basis. In light of the rapidly growing use of testosterone products, the committee declared that the risks and benefits of TRT have not been adequately tested, especially in older men. Furthermore, because some studies have indicated that TRT may increase the risk of prostate cancer, especially for men who are already in a high-risk group, the committee called for doctors to immediately take greater care in prescribing TRT. They did not support the idea of a massive study of testosterone for benefits and risks because such a trial should begin with an ability to tell men what benefits might be expected. The committee advised the National Institute of Aging rather to begin smaller trials in older men having sexual dysfunction or depression. In addition, the committee called for careful planning of any future trials in order to enable assessment of whether TRT does indeed increase the risk for prostate cancer in older men. This will require testing that excludes participants who are already at high risk for prostate cancer (Liverman and Blazer, 2004).

What mainline medicine denies or resists, a dietary supplement producer surely will see fit to provide. Thus, we find many products, at a more affordable price than those previously cited, that are claimed to act as either androgen precursor—a proandrogen—or a testosterone secretagogue. These have been touted as the answer to any perceived lessening of masculine features or actions, and they do not require the user to obtain a prescription from a physician. Although the major focus is on retaining or recovering sexual vigor, other major benefits would be to oppose a loss of muscle mass (along with an increase of fat), and a lowering of strength, energy, and sense of well-being.

The weakly androgen precursors known as andros can undergo (to a variable degree) chemical transformation to form the normal active male hormone, testosterone. The andros include 4-androstenediol (made famous by Mark McGwire of major league baseball), 5-alpha-androstenediol, 19-nor-4-androstenediol, and 1-androstenedione. Early in March 2004 the head of Health and Human Services announced that FDA was banning further distribution for androstendiol as a dietary supplement, which seemingly targeted only the first of the four compounds without explicitly indicating the action would apply equally to the others. However, the position of the FDA in mid-2004 was to shift the problem by passing off the whole lot of anabolics or anabolic precursors to the Drug Enforcement Administration for their warranting classification as scheduled drugs similar to Rx anabolic agents and androgens.

Without a physician being involved so as to provide monitoring of blood testosterone levels following self-medication with the andros, a person is flying blind. Many younger men are doing just that for the pursuit of bodybuilding. Excessive amounts of either testosterone or synthetic anabolic-androgenic molecules are believed to increase the risk for cancer of the liver, prostate, or breast (yes, a risk for men too), as well as the likely early onset of symptoms of benign prostatic hyperplasia (prostatism). These risks should be the greater for an earlier point in life that extra androgen exposure begins. Thus, warnings that health risks for men using androgenic hormones (or pro-hormones) outweigh their benefits are especially true for men who begin using hormonal supplements before 50 years of age. Conversely, initial use at or after age 65 should be of lesser concern. This issue, as for analogous risks of estrogenic HRT for women, has a direct bearing also on the later discussion of DHEA.

Regardless of the many physical aspects of aging that may respond to an androgenic hormone, especially interesting is a possible action to aid men in their retention of brain functions supporting cognition. In actuality, an opposition to memory deficits is thought to be mediated by estrogenic metabolites of the testosterone, i.e., estrogen is important for aspects of memory in aging men, just as it is said to be for women. Laboratory research showed that the replacement of testosterone restored impaired cognitive functions in aging mice. Moreover, intact older dogs were significantly less likely than same-age castrated dogs to develop severe cognitive impairment. One might wonder how soon we will see a veterinary product for companion animals titled "DHEA for Your Dog" (and Cats?) to reduce the risk for their loss of cognitive well-being. Moreover, it already has been seen that older men who undergo androgen replacement often report improvement in their memory. (Conclusion: "Old dogs" are indeed unlikely to learn "new tricks" since they tend to lose some of their "old tricks.")

DHEA

DHEA (prasterone) is a normal steroid hormone that is secreted by the gonads and adrenal cortex of both sexes. It also is found abundantly in the brain, being at least partly produced there from a precursor, pregnenolone (Zwain and Yen, 1999). The output of DHEA begins to decline as soon as people reach their late twenties and continues a long slump downward to merely 5 to 10 percent of its peak level by the age of 80 years. Many speculations exist as to the impact of this decline; it is easy to suppose that it might contribute to many age-related losses in physiological competence. As a consequence it has been proposed that replacement therapy is appropriate to reduce or reverse such deficits as may result from its decline with age. Oral administration of supplemental DHEA has been associated with various supposed antiaging benefits.

Many promoters outside of mainline medicine have arisen for replacement therapy with DHEA, which has been promoted openly as the "fountain of youth hormone." Indeed, it seems to be a mainstay of the physician members of "A4M"—the Association for Anti-Aging Medicine. The following are the generally well-accepted facts about DHEA:

- It is a normal constituent of the human body, secreted by the adrenal cortex.
- It is the most abundant steroid in the blood.
- It is present at even higher levels in brain tissue.
- It is a precursor to the sex steroid hormones (both estrogen and androgen).
- It shows an age-related lowering of secretion, falling 90 percent from ages 20 to 90 years.
- The trend downward is correlated with the various unwanted changes of aging (but correlation never proves causation).
- Data suggest that its use opposes or reduces age-dependent changes.

Aging-Related Conditions That DHEA Supposedly May Overcome

Conditions that might be helped by DHEA include the following:

- Andropause (decline of male gonadal hormone and libido, plus other features below)
- Chronic fatigue
- Depression
- Decline in memory
- Decline in muscle strength and reduced lean body mass
- Decreased immune function
- Difficulties of sleep

Further suggestions have been made that DHEA can oppose depression and reduce suicide among seniors. Some scientists believe the decline of DHEA secretion may be partly responsible for increased rates of depression with aging. Moreover, a number of studies point to an association in early adulthood between low levels of DHEA and occurrence of postpartum depression or anorexia nervosa.

That DHEA tends to be metabolized in the body to both testosterone and an estrogen could support the benefits reported upon taking of DHEA by persons suffering depression, since both sex hormones are linked to mood. Although doses of estrogen and testosterone may indeed benefit many people in certain circumstances, the practice is regarded as carrying a potential for increasing their risk for cancer. This is most true for persons who are genetically susceptible to some hormone-sensitive malignancies such as cancer of the breast, cervix, uterus, or prostate. Moreover, the possibility of increased risk for liver cancer with long-term exposure arises from an association between liver cancer and medical use of some semisynthetic androgens.

When taken in supratherapeutic doses, either the natural androgen, testosterone, or synthetic pharmaceutical anabolic-androgenic steroids may tend to increase violent, aggressive behavior. Moreover, they carry a risk for such serious mood changes as mania and/or depression to the point of psychosis (Markowitz et al., 1999). These effects have been reported to result in even homicidal behavior among nonmedical users of androgenic steroids by bodybuilders. Such incidents support the view that androgens can in some unknown fraction of users provoke brain activation leading to paranoia and violence (including homicide or suicide). Clearly, these inferences are not based on scientifically validated clinical research. Because of ethical and federal human research safety considerations, research proposals could not gain approval to be performed if they involved those excessive levels of steroids to which many bodybuilders or other users of andros eagerly (and often ignorantly) subject themselves. It is currently impossible to separate the degree of contributions to behavioral dysfunction in steroid abusers between their particular brain chemistry and the intrinsic effects of the steroids on the brain. Whether one can so overuse DHEA or andros as to provoke the same disastrous outcomes that occur after misuse of the pharmaceutical androgenic steroids is unknown.

MELATONIN

Melatonin is a normal hormonal secretion of the human pineal gland, which lies at the base of the brain above the soft palate. It has actions analogous to those of some of the major brain neurotransmitters, and it is chemically related to one of them, serotonin, from which it is synthesized by pineal cells. It has captured much attention since the 1980s because of its reportedly favorable effects on mood and sleep. In the latter case it has been promoted for overcoming jet lag as well as for general insomnia. It has also been proclaimed that melatonin stimulates the immune system and exerts antioxidant, anticancer, and antiaging activities. Because melatonin occurs naturally in plants and some foods, it can be sold as a dietary supplement without review or approval from the FDA. In contrast to the situation in the United States, only prescription sales of it are permitted in Great Britain and Germany. European melatonin has a quite different status because it is classified (correctly) as a neurohormone, which causes it to have Rx status. Although it is indeed a natural substance, it is more cheaply available from synthesis than by extraction from an animal or vegetable source.

More research, both animal and human has probably been done on melatonin than on all but a few other supplement items that are neither vitamins nor minerals, yet many uncertainties about its useful applications and its long-term safety exist. One question was raised about safety because of results of a mouse study suggesting that particular caution is needed regarding high melatonin intake by hypercholesterolemic patients (Tailleux et al., 2002). The researchers found that feeding of an atherogenic diet supplemented with melatonin to hypercholesterolemic mice led to high increases in the level of development of atherosclerotic lesions in the proximal aorta of the mice. Data suggested that a higher degree of LDL (low-density lipoprotein)-cholesterol oxidation was one reason for the difference.

The FDA has approved melatonin as an orphan drug for only one purpose: treating a rare clinical sleep disorder of some blind persons. Concern among scientists and public health workers over the discrepancy between the wide public use of melatonin and the paucity of evidence for its health benefits or its safety led to the convening of a workshop by the NIH in 1996. The conferees' general conclusion was that no evidence existed that use of melatonin has caused a medical catastrophe, but neither do adequate data exist on either its long-term safety or efficacy or its long-term benefits (Arendt, 1997). It may have short-term benefit for insomniacs or travelers crossing several time zones and thus developing jet lag. However, even this claim is subject to dispute.

Researchers looking for a way to make night shifts more bearable for residents in emergency medicine did a randomized crossover trial of melatonin as an aid to daytime sleeping, but they found melatonin to be ineffective (Jockovich et al., 2000). It had no more effect than did a placebo on sleep duration, sleep efficiency, mood disturbance, and nighttime sleepiness. This was the fourth trial of melatonin for people working shifts in hospital emergency departments, and all showed negative or equivocal results. Moreover, it is reported at times to cause side effects of gynecomastia (breast enlargement in men, but not in women), or seizures in children having a preexisting neurologic disease.

Melatonin may have a coordinating role in gonadal function for humans, but if so it is still poorly defined. Melatonin has a more certain role in the regulation of body rhythms, i.e., in sleep and body temperature (Sack et al., 1998). Indeed, its effectiveness as a sleep aid may occur because of its action to lower the core body temperature, which is a normal aspect of the onset of sleep, in a dose-related manner (Satoh and Mishima, 2001). A few observations suggest an abnormal pattern of secretion of melatonin in patients showing sleep or mood disorders. In one small study 20 patients with primary insomnia had significantly lower levels of serum melatonin than did an equal number of normal subjects. Some patients with depression have a less-than-expected rise of serum melatonin at night, but supplemental melatonin did not improve their mood.

Persons with chronic alcohol dependence undergoing withdrawal have also been found to show a low nocturnal serum melatonin level. Despite this apparent deficiency, which might contribute to their disrupted sleep in withdrawal, no significant improvement in sleep quality upon melatonin supplementation occurred. Melatonin is widely available, usually as tablets containing 3 to 10 mg to be taken once daily. However, the tablets are reported to show such wide variations in their bioavailability that the response to a given dose is likely to be delayed past the time needed for real benefit as a sleep aid. Variations in melatonin metabolism among persons may be another reason for the mixed findings in clinical response (Di et al., 1997). Cause exists to wonder whether all sources on the market are truly supplying the labeled content of melatonin per serving (Chapter 10).

Despite these uncertainties about the reliability and safety of melatonin even for its *short*-term use, persons still promote its *long*-term use as a cancer protective agent. This belief apparently is derived from very limited animal research data. Some sketchy preliminary results suggest that melatonin may help patients who already have cancer. The rationalization mainly given for such an application is that melatonin has antioxidant activity, but this is a weak argument.

Studies suggest that for most healthy people (at least men) levels of melatonin in their plasma probably do not decline with aging (Zeitzer et al., 1999). Scant evidence exists that a deficiency in melatonin secretion causes any illness. Hence, little support can be found for the conclusion that using melatonin as a replacement therapy would improve health. Correction of a doubtful or nonexistent deficit certainly may not be expected to provide a significant health benefit or an increase in lifespan.

Melatonin for Hypertension?

Neuroscientists at the division of sleep medicine at Brigham and Women's Hospital and Harvard Medical School evaluated the effect of melatonin after a single dose and after a longer treatment period of three weeks on blood pressure (Scheer et al., 2004). They gave 16 men having untreated essential hypertension (high blood pressure with no known cause) either a placebo or 2.5 mg of melatonin orally one hour before they went to sleep. Then they compared the effect of the three-week treatment to the response after melatonin taken once. The researchers found that patients taking melatonin repeatedly showed lower nighttime systolic blood pressure (the higher number in a blood pressure reading) by 6 mm Hg (millimeters of mercury) and lower diastolic blood pressure (lower number) by 4 mm Hg. One dose of melatonin showed no effect on blood pressure. Scheer and colleagues (2004) conclude that repeated but not single doses of melatonin before bedtime had a significant action to reduce blood pressure during sleep in male patients with untreated essential hypertension. Melatonin taken at night may be a gentle alternative or a complementary approach to the use of regular antihypertensive medicines.

Patients taking melatonin for other purposes also reported an improvement in their sleeping. This small study suggests that melatonin's ability to help regulate the body's biological clock might be responsible for its effect on blood pressure, because the biological clock may be a factor determining blood pressure or influencing its regulation. However, the researchers acknowledged that an improved sleep over three weeks might have helped to reduce blood pressure.

CONCLUSIONS

Although a decade has passed since the following conclusion was reached concerning melatonin, it probably is as valid now as then: "Melatonin is potentially useful but its safety and efficacy remain uncertain" (Lamberg, 1996).

The controversial nature of antiaging science and medicine was discussed in article published in the journal of the American Association for the Advancement of Science, *Science,* on February 8, 2003 (Juengst et al., 2003). A subsequent letter commenting on the topic came from seven active researchers in the field. The letter was devoted to emphasizing "that there are currently no scientifically proven antiaging medicines, but that legitimate and important scientific efforts are underway to develop them." Moreover, they warned against confusing research published in a peer-reviewed

Journal of Anti-Aging Medicine with "pretender" sources purveying "anti-aging quackery" to laypersons. The latter "literature" is likely to mislead the public. Two sources named as being pseudo-journals likely to confuse are the *International Journal of Anti-Aging Medicine* and the *Journal of Longevity.* The views of those seven researchers match those expressed by Taaffe et al. (1994), who were researchers at the VA Medical Center at Palo Alto, California. They stated: "There is no current 'magic-bullet' medication that retards or reverses aging."

Chapter 14

Antioxidant Supplements: Fountain of Youth Formulas?

BASIC SCIENCE

Over the past half-century major advances in physiology and biochemistry have been made through the study of energy metabolism within cells. For the potential energy of foods (carbohydrates, fats, and proteins) to be released in a usable fashion, a virtual burning (what chemists call "oxidation") must occur. This parallels the release of energy from wood or fossil fuels as they are literally burned to heat our houses. Just as the danger of the fire in our fireplace or furnace running wild exists, so does the danger of the release of energy by cells, which occurs at a vital intracellular structure known as the mitochondrion (plural, mitochondria). This power plant of the cell takes the two-carbon atomic units into which more complex carbohydrates or fats have been digested and reacts them with oxygen (O_2) to form carbon dioxide (CO_2) and water (H_2O). Utilizable energy is released and stored chemically in this process. Obviously, this is not done in a literal burning flame, but rather much more subtly through complex enzymatic mechanisms. These accomplish the transfer of electrons and protons between certain macromolecules (very large ones), especially the large enzyme molecules (proteins) that are present for this specific purpose.

A fundamental energized molecule that is generated by the release and transfer of energy is known as ATP, or adenosine triphosphate. Lacking an adequate intrinsic supply of ATP to power its vital functions a cell will soon die. A person will ordinarily die if their air and oxygen supply is cut off for a matter of minutes, as in suffocation or drowning. Cutting off the oxygen supply at the cellular level can be produced by a chemical action that blocks the use of oxygen that is available, and can cause death with nearly equal rapidity. Thus, carbon monoxide acts by blocking the ability of the red blood cells to carry oxygen to the cells of the brain and other vital organs. At a more fundamental level, the poison cyanide acts within the cell to prevent

Consumer's Guide to Dietary Supplements and Alternative Medicines

doi:10.1300/5698_14

the enzymatic processes of electron transfer (oxidative metabolism) necessary for generating ATP.

When a cell uses oxygen in the process of converting food into energy, important molecules are generated incidentally that are known as "oxidizing free radicals" or simply "free radicals" (also commonly known as reactive oxygen species or ROS; see Table 14.1). When produced at other proper places and times and in normal amounts, free radicals may serve a useful purpose, i.e., when released by immune cells as weapons to kill harmful microbes. However, when produced in greater amounts than can be kept under tight control, even as a side-aspect of energy metabolism, free radicals can damage the body's cellular machinery. They can cause injury or death to cells and damage to the function of tissues or organs. This adverse impact of oxidizing free radicals is often called *oxidative stress.* Certain vitamins, many other plant components, and some endogenous, normal biochemicals (e.g., urea, glutathione) serve a defensive function against free radicals so as to prevent their damaging effects, and thus they are known as antioxidants (Table 14.1).

The danger in the energy release reaction arises because the process of electron transfer regularly fails to keep all the electrons in the safe places where they belong. When some, to a small degree, "get loose" they are prone to react with O_2 molecules. The resulting product, superoxide, has been called "a molecular loose cannon" because of the bad consequences it can produce. Enough superoxide loose within a cell can cause irreversible damage, foremost because of lipid peroxidation that injures the mitochon-

TABLE 14.1. Major reactive oxygen species (ROS) mediating oxidative stress.

Free radicals[a]	**Nonradical active-oxygen species**
Hydroxyl radical (HO·)	Hydrogen peroxide (H_2O_2)
Superoxide radical (O2·)	Singlet oxygen ($^1O_2$)
Peroxyl radical[b] (ROO·)	
Alkoxyl radical (RO·)	

Source: Modified from Conklin (2000).

[a]Free radicals contain an unpaired electron (represented by dot) instead of usual pairs.

[b]Peroxyl and alkoxyl radicals arise from lipid peroxidation of polyunsaturated fatty acids and thus degrade the properties of fatty acids, as in cell membranes.

drial membranes. This reduces the ability of mitochondria to produce ATP and can bring cell death. In addition, oxidative damage of macromolecules—not only vital proteins but also nucleic acid molecules of the DNA and RNA within cells—can occur. If superoxide originates "on the loose" (outside the cell) by any process, it can cause the same sort of damage to lipoproteins of the external cell membrane and the breakdown of that membrane, which quickly causes cell death. The biological solution is to have a specific "antidote" of sorts to superoxide. This consists of an enzyme, superoxide dismutase, which is devoted specifically to changing and breaking down superoxide so as to neutralize is injurious potential.

How Cells Are Defended Against Oxidative Stress

Cells have several protective mechanisms for handling the hazards of ROS. It is only when these mechanisms are overwhelmed that oxidative stress occurs. A major means of defense is the enzyme known as superoxide dismutase (SOD) that changes superoxide to a less dangerous substance, hydrogen peroxide (H_2O_2) (yes, it's the same chemical likely to be present in your household!). Another enzyme, catalase, can convert hydrogen peroxide to harmless water molecules. However, if that is not accomplished quickly enough, a hydrogen peroxide molecule may instead capture free electrons and form two hydroxyl radicals, which are the most toxic form of ROS. If the defense mechanisms work correctly, the radicals will be captured and neutralized (scavenged) by antioxidant vitamins or by an internal scavenger, or antidotal molecule, glutathione. If the supply of either glutathione or dietary antioxidant vitamins or the enzymes SOD and catalase should be inadequate, susceptibility to oxidative injury exists.

A major reason for chronic alcoholism accelerating the aging of tissues and organs is thought to be that metabolism of alcohol generates extra amounts of superoxide. Moreover, alcohol-induced superoxide injury to the liver eventually will aggravate the danger by reducing the ability of the liver to synthesize enough glutathione.

A prominent theory to explain the physiological downhill slide of aging is that our defenses against oxidative injury become progressively less adequate with advancing age, especially after the fourth or fifth decade of life. An adjunct to this concept is that minor oxidative injuries to DNA tend to accumulate progressively throughout life, and that the cumulative toll of injury to the genetic materials is eventually too great for it to be counteracted. Then the oxidative stress becomes increasingly and progressively more responsible for continuing deterioration of the functions of various organs.

The positions outlined comprise the theoretical basis for a great many of the botanical and biochemical supplements being promoted for use in avoiding or opposing a variety of illnesses, especially cancer. Examples are listed in Exhibit 14.1. Proof for these ideas is very elusive, and the evidence favorable to them is either from animal experiments or is indirect, i.e., arising from epidemiologic correlations, which can never supply a proof.

Can Antioxidants Indeed Prolong Life Span?

Experiments published in *Science* by Melov et al. (2000) described some basic animal research attempting to answer this vital question in a much-studied, small, wormlike creature *(Caenorhabditis elegans).* This species has served as a model for research on longevity factors. In this case researchers tested whether synthetic substitutes for the enzymes superoxide dismutase and catalase could influence the life span of treated worms compared to untreated ones kept under identical conditions. They found that the treated worms had a life span increase of 44 percent. They next tested a mutated laboratory strain of worms that show premature aging and death. Treatment of such worms with the enzyme-mimicking chemicals restored their life span to normal. The authors made a quite significant conclusion: "It appears that oxidative stress is a major determinant of life-span and that it can be counteracted by pharmacological intervention." If this principle applies as far up the biological scale as human beings, and if supplemental antioxidant nutrients can do as the enzyme-mimicking molecules did, then one has an obvious way to pursue a longer life.

ANTIOXIDANTS AND CANCER

Multiple Antioxidant Nutrients

By now the reader will recognize that doing a double-blind placebo-controlled study over enough years to detect changes in rates of cancers would be an extremely difficult and costly undertaking. Thus, we must give much credit to those launching into such a daunting effort and completing it, even though it had imperfections. Indeed, that was done from 1995 for seven years with about 13,000 participants by the French Institute of Health and Medical Research, which designed the study called SU.VI.MAX (an acronym for Supplémentation en Vitamines et Minéraux Antioxydants) (Hercberg et al., 1999). It had the goal of evaluating the effectiveness of nutrition, especially of antioxidants, in preventing cancer and/or cardiovas-

EXHIBIT 14.1. Activities of antioxidant supplements relevant to cancer therapy.

Vitamins and vitamin-like compounds	
Vitamin C	Water-soluble antioxidant
Vitamin E	Chain-breaking, lipid-soluble antioxidant; inhibitor of protein tyrosine-kinases
Beta-carotene	Lipid-soluble antioxidant
CoenzymeQ10	Lipid-soluble antioxidant, cofactor for electron transport
Amino acids, peptides, and other metabolites	
alpha-Lipoic Acid	Lipid- and water-soluble antioxidant and radical scavenger
N-acetylcysteine	Water-soluble antioxidant, source of cysteine for synthesizing glutathione
Glutamine	Source of glutamate for glutathione synthesis, cellular fuel for intestinal epithelial cells and lymphocytes
Methionine	Necessary to formation of selenomethionine (*see* SELENIUM)
Glutathione	Water-soluble tripeptide radical scavenger antioxidant
Uric acid	Water-soluble nonenzymatic radical scavenger antioxidant
Minerals	
Selenium	Incorporated into selenomethionine and selenoproteins, which are strongly involved in antioxidant mechanisms
Isoflavones	
Genistein	Antioxidant, inhibitor of topoisomerase I and II, inhibitor of protein tyrosine-kinases
Daidzein	Antioxidant
Flavonoids	
Quercetin	Antioxidant, inhibitor of topoisomerase II, inhibitor of protein tyrosine-kinases

Source: Modified from Conklin (2000).

cular disease. Rather than regulating food intake, they devised a daily regimen of nutrients to be supplied via dietary supplements that contained the following:

- Beta-carotene (6 mg)
- Vitamin C (120 mg)
- Vitamin E (30 mg)
- Selenium (100 mcg)
- Zinc (20 mcg).

The trial comprised not a dietary test but rather a test of low dosage supplementation. The Hercberg et al. (1999) emphasized that foods containing antioxidants would do a much better job of delivering antioxidants than do supplements. SU.VI.MAX involved more than 5,000 men (ages 45 to 60) divided into two groups: one to receive the supplementation and the other to receive placebos. More than 7,800 women (ages 35 to 60) also were divided between two similar groups.

After following the subjects for seven and one-half years, men receiving the antioxidants showed a 30 percent lower cancer rate than did the placebo group, and a 37 percent reduction in overall mortality. Nevertheless, it was rather disappointing that no significant difference was found for the group of women receiving supplements. A representative of France's national cancer center attributed the difference between the results for men and women to their having different metabolic profiles, and to French women being more inclined to eat greater amounts of fruits and vegetables than are French men. Thus, French women are less able to benefit from the supplementation. In addition, neither the male nor the female supplemented groups had statistically significant differences from the placebo groups in their rates of cardiovascular disease.

At first glance this suggests that the antioxidants had no preventive effect, but it may simply be that French citizens are not so likely as are other nationalities to show an effect because they already tend to have a considerably lower rate of cardiovascular disease compared to others such as Americans and other Europeans. This is the so-called "French paradox," which is attributed to some dietary protective factor characteristic of France. This is thought rather widely to be an antioxidant bioflavinoid component of grapes and red wine, resveratrol. Thus, for a better test of how antioxidant supplements affect heart disease, it should be conducted in a country having a higher rate of heart disease than does France. Moreover, it seems very likely that the outcome would have been more positive if the research had used more substantial amounts of the supplements.

Vitamin C: Biologic Functions and Relation to Cancer

The title of this section was applied to a conference sponsored by the National Cancer Institute and National Institute of Diabetes and Digestive and Kidney Diseases on September 10-12, 1990, at Bethesda, Maryland. During this meeting Gladys Block (1990) gave a paper titled "Epidemiologic Data on the Role of Ascorbic Acid in Cancer Prevention." An excerpt from the abstract of her paper summarizing her findings is shown:

> Approximately three-fourths of the epidemiological studies (33 of 46) of the role of vitamin C in cancer incidence or mortality have found statistically significant protection effects . . . The evidence for a protective effect of vitamin C or some component of fruits is strong and consistent for cancers of the esophagus, larynx, oral cavity and pancreas, and there is strong evidence for cancers of the stomach and cervix . . . A major meta-analysis of breast cancer studies suggests a significant protective role for vitamin C in that cancer as well. While it is likely that ascorbic acid, carotenoids, folate, and other factors in fruits and vegetables act jointly, an increasingly important role for ascorbic acid (Vitamin C) in cancer prevention would appear to be emerging. (Kaufman, 1992)

ANTIOXIDANTS AND DEMENTIAS

> One of most frustrating failings of the human mind is its Lilliputian capacity for storing and retrieving important but infrequently used information.
>
> Haynes et al. (1986)

The most-feared scourges associated with aging other than cancer surely are first Alzheimer's disease (AD) and second the vascular form of dementia (from "hardening of the arteries"). The number of AD patients has been growing for several decades and will continue to do so in the next several decades. This trend is a result of greater longevity in the U.S. population, owing to the reduced rate of cardiovascular mortality and of deaths from infectious disease, which began by mid-twentieth century. Two types of AD exist categorized by age of onset, the early type may begin in the forties, and the more typical late-onset type is manifested after the age of 60 years. The early-onset form is called *familial;* it constitutes only 15 percent to 20 percent of cases and has a genetic basis arising from mutations of genes on certain chromosomes. The later-onset form is called *sporadically occurring,* it comprises nearly 80 percent of all AD cases, and it does not have a genetic origin. The delay of the development and manifestation in the vast majority of cases of AD means that formerly many persons who might have been biologically prone to develop AD did not survive to the appropriate age for it to be manifested.

Some older persons (more than 50 years) become highly worried when they experience memory difficulties, fearing that they may foreshadow AD. However, if such lapses have been present for five years, but still do not seriously interfere with or prevent work and leisure activities, little or no chance exists that AD is the cause. Instead, the problem should be labeled "age-related memory impairment." Whether an antioxidant is able to benefit even these age-related memory complaints, which represent a benign aging-related process, is another unanswered question. A book focusing on age-related memory impairment (Crook and Adderly, 1998) strongly endorses using an amino acid supplement, phosphatidyl serine, as having adequate evidence for its being a very effective intervention.

Even more recently, some are advocating another phospholipid, phosphatidyl choline, which simialr to phosphatidyl serine is an important component of nerve cell membranes. It is also a precursor of the very important neurotransmitter, acetycholine. This molecule may also be ingested in the form of lecithin, which is a larger molecule that contains the phosphatidylcholine. A newer alternative source of choline has been marketed, alpha-glyceryl phosphorylcholine (alpha-GPC), which is said to be an extremely bioavailable form of choline that readily crosses the blood-brain barrier. In fact, it is claimed that alpha-GPC is a "preferred" source of choline since it is one that is produced in the normal metabolic processes. Insufficient data on alpha-GPC are available to support or to disagree with this position.

The diagnosis of early AD in life (rather than at autopsy) is difficult and frequently uncertain, although contemporary physicians are much more willing to make that diagnosis than were those 30 to 50 years ago (Grundman et al., 2004). An accuracy of 90 percent or greater in clinical diagnoses is claimed to be possible, when later checked against autopsy findings. Not only do characteristic deficits of memory exist in AD, but also declines in language, spatial orientation (getting lost), and/or executive functions of the frontal lobes. These seriously hinder occupational and social activities. Moreover, for an AD diagnosis, no evidence suggesting a cerebrovascular (arteriosclerotic) cause can exist.

Great amounts of research have been directed to acquiring an understanding of the causes of AD through which preventive and/or therapeutic approaches could be devised. A strong consensus that AD arises from an abnormal excess in the production or the accumulation of a neurotoxic protein known as beta-amyloid (or A beta), which is somehow responsible for nerve cell death, exists. It is assumed that a buildup to a sufficient level occurs so as to kill brain neurons in critical pathways connecting different areas of the brain. Two mechanisms by which beta-amyloid accumulation might cause neuronal death are (1) a high level of oxidative stress and cell injury, and (2) an inflammatory state. The former may be preventable or at least opposable by the use of antioxidants, whereas the latter may be beneficially opposed not only by many plant antioxidants but also by the use of NSAIDS, the nonsteroidal anti-inflammatory drugs.

Susceptibility to this disease process is recognized to be highly gene related in early-onset AD, but it is not clear that this is true for even a majority of AD cases. One concept of the biochemical mistake leading to AD is that it arises from misfolding of newly synthesized proteins. It is not evident that this sort of error can readily be preventable or reversible. However, it is not essential to know fully how the end results of a dementia process occur if good evidence can be obtained that a certain therapy interrupts or opposes the process. One line of research is attempting to employ an artificial antibody to interrupt the disease progression.

The oxidative stress hypothesis for the development of not only AD, but also other dementias (especially alcoholic dementia), is especially embraced by CAM practitioners. It supposes that excess oxidative activity exerted by ROS contributes to an accelerated rate of brain cell death as a consequence of excessive lipid peroxidation of brain cell membranes. The resulting loss of cells becomes the fundamental basis for the cognitive deficit characteristic of dementias. Note that this is a hypothesis, not a relationship that has been established. A stronger basis may presently exist for explaining alcoholic dementia this way than is true for AD. However, some AD researchers combine the ROS-mediated injury hypothesis with the toxic protein hypothesis as the means for amyloid causing brain injury leading to dementia.

Dementia Prevention: Vitamin E

Although not following subjects for seven years, other significant studies have shown a value of the major antioxidant vitamin E (Morris et al., 2002). This project was conducted at the Rush Institute for Healthy Aging, Rush-Presbyterian-St. Luke's Medical Center in Chicago, and it followed 2,889 community residents, aged 65 to 102 years, for an average of 3.2 years. The research found that higher levels of vitamin E intake, either from foods or dietary supplements, are associated with less cognitive decline with age. A 36 percent reduction in the rate of decline occurred among persons in the highest quintile (fifth) on total vitamin E intake compared with those in the lowest fifth after adjusting for age, race, sex, educational level, current smoking, alcohol consumption, total caloric intake, and total intakes of vitamin C, carotene, and vitamin A. Little evidence of an association between cognitive decline and intake of vitamin C or carotenes existed.

In 2002 a favorable review came from the Neuroscience Laboratory of the Jean Mayer USDA Human Nutrition Research Center on Aging (HNRC) at Tufts University, Boston (Martin et al., 2002). The authors declared plainly that diets rich in fruits and vegetables have been shown to improve human well-being and to significantly delay the onset of pathologic processes including neurodegenerative disorders such as dementias. Foods are described as important sources of micronutrients, especially vitamins E and C, which play crucial roles in optimal cellular functioning. Vitamin E serves as an important component of biologic membranes, and vitamin C acts as a cosubstrate for several enzymes. Both E and C are involved in the antioxidant defense of cells generally. Vegetable oils, nuts, and seeds are the major dietary sources of vitamin E, and fruits and vegetables are primary sources of vitamin C. However, the fact is that the levels of vitamins E and C provided by diets vary significantly. Human trials of varying doses of vitamins E and C, including low, supplemental, and pharmacologic doses, have found that these two nutrients may improve immunity, vascular function, and brain performance. Therefore, it is not surprising that an optimal intake of these nutrients has been associated with decreased risk of the cognitive impairments associated with aging.

Nevertheless, some researches have failed to detect cognitive benefits. The one by Luchsinger et al. (2003) investigated the relationship between AD and the intake of carotenes, vitamin C, and vitamin E in 980 elderly subjects. The study found 242 cases of AD in an average follow-up of 4.1 years. Higher intake of carotenes and vitamin C, or vitamin E in supplemental or dietary (nonsupplemental) form, or in both forms, was not correlated to a decreased risk of AD. A review by Delanty and Dichter (2000) acknowledged that

> the results of clinical trials using various antioxidants, including vitamin E . . . have been mixed. Potential reasons for these mixed results include lack of pretrial dose-finding studies and failure to appreciate and characterize the individual unique oxidative processes occurring in different [neurologic] diseases.

More recent researches have attempted to quantify seniors' intake of vitamin E and follow them over years to determine whether their level of intake shows a relationship with the AD rate. Two studies of this sort (Wu et al., 2004; Zandi et al., 2004) indeed found that higher intake of vitamin E was associated with a lower rate of AD. Another study, a prospective randomized trial, tested the antioxidant hypothesis on patients in later stages of AD using a 1,000-IU (international unit) dose of vitamin E twice a day. This treatment group showed a delay in such endpoints as time to institutionalization, loss of ability to perform basic activities of daily living, becoming classified as in severe dementia, or death. However, a defect in the random allocation of patients to a placebo group or to the vitamin E treatment groups led to criticism of the results, with experts deciding that high-dose vitamin E was not validated by this study to be an effective treatment for AD.

One reason for physicians preferring the use of other antioxidants besides high doses of vitamin E is a concern that its tendency to show anticoagulant effects could increase the risk for stroke. This comes from observations such as dental patients who took more than the RDA (recommended daily allowance) (400 IU) of vitamin E being slower than normal to heal from dental surgery and tending to hemorrhage excessively, which was attributed to their taking supplemental vitamin E.

A retrospective human research was reported by Morris et al. (2002). During the course of the study more than 60 percent of the nearly 3,000 study participants displayed some degree of decline in their mental functioning, whereas 39 percent had no decline or even improved. No diagnosis of Alzheimer's disease occurred. The group that reported the highest intakes of vitamin E had less fall in mental function than those whose vitamin E intake was lowest. A 36 percent lower rate of cognitive decline occurred for persons in the highest fifth of intake of vitamin E compared to those in the lowest fifth of intake. Estimates of vitamin E intake included both food and supplements. Those with the highest intake of vitamin E in food had a 32 percent lower rate of mental decline versus those having the least vitamin E in their diets.

For those who took vitamin E supplements, the cognitive benefit was seen only among those who received little vitamin E from their diet, not in those who already received a plentiful amount of the vitamin in their food. This may represent a ceiling effect, meaning that increases beyond a "good supply" of vitamin E cannot be helpful. By contrast, vitamin C seemed to show little effect on mental function. The team recently reported similar findings for vitamin E and development of AD. High intake of the nutrient was linked to a 70 percent lower risk for receiving a diagnosis of AD in a four-year period. Taken together the two studies strongly suggest that vitamin E has some protective effect toward the brain with respect to cognition. A point of emphasis made by some commentators is that *dietary* vitamin E may be superior to vitamin obtained in supplements, as no additional benefit to cognition was seen from supplements in people who had a good amount of vitamin E in their diet.

A research team headed by the Johns Hopkins School of Public Health tested the effects of vitamins E and C on Alzheimer's disease risk level (Zandi et al., 2004). They analyzed data from a large AD study of more than 4,700 subjects, age 65 or older. Study participants were asked at their first contact (1996) for detailed information about their use of vitamin supplements. The researchers then compared the subsequent risk of developing AD over the study interval (to 1999) among supplement users versus nonusers to reach their conclusions. About 17 percent of the participants were taking supplements of vitamin E or C. The were significantly more likely to be female, they were younger and better educated, and they reported better general health compared to nonusers.

Besides those who took vitamin supplements, another 20 percent of study participants used multivitamins, but without a high dosage of vitamin E or C. The analysis revealed a trend toward a reduction of rate for Alzheimer's disease with supplementation of both vitamin E and C, even after controlling for age, sex, education, and general health. However, no reduction in the risk of AD occurred with either vitamin alone or with multivitamins. Furthermore, use of vitamin E supplements along with multivitamins containing vitamin C also reduced AD risk. The study director, Dr. Peter Zandi said,

> Further study with randomized prevention trials is needed before drawing firm conclusions about the protective effects of these antioxidants. Such trials should consider testing a regimen of vitamin E and C in combination. If effective, the use of these antioxidant vitamins may offer an attractive strategy for the prevention of Alzheimer's disease. (Zandi et al., 2004)

Typical multivitamin products seldom contain much more than the RDA of vitamins E and C, and in both of these cases the RDA is very low according to natural physicians. In contrast, products that provide the individual vitamins tend to contain considerably higher amounts per serving, which would help to account for effectiveness of the vitamins taken together in contrast to failure of the smaller amounts in multivitamins. The Food and Nutrition Board of the National Academy of Sciences (the top U.S. source of recommendations on nutrient levels) in 2000 set new daily "safe upper limits" for vitamin C at 2,000 mg and 1,000 IU for vitamin E.

Developing methods for the prevention of Alzheimer's disease is an urgent priority because of the impending epidemic of AD as the baby boom generation reaches the age for high risk of AD. But study of modifiable (i.e., nongenetic) risk factors for the illness is still at an early stage. The severe impact of the disease and the current absence from mainline medicine of any proven *preventive* strategy favors persons using whatever available recourse they hope might be helpful. This leaves the field open to promotion of natural remedies on the basis of both the oxidative stress and inflammation concepts of the disease mechanism(s).

Because an expected protective effect from using supplemental antioxidants is likely to be small to moderate, a quite large-scale (tens of thousands of subjects), randomized, placebo-controlled clinical trial for prevention of AD would be required to resolve the issue of efficacy for antioxidants. A major question is who will finance time-consuming and expensive trials needed to provide a definite answer. Obtaining an informed consent, as is requisite from clinical trial participants, might also be difficult, as would be the long-term compliance issue.

However, some clinical researchers suggest that placebo control groups have been outmoded by the advances represented by donepezil (and vitamin E) as therapies having significant value. Karlawish and Whitehouse (1998) of the National Institute on Aging and Center for Bioethics at the University of Pennsylvania declared as early as 1998 that the use of placebo control designs was made obsolete because of the benefits possible from those two therapies, rather than the former lack of any accepted beneficial therapies. Clearly they were not awaiting a meta-analysis for their position on vitamin E. Another similar paper from the University of Minnesota (Knopman et al., 1998) in the same issue went further to propose that future trials of other new agents should consider combination therapy as a likely strategy for their design. Moreover, they declared that, "The long duration of future AD trials also will make placebo-controlled trials more difficult to justify and more difficult to recruit for. Add-on or active-control designs represent the alternative approaches."

A possible end to uncertainty in some minds regarding antioxidant vitamin value may be reached through a National Institute of Aging–funded study begun in 2000 to compare the safety and efficacy of vitamin E (1000 IU twice a day) with the standard anti-AD pharmaceutical, donepezil (10 mg per day), or placebo in an elderly population of persons who initially had mild cognitive impairment. The end point of the study is onset of diagnosed AD (Knopman et al., 1998). This was a multicenter (U.S. and Canadian) study designed to test these two preventive strategies against AD. Other candidates for future testing might include agents having a selective estrogen receptor activity, those acting as selective inhibitors of the COX-2 enzyme, which are hoped to be agents acting specifically against production and deposition of amyloid in the brain. However, more recent concerns about safety of COX-2 inhibitors diminish interest in their capacity for acting against AD. Meanwhile, many and varied botanical materials are touted as preventives for AD because they have "more power" than vitamins C and E as antioxidants. This continues despite neither vitamin has yet been classed as evidence-based for slowing the progression of AD, much less preventing it.

Nonvitamin Dementia Prevention

Curry/Turmeric/Curcumin

Curcumin is a substance found in the spice turmeric that long has been commonly used in Asia for preparing curries, and it is a prominent component of the diet in India. It has been hypothesized that eating curry may be at least part of the reason why AD is supposedly uncommon in India in contrast to rates in Western countries. Studies in Indian villages found a lower incidence of AD than the expected rate for persons older than 65 years. Curry/turmeric seems clearly to be safe even in large amounts in foods. It also is known to be an antioxidant. Researchers at UCLA decided to examine curcumin, the active component of turmeric, that has well-known anti-inflammatory properties (Lim et al., 2001). Their rodent studies found that curcumin reduced the level of brain amyloid, the abnormal protein deposited in the brain of Alzheimer's patients. Curcumin appeared also to reduce the inflammatory responses to amyloid in the rat brains. The laboratory model used was older rats that received injections of amyloid directly into the brain. The rats that received curcumin by mouth performed better in a maze and in similar behavioral tests than did placebo controls. Whether this is a good model of the human disease is unclear.

Lim and colleagues (2001) further tested curcumin on mice that were genetically engineered to develop brain lesions consisting of amyloid plaques. They found that the plaque rate of mice eating food supplemented with curcumin was 43 percent less than for mice that did not receive the spice. Eating curcumin also reduced inflammation and free radical damage in the mouse brains. Adopting a curry-containing diet would seems to be a safe step, even though the possible long-term payoff is still uncertain at the present.

Polyphenols

Numerous botanicals contain flavonoid constituents, which are a major subgroup of polyphenols, that exert high levels of antioxidant activity (see also Chapter 24). One that first had great publicity as a potential opponent to dementia in the early 1990s was best known as Pycnogenol. This was originally obtained from the bark of maritime pines of France and northeastern North America, but later, equivalent preparations were obtained as an extract of grape seeds. Products based on both sources are widely available, but their ability to benefit a patient with possible or probable Alzheimer's dementia is still unproven.

Ginkgo biloba

On August 19, 2004, there was a public announcement from the Imperial College of London and St. Mary's Hospital concerning the launching of research to determine if use of *Ginkgo biloba* can help patients with early memory loss. The study of 250 patients of ages over 55 years will test whether general practitioners by prescribing the supplement for those who are still living in the community may provide the advantage of a "sooner the better" effect. It will be the first study to test gingko as therapy for patients who are showing only early symptoms (presumed) of dementia. Prior studies have concentrated on patients receiving hospital care, for whom the dementia is at a much more advanced stage. The participants in the double-blind trial will take their conventional medicines for their age-associated memory loss, and for six months they will also take either 60 mg of a gingko extract or a placebo twice daily (Alzheimer's Research Forum, 2004).

Ginkgo is believed to cause blood vessels to dilate and so improve blood flow to the brain, as well as making the blood less likely to form small clots that may damage the brain and its functions. Ginkgo also is known to have antioxidant activity, which may serve to protecting nerve cells against oxidative injury. The leader of the research, psychiatrist Dr. James Warner, said that ginkgo could provide an inexpensive alternative to the current Rx medicines for dementia, and with fewer of their potential side effects such as nausea, loss of appetite, tiredness, and diarrhea. Quality ginkgo extracts currently are available over the counter in the United Kingdom, most European countries, and the United States (Alzheimer's Research Forum, 2004).

Omega-3 Fats

Dietary omega-3 polyunsaturated fatty acids are found to improve brain functioning in animal studies, but limited data exists on the question of whether this type of fat has a protective action relative to AD. Morris and co-workers (2003) reported on their prospective study conducted from 1993 through 2000 to test whether consumption of fish and intake of other sources of omega-3 fatty acids would be protective against AD. The observed population was 815 residents, aged 65 to 94 years, who were initially unaffected by AD and who completed a dietary questionnaire on average 2.3 years prior to clinical evaluation of disease. A total of 131 sample participants developed Alzheimer's disease. Participants who consumed fish once weekly or more had a 60 percent lower risk of AD compared to those who rarely or never ate fish. Their total intake of omega-3 polyunsaturated fatty acids also was correlated with a reduced risk of AD, as was intake of docosahexaenoic acid (DHA). Eicosapentaenoic acid (EPA) intake was not correlated with incidence of AD. The associations were unchanged after further adjustments for the intake of other dietary fats and vitamin E, and for cardiovascular conditions.

A METABOLITE USEFUL FOR FAILING MEMORY

Phosphatidylserine

In this instance we will deviate from antioxidants to include a metabolite for which value as a restorer of age-related memory problems is reported. Phosphatidylserine (PS) is a normal metabolite, a phospholipid, found in human tissues and synthesized from dietary sources of the amino acid, serine. PS may be obtained preformed in small amounts from fish, rice, soy products, and green leafy vegetables. It is a member of the chemical group called phospholipids, because every molecule includes a phosphate and two fatty acids attached to glycerol (this is the basic structure of a fat or lipid). The serine is attached through the phosphate group. Phospholipids are normal, fundamental components of all cell membranes, and are especially abundant in nervous tissue, which explains their being influential toward brain functions. Phosphatidylcholine is another example of important lipid of the nervous system.

PS has been derived from both animal and vegetable. Early studies used PS derived from bovine brain cortex, for which human tolerability of treatment with 300 mg daily was shown in 130 patients. More recently, because of the "mad cow" scare about using organs, especially brain tissue or spinal nerves, from cows, PS has instead become available from soybeans (Suzuki et al., 2001). A study by Jorissen et al. (2002) examined the human tolerability of two dosages of soy phosphatidylserine (SPS). Study subjects were 120 elderly persons of both sexes who fulfilled either the more stringent standards for a diagnosis of age-associated memory impairment or the lesser criteria for age-associated cognitive decline. Subjects were assigned at random to one of three treatment groups: placebo, 300 mg, or 600 mg SPS daily. Standard measures of safety in terms of biochemistry and hematology, blood pressure, heart rate, and adverse events were assessed not only at baseline but also after six and 12 weeks of treatment. No significant differences were found in any of these outcomes between the three groups. Thus, soy-derived PS is judged to be a safe supplement for older persons if taken at doses up to 200 mg three times daily.

Soybean-derived phosphatidylserine was tested by Suzuki et al. (2001) for its effect on age-related memory impairment in rats by a maze test. In their 2001 report, they found that continuous oral administration of SPS (60 mg per kg per day for 60 days to aged male rats (24 to 25 months) significantly improved performance in the maze escape test. They described the outcome as similar to those with bovine brain cortex–derived PS, which they say "restores cognitive function in human patients with senile dementia." SPS also increased acetylcholine release and other biochemical measures of brain preparations from aged rats relative to the level in young rats. The memory effects of SPS in the rats can be partly explained by the changes found in these biochemical activities. These and other studies in rodents provide a foundation and rationale for human usage. Although PS became available first in Europe, a considerable number of studies in the United States have found benefits of PS for age-memory impairment. These studies are summarized and reviewed at length in a book by Thomas H. Crook, PhD, and Brenda Adderly (1998) of Memory Assessment Clinics Inc. in Bethesda, Maryland. Needless to say, these reported benefits seem not to have been widely noted or accepted by scientific medicine.

ANTIOXIDANTS VERSUS KIDNEY DISEASE

A review on antioxidants in the prevention of renal disease by Dr. E. N. Wardle (1999) considered the role of oxidative processes in kidney damage that can occur in severe diseases—glomerulosclerosis and renal medullary interstitial fibrosis. Speaking generally, atherosclerosis is an important causative factor for such chronic renal diseases. Wardle concluded that more attention should be paid to usage of antioxidant food constituents or dietary supplements having a recognized antioxidant potential, and that a wide choice of foods and supplements are available that could confer protective benefits. Supplementation with vitamins E and C, use of soy protein diets, and drinking green tea could even bring remarkable improvements.

However, kidney disease may occur at any age. A paper from the Institute of Nutrition in Moscow reported their finding value for pediatric practice in dealing with glomerulonephritis to be obtained from use of the polyunsaturated omega-3 fatty acids. These were found to oppose renal injury. Treated patients achieved better clinical remission, as well as a more rapid fall of hypercholesterolemia, and hypercoagulation than did patients from a control group.

ANTIOXIDANTS FOR "MYSTERY MALADIES"

The second half of the twentieth century saw a number of puzzling and controversial illnesses that raised such questions as what causes them, how to treat them, and even do they really exist? These include fibromyalgia (FM), chronic fatigue syndrome (CFS), multiple chemical sensitivity (MCS), and Gulf War syndrome (GWS). Efforts to tie them to an infection have failed, generally speaking, but evidence exists that something (perhaps a past infection, or a chemical injury?) has provoked adverse changes in some immune system activities. It has not proven possible to treat them successfully via anti-infective drugs, with a possible exception of isolated cases of GWS.

A prooxidant activity of certain WBCs (white blood cells), consisting of a release of highly reactive free radical molecules (ROS), is normally directed toward killing of bacteria or intestinal parasites. When this action becomes misdirected, injury or death of normal cells can result. This is well accepted as a basis for some autoimmune diseases, but it is only hypothetical as the mechanism responsible for some of the mystery maladies.

In a recent research 85 female patients diagnosed with fibromyalgia and 80 healthy women matched for age, height, and weight were evaluated for oxidant-to-antioxidant balance (Bagis et al., 2003). The researchers measured the women's level of production of the chemical malondialdehyde, which is a toxic byproduct of lipid peroxidation and serves as a useful marker for the ongoing occurrence of free radical damage. Also measured were levels of a protective enzyme against ROS, superoxide dismutase. Pain was assessed by use of a visual analogue scale. Tender points characteristic of FM were assessed by palpation (probing with the fingers). Age, smoking, body mass index (BMI), and duration of disease were also recorded.

Malondialdehyde levels were significantly higher and superoxide dismutase levels were significantly lower among FM patients than for the healthy controls. Age, body mass index, smoking, and duration of disease did not affect the measures. The results offer support for the hypothesis that FM symptoms reflect an abnormal process comprising tissue oxidative injury. Elevated levels of free radicals may indeed be responsible for the state of fibromyalgia. Currently, no recognized therapeutic diet exists for patients with FM, but several reports indicate that fish oil, magnesium, and malic acid combinations, or vitamins, especially B12, may be beneficial. Experimental diets have contained a high level of antioxidant vitamins and minerals.

Other therapeutic approaches being studied include S-adenosylmethionine (SAMe), an antidepressant, anti-inflammatory, antioxidant, and methyl donor. A report from Italy by DiBendetto and colleagues (1993) found that SAMe significantly reduced the number of tender points by 28 days treatment compared to a randomly assigned group that received an electrical stimulation rather than drug therapy. Among earlier positive reports on SAMe in FM were two double-blind placebo-controlled studies.

FUNCTIONAL FOODS THAT MAY FIGHT AGING

Blueberry

The European wild blueberry, known as bilberry, long has been reputed to have value against such ocular problems as cataract or macular degeneration. More recently it has been supposed that this benefit derives from bilberry ingredients that serve as strong antioxidants. Indeed, cultivated American blueberries have been found to contain various biologically active compounds, including the antioxidant vitamins A, C, and E as well as anthocyanins (also potent antioxidants), anthocyanosides (which may act as bacterial inhibitors), folic acid, carotenoids, ellagic acid (possible inhibitor of cancer initiation), and dietary fiber. Unfortunately, adequate confirmation of the claims of protective action for vision is currently still lacking.

The same must be said for the claim that a heart-healthy benefit is available from blueberries, which is attributed to their providing a compound that acts similarly to resveratrol against cholesterol-related cardiovascular problems. However, substantiation for this came from laboratory findings (Rimando et al., 2002, 2004) from the USDA Natural Products Utilization Research Unit in the National Center for Natural Products Research at the University of Mississippi, Oxford. The studies found that a blueberry antioxidant called pterostilbene was able to suppress carcinogen-induced lesions in mouse mammary gland cells, as did also resveratrol from grapes.

Pharmacologist James Joseph, PhD, and his colleagues at HNRC reported striking benefits toward brain function for aging rats fed a blueberry supplement (Joseph et al., 1999). Other groups of rats received supplements of either strawberry or spinach extracts. The rats were 19 months old upon beginning the research, which is age-equivalent to humans at 60 to 65 years old. They were fed the blueberry supplement for two months, which brought them to an equivalent of 70 to 75 years old. The rats fed blueberries, in addition to normal diet, performed better than did equal-aged rats on the standard control diet in behavioral tests, e.g., swimming a water maze or finding an underwater platform in murky water. On these two tests of so-called "working memory," all three groups getting supplements outperformed the animals that were not receiving supplements.

Moreover, the supplemented rats also did better on motor tests involving a rotating rod or an inclined rod used to test the animals' motor coordination. Young rats, six months old, could stay on a rotating rod for an average of 14 seconds. Old rats fell off after merely six seconds, but the older rats that were blueberry supplemented could stay on for ten seconds. When the rats' brains were examined, evidence suggested that the brain cells communicated better and neural messages were transmitted more effectively for rats receiving blueberries. Retaining good motor control would be an important aid to elderly persons being able to avoid critical falls and bone fractures that can be "the beginning of the end."

In further studies using in vitro cultured cells, Dr. Joseph's team (Joseph et al., 2000) determined that the most effective components of the blueberry extract was the polyphenolic anthocyanins, which also showed the most ability to penetrate the cell membrane. They provided not only antioxidant but also anti-inflammatory protection. It was suggested that these effects were highly relevant to matters of Alzheimer's disease susceptibility. He found that feeding a blueberry-supplemented diet for 12 months enhanced the Y-maze performance of mice that were double transgenic, meaning that they carried two mutations that made them genetically predisposed to show pathology and behavioral deviations resembling those seen in Alzheimer's disease. The mice had a favorably increased adaptability as compared to controls not receiving blueberry supplement. Thus, the Tufts researchers have shown for the first time that polyphenolic compounds found in fruits and vegetables have a positive action against brain aging in normal mice and even in a mouse model of Alzheimer's disease.

Attempting to confirm possible benefits of blueberry (and strawberry or spinach) to the aging human brain is the next step needed. Although support for this may be claimed in the tradition of bilberry's healthfulness, it would be an unwarranted assumption. Until confirmatory human data are obtained, the expected health value of bilberry extracts in dietary supplements or blueberries in the diet must be seen as scientifically unconfirmed. What could or should be done in the meantime? Why not elevate your intake of blueberries and strawberries? Eat blueberries—fresh in season, canned, frozen, juice concentrate, jam, or jelly. For those who enjoy gardening, why not cultivate blueberry bushes (perennials) in your own yard or garden?

Selenium

Selenium has important antioxidant properties. It is thought to influence favorably the immune system and tissue anti-inflammatory responses by facilitating production of the enzyme glutathione peroxidase and thus synthesis of glutathione, which detoxifies free radicals. However, when selenium supplements were given to people with rheumatoid arthritis in a double-blind, placebo-controlled trial over three months, selenium treatment did not show any objective clinical benefit (Peretz et al., 2001). One might question whether this trial was of sufficient duration. Regardless, the selenium supplement did improve subjective quality-of-life measures for patients in the treatment group. Nevertheless, a trial for reduction of the risk for gastrointestinal cancer recently showed a positive benefit, and the authors called for further evaluation of selenium in this regard.

GOOD EATING FOR A GOOD INTAKE OF ANTIOXIDANTS

A team of USDA nutritionists published a study that supplied a list of the Top 20 antioxidant-rich foods (Wu et al., 2004). The USDA scientists assayed more than 100 different kinds of fruits, vegetables, nuts, spices, cereals, and other foods using a method for measuring oxygen radical absorbance capacity (ORAC). This enabled them to detect both lipid soluble and water soluble antioxidant activities of the foods sampled. They also singled out certain foods for testing the impact from different processing actions, such as peeling without or with cooking. Fruits, vegetables, and beans claimed nearly all the ranks in the top 20, which includes the following (1 = best):

1. Small red beans (dried)
2. Blueberries (wild)
3. Red kidney beans
4. Pinto beans

5. Blueberries (cultivated)
6. Cranberries
7. Artichokes (cooked)
8. Blackberries
9. Prunes
10. Raspberries
11. Strawberries
12. Red delicious apples
13. Granny Smith apples
14. Pecans
15. Sweet cherries
16. Black plums
17. Russet potatoes (cooked)
18. Black beans (dried)
19. Plums
20. Gala apples

The champion, small red beans, look similar to kidney beans—same color and shape—except for being smaller. They are sometimes identified as Mexican red beans, but actually are grown only in Washington, Idaho, and Alberta, Canada. As you might suppose, most antioxidant foods lose some of their antioxidant capacities in processing. A notable exception was the tomato, a source of the excellent antioxidant lycopene, levels of which are actually enhanced by cooking. Otherwise, fresh is the best choice over frozen, cooked, or any other form of processing. Although a blueberry pie may seem to be a rather healthful treat, it can't begin to match a bowl of freshly picked blueberries. Moreover, blueberry bushes could be grown for picking in your own yard almost anywhere in the lower 48 states, except in the deserts and the higher mountains.

Rather than focusing on only one source, however, one should choose a variety of these 20 sources, which could supply more different healthful components than would be obtained from merely one. Blueberries deliver a chemical type called anthocyanins, which are said to help protect brain cells, and raspberries and strawberries are excellent for their delivery of ellagitannin, a substance that has been found to prevent the growth of cancerous cells in laboratory researches. Besides antioxidants, pinto or kidney beans are good sources of the B-vitamin, folate, which favors cardiovascular health by helping to lower homocysteine levels. Similarly, pecans will add copper and potassium to your diet as well as antioxidants. Thus, it's "the more the merrier" when choosing to get many different items from this list into your diet.

NONSUPPLEMENTAL APPROACHES TO FIGHT AGING

From the anonymity of e-mail forwarding chains came these thoughts.

How to Stay Young

1. Throw out nonessential numbers. This includes age, weight, and height. Let the doctors worry about them. That is why you pay them.
2. Keep only cheerful friends. The grouches pull you down.
3. Keep learning. Learn more about the computer, crafts, gardening, whatever. Never let the brain idle. "An idle mind is the devil's workshop." And the devil's name is Alzheimer's.
4. Enjoy the simple things.
5. Laugh often, long, and loud. Laugh until you gasp for breath.
6. The tears will happen. Endure, grieve, and move on. The only person who is with us our entire life is ourselves. Be *alive* while you are alive.
7. Surround yourself with what you love, whether it's family, pets, keepsakes, music, plants, hobbies, whatever. Your home is your refuge.
8. Cherish your health. If it is good, preserve it. If it is unstable, improve it. If it is beyond what you can improve, get help.
9. Don't take guilt trips. Take a trip to the mall, to the next county, or to a foreign country, but not to where the guilt is.
10. Tell the people you love that you love them, at every opportunity.

And always remember that life is not measured by the number of breaths we take, but by the moments that take our breath away.

CONCLUSION

In short, help may be on the way from pharmaceutical and biotech industry activities in the fight against the fundamental factors of the bodily ravages of time, but the help will not likely arrive soon. Perhaps greater short-term hope may come from better dietary choices and lifestyle practices.

Chapter 15

The Soya Saga: Are Soy Products Safe and Effective?

HEALTH PROBLEMS ASSOCIATED WITH SOY FOODS

> Far from being the perfect food, modern soy products contain antinutrients and toxins and they interfere with the absorption of vitamins and minerals.
>
> Sally Fallon and Mary Enig (2000)

Soya, soy, or the soybean all refer to a member of the pea family *(Leguminosae),* which is an annual plant that grows from one to five feet high. Its wild ancestor was domesticated in China before recorded history. Although soybeans have been cultivated by Asian cultures for thousands of years, about 50 percent of worldwide soybean production now occurs in the United States where health and nutrition magazines have touted the benefits of soy as a cure-all valuable for weight loss, hormonal difficulties, women's health, cancer prevention, and other problems. It is easy to conclude that such claims for soy represent sales promotion propaganda more than they reflect valid nutritional advice based on sound scientific evidence. A critical examination of health issues arising is essential.

BIOLOGICAL QUALITY OF SOY PROTEIN

Soybeans are rich in protein, vitamins, minerals, and fiber. The major varieties of soy nutritional products include soy protein concentrates, soy lecithins, soybean meal, and soy oil. The term *soy* generally is applied to products made from whole soybeans; *soy protein* is the product derived by extracting the protein from soybeans. A major feature of whole soy and most of its processed forms is its content of worrisome nonnutrient components. Most widely known are the isoflavones, the key components of soy

Consumer's Guide to Dietary Supplements and Alternative Medicines

doi:10.1300/5698_15

that make them a possible basis for hormonal actions by their acting on mammalian estrogen receptors as weak agonists (activators). Consequently they are known as phytoestrogens. They are important because although marketed as important nutritional substances they often are used intending for their action similar to hormonal drugs.

It may be important to recognize that rice was and is the staple grain in China and Japan, with soya playing a considerably lesser dietary role, thus the arguments that any safety and health concerns are trumped by the long history of soy use in Asia are open to question on this account. It is also noteworthy that much selective breeding of soy has occurred since its initial cultivation in North America, and that recent genetic engineering has produced herbicide-resistant GM (genetically modified) strains. Indeed, William Hawks, an undersecretary at the Department of Agriculture, made a statement in late 2003 in Memphis, Tennessee, "More than 80 percent of all soybeans we produce come from transgenic seed" (Roberts, 2003). This fact lends additional support for the proposition that the soy products Americans are now eating cannot be validated for their healthfulness by past experience in Asian peoples, who ate no GM soy. The soy that they ate is not identical to the soy being delivered to the U.S. population. Uncertainty remains as to whether the difference could be dangerous or indifferent.

Furthermore, critics state that soy-based foods eaten in Asia are mainly derived from soy that has been fermented, which is not at all true of American products, therefore any direct comparisons are invalid also on this account. Fermented soy forms are somewhat available now, but most if not all soy food components or additives for use in American food products are not derived after fermentation.

SOY AS A PROTEIN CONCENTRATE SOURCE

Soy protein concentrates, although supplying a high quality protein in terms of the amino acids that it provides, is difficult to digest. Some authorities state that only those fermented forms known as miso and tempeh actually supply any readily absorbable nutrients. Moreover, some warn that soy protein is relatively poor in content of the vital amino acid tryptophan, as also is true for corn. An excess dependence on corn in the American South a century ago was found to be responsible for the disease known as pellagra because of inadequate dietary tryptophan. It also is being said that overdependence on soy as a source of protein, e.g., by vegetarians, could cause such persons to become deficient in the crucial brain neurotransmitter serotonin, for which tryptophan is the necessary precursor.

The usual level of tryptophan in the protein of breast milk is significantly higher than that found in unsupplemented soy protein. This would indicate that reliance on soy protein in infant formulas could be detrimental to the development of the nervous system for infants.[1] No doubt should exist that human breast milk is the optimal diet for any infant.

Despite these factors in the year 2000 such questionable endorsements as the following were still exclaimed: "Unlike concentrated supplements, foods rich in phytoestrogens, such as vegetables, grains and legumes, are also excellent sources of fiber, unsaturated *[sic]* protein, vitamins and minerals, and their consumption should be encouraged" (Murkies et al., 2000).

Furthermore, a question has been raised whether too much soy protein in the diet might have the same injurious potential for the intestinal tract of human infants as was found for weanling piglets (Ross, 2002).[2] Thus, although acknowledging that the overall nutrient quality of soy protein is fairly good, but not excellent, its main advantage over other sources of protein concentrates is economic—it is cheap. *Profitability* is the central reason for the U.S. food processing industries moving to adopt soy so extensively and to promote its use rather than soy having a particularly healthful nature. However, the idea that soy falls short of being an ideal nutrient would never be inferred from the laudatory propaganda used to multiply its acceptance.

A Soy Alternative, Whey Protein

Some researchers would declare that a superior choice for a protein supplement is readily available in the form of whey protein. If it were more widely used it would for certain boost the U.S. dairy industry. This fraction (20 percent) of milk protein that is left after the making of cheese is acclaimed as being more nutritious than the protein provided by eggs, pork, beef, or chicken. It may soon compete for use in the manner of soy protein. It is said the history of whey usage dates to the mid-seventeenth century in Italy. Its reputation for being a "complete protein" because of its supplying all the essential and nonessential amino acids, and being favorable to muscle proteins synthesis (Borsheim et al., 2004), have made it very popular among athletes. Whey's ready utilization of in contrast to that of soy protein gives it a much superior biological value. Moreover, whey supplies a superior level of branched-chain amino acids, which are very favorable to muscle repair metabolism, as well as being a source for glutamine and its positive effect on immune system activity and on levels of glutathione. A report from Australia (Belobrajdic et al., 2004) states that a diet high in whey protein is more favorable than high meat protein for weight reduction by lowering excess insulin secretion and appetite. In Japan researchers have isolated peptides from whey that exert an antihypertensive action. One drawback of whey is its possible contribution to milk allergies.

THE PHYTOESTROGEN ASPECT

Perimenopausal women have been encouraged take to soy products for relief from their hormonal-deficit symptoms because of the phytoestrogen content of soy. Both soy and soy protein contain the several isoflavones that act as phytoestrogens—genistein, daidzein, and glycetein—as well as other nonprotein phytochemicals (protease inhibitors, lectins, phytate). The isoflavones exert estrogenic and antiestrogenic effects as well as nonhormonal activities. Soy and soy-derived isoflavones in the past decade have gained much attention and usage for their phytoestrogenic activity because of its supposed benefits on cardiovascular health, for its relief of menopausal symptoms, and for opposition to postmenopausal osteoporosis. Because of their status as natural agents, some advocates promote a view that phytoestrogens are more safe than equine estrogens or synthetics women have used in pharmaceuticals for hormone replacement therapy.

It must be noted that the foremost pharmaceutical products that supply estrogen to mature women for use before, during, and after menopause have been Premarin and Prempro. The estrogen components of these are natural products, not synthetics, being a mixture of natural estrogens prepared from pregnant mare urine. Synthetic estrogens presently are mainly encountered in oral contraceptive products. However, the advocates of "strictly natural" now allege that the equine hormone should not be used in place of human estrogens. Specially formulated "bioequivalent" products of human hormones are being marketed, but they are made available only through a few pharmacy outlets.

Research to date is inadequate to show conclusively whether the supposed positive health effects of soy are real and whether they can be attributed to the isoflavones alone or to isoflavones in conjunction with other soy components.

Controversies continue as to whether the apparent or supposed benefits of soy outweigh the potential for detrimental effects. The benefits and risks are shown in the following list:

Benefits	**Detriments/Risks**
Women experience activation of their tissue estrogen receptors,	Women may be at higher risk for breast cancer; increased gallbladder disease;

possibly an alternative to pharmaceutical hormone replacement therapy to oppose peri- and postmenopausal symptoms, protect blood vessels.	higher rate of blood clots, which may increase the risk of heart failure; young women may show menstrual deviations.
Men, no known benefits.	Men, or women, may have a higher risk for brain aging or dementia.
Children, no known benefits	Male children may show feminizing of body Female children may show premature sexual development
Fetuses, no known benefit	Sexual development of male fetuses may be abnormal (e.g., hypospadias)

Epidemiologic data show that women from Asia, where soy is a component of the diet, have a lower rate of breast cancer than non-Asian women who eat a Western diet. This has encouraged the view that American women may reduce their rate of breast cancer by incorporating soy into their diets. Indeed, when Asian women immigrate to North America they are said not to lose their breast cancer resistance, although their daughters do lose the advantage. This suggests that an early-life exposure is critical to the difference, and experiments in rats support the hypothesis that early exposure is critical. If so, exposure to soy begun after the age of child-bearing may not reduce breast cancer risk, but other benefits may still be possible.

However, concentrated phytoestrogen supplements may have strong enough estrogenic action on the breast to interfere with therapeutic use of tamoxifen (an antiestrogen) as an Rx preventive agent for breast cancer. Some authors believe that the phytoestrogen show such weakness of their receptor action in some observations as to suggest that if they should provide relief of menopausal symptoms it would have to be through another mechanism than that of conventional HRT.

Huntley and Ernst (2004) conducted a systematic review of randomized clinical trials of soy for HRT. Ten of the trials located fitted their inclusion criteria, but the results of the studies were inconclusive. Four of the controlled trials were positive, suggesting soy preparations had benefit for perimenopausal symptoms, but six were negative, with only one of those showing a positive trend. They concluded that some evidence exists for efficacy of soy preparations for reducing menopausal symptoms, but not clearly enough for a definitive judgment. Adverse event data of the trials showed no serious safety concerns for soy products in short-term use. They could make no judgment regarding possible long-term risks.

The supposed cardioprotective effects of soy products, if real, could be produced through a variety of possible actions. These include a favorable effect on the blood lipid profile and inhibition of low-density lipoprotein (LDL) cholesterol oxidation. The precise mode of action for soy improving the blood lipid profile is uncertain. Another possible means is by altered liver metabolism increasing the removal of LDL cholesterol and very-low-density lipoprotein (VDL) cholesterol by hepatocytes. Soy also is suggested to lower blood pressure, reduce atherosclerosis, and raise arterial elasticity. Unfortunately, presently little confirmation of such hypothetical actions exists. A most recent clinical study reported the conclusion that in postmenopausal women neither the phytate nor the isoflavone contents from soy protein exert a significant effect to reduce oxidative damage or to cause a favorable alteration of blood lipids (Engelmann et al., 2005).

NONESTROGENIC ADVERSE RESPONSES TO SOY

Protease Inhibitors, Lectins, and Phytate

The raw soybean contains numerous antinutrients and toxic components. Although processing can reduce them, it does not entirely eliminate them. For example, raw soybean has an anticoagulant action that is attributed to its antitrypsin activity. Trypsin is a special enzyme, a protease needed to digest proteins. In addition, trypsin is needed to allow vitamin B12 to be freed from its complexes with other food constituents and assimilated. Thus, if this trypsin activity is blocked by a soybean component acting as an antitrypsin agent, the person so affected has a decreased availability of vitamin B12. The risk of a person developing an actual vitamin B12 deficiency could be raised by excess use of soy.

Raw soybean contains several "antinutrients," mainly phytic acid (as phytates), which bind and prevent mineral absorption—especially zinc, calcium, and magnesium, and even iron. Because phytic acid also is present in grains, vegetarians who depend on soybeans, soy-containing products, and phytate-containing grain products could be at even higher risk for deficiencies of these minerals. Phytates are present only in plants, not in animal foods.

Hemagglutinins are another class of antinutrients in the raw soybean that have an ability to agglutinate (cause to clump together) the red blood cells in humans, and to significantly suppress growth. These antinutrients are known also as "phytoagglutinins" or "lectins." Processing is intended to remove them.

Soy Allergy Concerns

People becoming allergic to certain components (antigens) of common foods is not a rare happening, but one that may cause considerable distress and difficulty of obtaining a correct diagnosis and effective management. Soy is no exception. Some sources say it is among the leaders in proallergic properties and suggest that genetic modification may magnify that feature. Soy allergy is manifested as symptoms involving the respiratory tract (asthma), skin (contact dermatitis), and probably other parts of the body. Concern is warranted that contact with infant formulas containing soy components may be an excess risk for babies who may be at elevated chance of becoming allergic. Acquiring a soy hypersensitivity in adults is clearly possible as well. Spectacular instances of large-scale, inhalation-related allergic sensitization have been described from Barcelona, Spain, and elsewhere.

SOY AS A PHYTOESTROGEN

Soy is being widely promoted as a natural alternative to pharmaceutical estrogens for HRT. Indeed, some women take soy products as a nutraceutical for alleviation of menopausal symptoms as an alternative to pharmaceutical estrogen replacement therapies. This is based on the supposition that soy can provide a phytoestrogen activity that is similar in physiological effects to those of the normal estrogenic hormones in women, except that it is significantly weaker.

A report in the prestigious journal *Proceedings of the National Academy of Sciences of the United States of America* raised questions about the safety of soy-based infant formulas (Yellayi et al., 2002). It presented animal data showing that genistein-treated mice experienced shrinkage of their thymus gland by as much as 80 percent below its normal weight. Their blood levels of the compound were similar to those found in human infants fed a soy-based infant formula. Because this gland serves in early life to "set up" the T-cells of the immune system for their lifelong functions, it is possible to project such findings as being a threat to normal immune system activity and source for a variety of possibly consequential abnormal states.

A British study on pregnancy and childbirth from 1991 to 2000 found among boy babies an unusually high rate of a congenital maldevelopment, hypospadias, a malformation of the penis that requires difficult surgery for its correction. However, no significant differences in the rate of hypospadias cases were found from the control group among mothers who smoked or consumed alcohol, or with respect to any aspect of their previous reproductive history, including number of previous pregnancies, number of miscarriages, use of oral contraceptives, time to conception, and age at menarche. The ruling out of those factors left the puzzled researchers seeking an explanation when they noted that mothers who were vegetarians during pregnancy were five times more likely than meat eaters to have a son with hypospadias. It seemed possible to them that phytoestrogens in vegetables, especially dishes based on soy, had interfered with the embryonic development of the urogenital tract of the boy babies.

An alternative possibility raised by the researchers is to blame pesticide residues, some of which may exert estrogenic effects, but this seems a much less plausible cause than the phytoestrogens, which are known to be capable of exerting significant hormonal effects even in adult women. Additional data will be needed to refute or to establish the role of phytoestrogens in this maldevelopment problem of boy babies (North and Golding, 2000). Until that time, it seems clear that caution should dictate an avoidance of soya-based food items during pregnancy, or (better yet) by the time that efforts to conceive are begun. Certainly women should de-emphasize soy in their diet during pregnancy.

CONCLUSION

The current degree and usage pattern of soy-related food materials in the U.S. diet comprises a vast uncontrolled nutritional experiment, the full outcome of which no one can foresee. The widespread use of soy products is a testimonial to the powerful influence of marketing and promotional know-how, while nutritional and biomedical scientists must play an underfunded "catch-up" game in attempting to discern what outcomes are being produced by a revolutionary dietary change. What unforeseen costs of this experiment may be uncovered is a critical subject for researchers to continue pursuing in the years ahead. For those who wish not to be an unwilling, unwitting participant in this experiment, opting out will require much tedious effort to avoid the ubiquitous soy materials in the multitudes of processed foods. However, some will view it as not merely worthwhile, but also quite necessary to avoid being manipulated into ill health.

Chapter 16

Supplements and Superior Sex

BASIC SCIENCE

Sexual arousal for men occurs not just in the genitalia but in the whole body, and certainly begins at the brain level in response to sensory input, especially vision and touch and very likely also the sense of smell. Nerve impulses from the brain must travel down the spinal cord and out to the nerve ends that control the blood vessels serving the penis. There the impulses trigger production of a short-lived neurotransmitter known as nitric oxide (NO). Without those nerve impulses there can be no release of NO and no erection. That is why traumatic injury to the spinal cord generally will prevent a man from manifesting peripheral sexual arousal. Hindrance to the passage of the nerve stimuli to the sexual organ can arise from the adverse effect of beverage alcohol, either on an acute or chronic basis. This inhibitory effect of alcohol was recognized as long ago as the time of William Shakespeare, as shown by these famous lines (to students of pharmacology) from *Macbeth* (Act 2, Scene 3):

> Macduff: What three things does drink especially provoke?
>
> Porter: Marry, sir, nose-painting, sleep, and urine. Lechery, sir, it provokes and unprovokes; it provokes the desire, but it takes away the performance.

The neurotransmitter that carries the sexual arousal message in the central nervous system (brain and spinal cord) is acetylcholine. However, acetylcholine (ACh) seems to be too widespread and its function overly broad for a modification of its levels to be capable of significantly influencing sexual behavior. Despite the illogical basis, some supplement products recently have incorporated dietary factors designed to elevate the production of ACh. It can hardly be supposed that this would achieve the goal of improving libido and copulatory performance.

Consumer's Guide to Dietary Supplements and Alternative Medicines

doi:10.1300/5698_16

Normally, the presence of sexual stimulation causes blood flow to be directed into sinuses called the corpora cavernosa within the shaft of the penis. The inflow of blood leads to the enlargement and hardening of the penis—erection, or tumescence. This engorgement depends upon the NO being synthesized through enzymatic alteration of the amino acid arginine. NO in turn activates an enzyme that causes the production of cyclic guanosine monophosphate (cGMP), which is an intracellular signaling molecule. The normal action of cGMP then is to cause the smooth muscle cells in the wall of the arterial blood vessels to relax leading to dilation and the onset of an erection.

However, immediately following release of NO and the consequent production of cGMP, another enzyme, cGMP phosphodiesterase type 5 (PDE-5), becomes activated. It has its main role in the breakdown of cGMP nearly as quickly as it is formed. The result of the breakdown of cGMP by PDE-5 is a rapid reversal of the relaxation of the arterial smooth muscle, and consequently a reduction of blood flow to the penis, which allows a return to its flaccid state, detumescence.

IMPOTENCE AND THE VIAGRA ERA

In March 1998 the FDA approved a New Drug Application for sildenafil, soon to be world famous as Viagra. Sildenafil was initially investigated clinically in Europe as a medication for alleviating the pain of angina pectoris resulting from inadequate blood flow to the heart muscle through the coronary arteries. This was based upon laboratory data showing that it increased the release of the arterial-dilating chemical NO. The outcome of those experiments was discouraging, but London researchers became quite intrigued when many of the older men in the clinical trials insisted they did not wish to cease taking the drug because of their experiencing fully adequate erections, which they were no longer accustomed to having, and thus receiving a restoration of their sexual performance.

With certain types of disease or with aging the availability of cGMP decreases and become insufficient to support a normal level of response to sexual-arousing stimuli. Viagra acts to restore and maintain a capacity for responding with an erection by enhancing the level of production of NO and thus producing higher levels of cGMP. Viagra does this by a selective inhibition of the enzymatic action of PDE-5 so as to prevent its destruction of cGMP. This results in an elevated cGMP level in the corpora cavernosa. In turn, this maintains relaxation of the smooth muscle in the arteries of the corpus cavernosum, increases blood flow to the genitals during sexual stimulation, and leads to stronger erections of longer duration.

Five years after this unexpected finding Viagra was approved as a treatment for men suffering from difficulty in achieving erection (erectile dysfunction or ED). Men having a physical need for a PDE-5 inhibitor may also suffer from atherosclerosis, hypertension, and possibly heart disease. Thus, such men may have a heightened risk for acute adverse cardiovascular events. Prospective users taking certain vascular Rx drugs are warned against taking Viagra.

Aside from a possible risk of dying from an acute cardiovascular accident, a very small risk exists for the rare experience of priapism, an erection that may be sustained for hours and require medical attention because of the possibility for permanent damage. Also possible is a temporary retinal dysfunction consisting of an alteration in color vision. Otherwise, the main drawback for Viagra is its cost. However, this seems not to have been a serious impediment to sales. Free "starter packs" have been available through physicians to "prime the pump" for prescription purchases. Naturally, competing, supposedly improved items vardenafil (Levitra) and tadalafil (Cialis) were marketed by 2003.

IMPOTENCE AND THE PLACEBO EFFECT

Complaints of ED are common among men treated with Rx drugs known as beta-blockers for hypertension or other cardiovascular disease problems. However, evidence suggests that a high rate of sexual dysfunction exists in untreated men with cardiovascular disease compared to men of a similar age, which leaves the actual cause of ED with beta-blocker usage unclear. A study was designed by physicians in Italy to test whether this apparent side effect of beta-blockers might be related to patients' knowledge of drugs having a reputation for such unwanted effects (Silvestri et al., 2003). It involved 96 men of an average age of 52 years who were newly diagnosed with either hypertension (40 percent) or angina pectoris (60 percent), but without ED. The International Index of Erectile Function questionnaire was utilized at the outset and twice between phases of the study.

In the first phase of the research all patients received a beta-blocker (Atenolol 50 mg per day) for 90 days. However, they were divided into three equal-sized groups: group A was unaware of the drug given and uninformed of possible side effects, group B was informed of the nature of the drug but not of potential side effects, and group C was informed of the drug and its potential side effects. After the three months the rate of ED was 3.1 percent in group A, 15.6 percent in group B, and 31.2 percent in group C (significantly different). Thus, it appears that expectancy of an ED problem was responsible for a doubling of the experienced (or at least reported) ED rate. Those men who reported ED entered a second-phase study in which they were randomly assigned to receive sildenafil citrate (Viagra) at 50 mg or a placebo. The two treatments proved to be equally effective in reversing their ED. The researchers concluded that the occurrence of erectile dysfunction on beta-blockers is low, much lower than was commonly thought (only 3.1 percent). The results also suggest that not only the patient's but also doctor's expectations (through cues he may give to the patient) concerning the chance of experiencing ED as an unintended response may greatly influence reports of this bothersome side effect.

The Italian research illustrates how difficult it may be to obtain valid data that are uncontaminated by cognitive/psychological/mental influences. This display of the high importance of psychological factors, as in the placebo effect, should be kept in mind regarding aspects of the subject to be discussed in the following sections. Especially, one must consider that data could be quite misleading if not obtained within operation of a carefully designed research project. Anecdotal reports must be viewed as not certain to be reliable, if not certain to be unreliable.

THE VIAGRA-SUBSTITUTE ERA

Supposed Natural Alternatives for Viagra

"Safe, all-natural" products for treating impotence have proliferated in the wake of the launching of Viagra, especially after the reports of fatal reactions experienced by some men using it. It has been pointed out that the intrinsic cardiac acceleration entailed with sexual intercourse may by itself be the main risk for some men who might have no need for sildenafil if it were not for the presence vascular disease. This would be more so for men of advancing age, a factor that correlates with the greatest deficit in sexual function. Because of their age-related risk factors, elderly men may be living with atherosclerotic heart disease. Moreover, the risk has been deemed greatest for men using a therapeutic vasodilator for coronary insufficiency, nitrite, or nitrate-containing Rx drugs. Another high risk that is a contraindication for the use of Viagra is taking a drug of the alpha-blocker class for treating hypertension within the previous four hours.

However, if the natural formula really acts as often is claimed, by the exact same biochemical-pharmacological mechanism as Viagra, it makes no sense to claim that the formula is free from the unwanted side effects seen with Viagra, the most common of which are headaches, flushing, dyspepsia, nasal congestion, and transient disturbance of color vision/discrimination. Up to 30 percent of Viagra users experience a side effect, but those are usually described as transient. Most important, use of an Rx cardiovascular drug should be equally a contraindication for those formulas claiming to be its "natural equivalents;" their claims of greater safety than with a synthetic agent are not plausible.

L-Arginine

The supplement industry declares that a safer, less expensive, and more natural way to achieve the benefits of Viagra exists. In the 1990s, scientists discovered that L-arginine, a nonessential amino acid commonly found in protein foods, is the usual precursor for endogenous production of nitric oxide. Under conditions in which NO is synthesized for a specified physiologic purpose, the level of available L-arginine might in theory be a limiting factor. Taking of supplemental arginine serves to ensure that adequate supplies of the source for NO exist, and *may* ensure that adequate synthesis occurs.

Yohimbe (Yohimbine)

Another, much older approach involves the alkaloid yohimbine from the inner bark of the tropical West African tree *Coryanthe yohimbe.* For centuries a tea distilled from the inner bark of this tree has been used to amplify male sexual activity and pleasure and also as an aphrodisiac also for women according to some claims. Yohimbine blocks receptors in the blood vessels called alpha-2-adrenergic receptors that mediate vasoconstriction. When yohimbine shuts off their function it allows increased blood flow through arteries into the penis, and at the same time decreases blood flow exiting by way of its veins. Although this botanical material had been used at least since mid-twentieth century in pharmaceutical form "under the counter" in the United States before DSHEA, it was regarded by medical science as merely a placebo. No clear justification for the idea existed, as documentation of the effects of such shadowy products wasn't available.

An adverse aspect of such use for yohimbe might arise from a synergistic interaction with Rx medicinals for hypertension, leading to a dangerously excessive fall in blood pressure. Moreover, a user might experience synergism of other drugs being taken by virtue of yohimbine acting as a potent competitive inhibitor of a liver enzyme, CYP 2D6. This enzyme has been listed for fifty or more Rx drugs as the basis for their metabolism. Thus, interactions to amplify (or, less likely, to reduce) the effects of those compounds are theoretically quite possible (Klaasen et al., 1996). Some authorities regard yohimbine use as excessively risky.

Other Botanical Components

Those of us who studied pharmacognosy in the mid-twentieth century never heard about or dreamed that so many sex-enhancing plant materials could exist as are now being offered in the United States. The trend has clearly developed to cash in on the greater acceptance of remedies for ED that was created by the advent of Viagra. Being made more ready to believe by this advance of scientific medicine, men are offered numerous "natural alternatives" to Viagra that are, of course, touted to be more safe. These products are cloaked with an aura of reliability or believability by their having been discovered and brought to civilization from remote corners of the earth about which most of us have little or no knowledge. Who can judge whether it is true that this or that herb provides a potion that prevented an Amazonian jungle tribe from going into extinction? Besides arriving through the U.S. Postal Service, solicitations for erotic enhancement products now besiege our e-mail in-boxes as well. Let it be noted at the outset that the Western medical literature contains essentially no validation for clinical efficacy across the whole array of botanicals (as well as one mammalian material).

Ginkgo Extract

Ginkgo biloba leaf reputedly has been used in traditional Chinese medicine for more than 5,000 years. It is described as an energizer of the central nervous system, which may include an ability to enhance sexual urge (prolibido) and sexual vigor. It is said to improve circulation in a manner that may overcome ED through enhanced blood flow. A clinical study by Cohen and Bartlik (1998) found that *Ginkgo biloba* had benefits to 78 percent of men with ED problems concurrent with, and possibly caused by, use of an Rx antidepressant. The hindrance of sexual function by the SSRI group of antidepressants is a well-known and serious side effect for persons needing such medicines.

Korean Ginseng/Panax Ginseng

Similarly, *Panax ginseng* has traditionally been used to overcome conditions of general weakening by enhancing the persons' energy broadly. This is applied more specifically to a lack of vigor producing weakening of sexual power. It is said to oppose impotence, premature ejaculation, and even infertility (which should not relate to the former two). USSR physicians reportedly detected a stimulation of physical and mental activities that can improve both athletic performance and sexual behavior.

Maca Root

Derived from *Lepidium meyenii* (now *L. peruvianum*), maca is an Andean crop that is touted as the answer for female infertility and impaired male sexual vigor at extreme altitudes of human habitation in the Andes mountains of South America. It is also said to improve energy and vitality in general. These benefits were "confirmed" by a testimonial from a physician and former president of American College for Advancement in Medicine (ACAM) in one product's promotional piece. The plant is said to have as its active ingredient *p*-methoxyisothiocyanate, but other components might also be responsible, such as prostaglandins and sterols. The level of interest from Japan, Europe, and North America is so great that the Peruvian government has taken steps to ensure the country's monopoly on the source material.

Preparations containing maca in Peru range from soft drinks to pills or capsules, to liquid tonics, candies, and even mayonnaise! Another important biological activity claimed for maca is chemoprotection against carcinogenic chemicals. The lack of a recognized basis for its standardization, and thus for marketing a reliable, effective dosage, makes it very difficult to know if a product is worthy of trust. In short, some validity for maca being a sexual enhancer might exist, but for it to be promoted as enabling men to "feel the strength and virility of an Inca warrior flowing through your veins" is an outrageous example, although surely imaginative, of advertising hype. However, yet it does not go so far as to become a disallowed therapeutic claim.

Muira Puama Extract

This plant extract from the tree *Ptychopetalium olscoides* is another one new to the North American scene, but it actually was first known to Western scientists by 1925. It grows in the jungles around the Amazon River where the indigenous people reportedly have called it "potency wood" and used it for centuries to deal with impotence.

Sexual desires, actual sexual intercourse, and sexual fantasies was reported, as well as in satisfaction with the sex life, intensity of sexual desires, excitement of fantasies, ability to reach orgasm, and intensity of orgasm. Reported compliance and tolerability were good. These initial findings conform with the strong anecdotal reports of benefits of Herbal vX on the female sex drive. (So why is it being promoted in products for men?)

Puncture Vine (Tribulus terrestris) and DHEA

Tribulus, another "powerful plant extract," is said to act as a secretagogue to elevate the level of testosterone secretion via an increased output from the anterior pituitary of intersitial cell stimulating hormone (ICSH), a hormone that acts to stimulate certain cells of the testes to secrete testosterone. If the claims for (nonerect) phallic enlargement made by various products were correct, which is surely questionable, a supposed prohormonal action of this component would seem to be the most likely mechanism. Experiments in primates have supported an ability to increase testosterone, and research in rats has shown that the Tribulus-treated rats had an elevation of sexual vigor and performance (Gauthaman et al., 2003).

Avena sativa *(Wild Oats)*

With a popular name of "wild oats" how can a plant *not* have an erotic reputation?[1] But where are the facts to justify such a reputation? Based on a lack of published clinical papers, its reputation may indeed derive merely from its name. A 37-year search PubMed search showed not one paper relating this plant to sexual behavior. Supplement makers saying that *Avena* has been known to heighten libido, thoughts, and pleasure associated with sex seemingly must be relying on folklore. They go so far as to state a mechanism, saying that *Avena* acts on the hypothalamus to stimulate release of LH (the luteinizing hormone), which then stimulates production of testosterone, making the male sex hormone more available, especially for men over the age of 50 years.

Cordyceps Mushroom

Cordyceps sinensis is one of the most rare and treasured of natural products. It has been an important ingredient in Chinese medicine for thousands of years. Cordyceps is primarily collected from the wild because the cultivated type is of lower quality, but the wild cordyceps is very expensive, costing up to $1000 for 100 grams. Wild cordyceps from Tibet is supposedly the best in the world. Research reportedly has shown that the wild cordyceps is richer in certain components and also that the proportions of active components are different from those in the cultivated mushroom.

This might cause some differences in its activity. Nevertheless, even cultivated cordyceps is rather costly.

Cordyceps became famous because of its reputedly powerful anti-impotence as well as general tonic actions. It is said that recent studies performed in China and Japan have shown a 64 percent success rate among men suffering from impotence versus 24 percent in a placebo group. Such supposed findings seem not to have appeared in a western peer-reviewed journal.

A Nonbotanical Component: "Velvet" from Deer Antlers

This represents the epithelial covering of newly grown antlers, an ancient component of the Chinese traditional medicines that are directed at restoring of male potency and another example that "traditional components" can mean "animal" rather than "herbal" in such remedies. The growth of the antler is a remarkable physiological feat for which the velvet is a sustaining element. Some extraordinary level of growth factors supplied through the velvet must exist, but how or why should such activity transfer to a desired effect upon the genitalia (of either sex) as it does to the buck's fancy head adornment? No relevant sources were obtained from a search of the PubMed database.

Overview of Natural Products for Erectile Dysfunction

A review of this topic by McKay (2004) is worthy of note. Six of the 11 items previously described were covered. This did not involve meta-analysis for lack of an adequate database. Of the six it was concluded that L-arginine, yohimbine, *Panax ginseng, Ginkgo biloba,* and maca root "may provide moderate benefit," which might be derived from an enhanced nitric oxide action quite comparable qualitatively but not quantitatively to the action of the Rx inhibitors of PDE 5—Viagra and its competitors. Neither *Tribulus terrestris* nor its supposed metabolite, DHEA, were found to have been clinically evaluated sufficiently to support any conclusion on the issue of efficacy.

EROTIC ENHANCEMENT FOR WOMEN

Viagra was quickly seen as possibly providing similar benefits of enhanced sexual sensation and orgasmic enjoyment for women; it was reported to be in clinical trials for that purpose already by 2000. Dr. Myron Murdoch, clinical instructor of urology at George Washington University Medical Center (and national director of the Impotence Institute of America) has said "it's not for all women," but that a Viagra-like drug may aid the 20 percent of women who have a deficient lubrication because blood flow to the glands associated with the female genitals influences lubrication. It is unknown to what extent such a vascular action might benefit those women who report experiencing sexual dissatisfaction, female sexual dysfunction, because either they lack interest in intercourse or intercourse provides them little pleasure. However, this may change in a few years as drug companies are racing to develop a libido-enhancer for a very large, underserved female market. Survey results have supposedly suggested that 43 percent of women suffer from sexual dysfunction, compared to 31 percent of men. Some have projected a $2 to $3 billion level of spending during the next ten years for new pharmaceutical products serving to improve the sex lives of these women (Gearon, 2006). However, the Viagra source, Pfizer, announced on February 27, 2004, that trials involving about 3,000 women had been inconclusive, and thus no further research would be done on this line.

Some supposed authorities on female sexual dysfunction allege that, in contrast to most male ED problems, women's sexual dysfunctions are probably more psychological than physical in origin. However, as for men, adverse factors for women may include Rx drugs, especially the antihypertensives and antidepressants, and some OTC medicines, as well as abuse of alcohol and illegal drugs.

The new philosophy of the age is that women deserve equal rights to erotic enhancement. Physicians, psychiatrists, and sexologists have begun to recognize and name such female sexual problems as hypoactive sexual desire disorder (HSDD), female sexual arousal disorder, and female orgasmic disorder. An NCCAM project is underway to determine whether such conditions occurring consequent to the use of selective serotonin reuptake inhibitor antidepressants can be reversed by *Ginkgo biloba.* Some Rx agents are likely to be available from the pharmaceutical industry soon, if not already. However, supplement makers will probably have been there first.

These products may contain some 30 botanicals and nutrient components, making it impossible to foresee what interactions among them and between the formula's ingredients and any regular medication might occur. All of this and not a shred of evidence of results from testing for efficacy or safety. Bald-faced assertions such as this are to be accepted on the reputation of the (unnamed) MD who is purveying this breakthrough.

Testosterone to the Rescue!

Most recently tested was a patch for delivery of testosterone continuously through the skin at a lower dosage than the one used for men. A 24-

week, randomized, double-blind, multicenter study enrolled 533 women who all had undergone surgery-induced menopause and who were taking oral or transdermal estrogen replacement (Buster, 2004). Patients averaged 49 years old, were in stable relationships (mean of 18 years), and had experienced ovariectomy an average of nine years prior to the study entry. The patients were randomized to receive either a placebo patch or the female testosterone patch, which delivers 300 μg per day of testosterone. Patches were changed twice weekly.

The group getting the testosterone patch showed a 51 percent increase in frequency of "totally satisfying sexual activity," and a 49 percent increase in sexual desire relative to those measures for the placebo group. Significant increases were also seen in arousal, orgasm, pleasure, responsiveness, and self-image as well as decreases in level of distress and concerns for women using the female testosterone patch. Adverse events were similar between the testosterone and placebo groups. Although the overall incidence of androgenic events was low, the incidence was slightly higher in the testosterone group; however, these events were mild and did not lead to withdrawal from the study. More than 90 percent of adverse events were mild to moderate in intensity. It is estimated that one-third of surgically menopausal women experience low sexual desire and nearly half of the women in the study reported being distressed about it. Low desire is the most commonly reported sort of female sexual health complaint.

The study was conducted at the Baylor College of Medicine and 50 other centers in the United States, Canada, and Australia. Its sponsor was Procter & Gamble Pharmaceuticals, the developer of the testosterone patch for women, which was not yet approved by FDA. (On September 21, 2004, it was announced that the testosterone transdermal system for women, to be called Intrinsa, was granted priority review status by the FDA. It is foreseeable that when it is approved for surgically menopausal women, a considerably broader demand for the prescribing of it will occur on the part of pre- as well as postmenopausal women. Who knows? It may cause women more commonly to look and act as eager as the models performing in TV or print commercials for Viagra and company or other male sexual restorers!

On September 8, 2004, Cellegy Pharmaceuticals Inc. announced positive results from analysis of the Phase 2 study data using its topical gel product, Tostrelle, and having begun preparations for Phase 3 clinical trials. This product contains testosterone (0.5 percent) for topical treatment of postmenopausal women with low testosterone levels who are distressed by the symptom of diminished sexual desire. The study showed Tostrelle was safe, produced testosterone levels within the normal range for young women, and produced a 65 percent improvement over baseline in the number of satisfying sexual events (a 30 percent greater increase than for the placebo group). These findings were presented to the International Society for the Study of Women's Sexual Health meeting in October 2004 (www.centers watch.com). Moreover another gel product, LibiGel, of BioSante Pharmaceuticals Inc. is also in the offing for the same use.

Female Bodybuilding

In former times, bodybuilding, and the magazines catering to that interest, were a male domain. No more! The highly illustrated purveyors of bodybuilding products are out for the feminine market as well. Their up-to-date formulations for eliminating body fat for either sex while enlarging muscles have now changed their labeling to "ephedra free." Furthermore, formulas are now available that promise to enhance a "natural" level of gender-specific breast endowment for women. Many analogous promises have flooded e-mails with promotions for men concerned with their inches. Once again skepticism should prevail when bold assertions rather than objective evidence are the only basis for claims.

FATAL PURSUIT OF EROS (DEATH BY APHRODISIAC)

If the previously described formulations represent the up-to-date, high-tech sex enhancers, be reminded that older "low-tech" efforts in this area have been around for a long time. Moreover, their utilization likely was more hazardous than for the contemporary crop. The pursuit of sexual satisfaction can result in great risks, and at times a rapidly disastrous outcome. The use of a plant material that is represented as an enhancer of sexual desire or receptivity, i.e., a compound known as an aphrodisiac can have a negative result. Although a few foods have a folk reputation for erotic enhancement, it is rather clear that the intended action of most aphrodisiacs is one that is properly classified as pharmacological in its nature. Moreover, some agents used for this purpose turn out to show a definite toxicologic hazard. Our first example of this sort was reported in New York City in 1995 by the Centers for Disease Control and Prevention in the publication, *Morbidity and Mortality Weekly Report.*

Encounters with Chan Su

Between February 1993 and May 1995 the New York City Poison Control Center learned of illness in five previously healthy men after they swallowed a substance they had purchased, which was marketed as an aphrodisiac for *topical* use. As a consequence of their illness, four of the five men died from disturbed cardiac rhythms that progressed to the fatal outcome of ventricular fibrillation. A strange feature was that all five patients showed measurable blood levels of what seemed to be the heart drug digoxin, despite that none of them had been prescribed digoxin for therapeutic purposes. Considered in the following case reports for three of the five victims are the results of chemical analyses of the five initially mysterious cases (Brubacher et al., 1995). The severe potential hazards from using a botanical product without knowledge of its nature or its grounds for being regarded as safe are well illustrated by these cases. Such "street" products are unregulated, are not likely to have been tested, and the label (if any) may not show their contents, intended mode of use, or dose (Centers for Disease Control, 1995).

Case Report 1

A 26-year-old man swallowed one piece of the purported aphrodisiac material intended for topical application. Several hours later he developed vomiting, abdominal pain, and weakness. Sixteen hours after ingestion he sought medical care at an emergency room (ER). From an examination and the initial laboratory test results, including an elevated plasma level of potassium (hyperkalemia), a toxic ingestion was diagnosed, and the patient was treated for hypotension and hyperkalemia. However, his cardiac rhythm deteriorated from normal to atrial fibrillation, then to progressive sinus bradycardia. Ventricular fibrillation developed and the patient died in cardiac arrest seven hours after being admitted and about 20 hours after taking the purported aphrodisiac. Because of the hyperkalemia and cardiac dysrhythmias, blood taken before death was analyzed and found positive for digoxin (Centers for Disease Control, 1995).

Case Report 2

A 23-year-old man ingested a topical aphrodisiac purchased in a smoke shop. About 30 minutes later he began to show persistent vomiting and diarrhea. About 12 hours after ingestion he sought care at an ER. Upon examination he was alert and not severely agitated, but he was also sweating and in respiratory distress. Initial laboratory test results were not helpful, but an electrocardiogram showed an abnormal pattern, a right bundle branch block. Because of his respiratory failure, he was intubated and ventilated. During intubation his heart rate declined to 20 beats per minute, but after 1 mg of atropine it increased to 150 beats per minute. About three hours after arrival, he had onset of ventricular fibrillation. The patient died despite aggressive efforts to resuscitate, including injection of an antibody preparation acting as an antidote for digoxin. His blood tested positive for digoxin (Centers for Disease Control, 1995).

Case Report 3

A 17-year-old male ingested a dark brown cube sold as a topical aphrodisiac. One hour later he had onset of sustained vomiting. About 24 hours after ingestion he sought care at an ER, when his heart rate was slow, 48 beats per minute, and irregular. Because initial laboratory test results showed similarities with the prior cases, toxic ingestion was presumptively diagnosed. Tests showed an elevated serum digoxin level. He continued to have a slow heart rate and to vomit. Thirty-six hours after ingestion and 12 hours after admission the patient was treated with the antidotal antibody, and subsequently the vomiting ceased and the heart rate increased to as high as 70 beats per minute. The patient improved and was discharged (Centers for Disease Control, 1995).

Follow-Up Investigation

The New York City Department of Health and Mental Hygeine obtained three samples of the supposed aphrodisiac from family members of the ill persons and other sources. The substance was a hard, dark brown, roughly square piece of material measuring about 1 cm by 1 cm by 0.5 cm. Labels or instructions for use were not always provided when the material was purchased. Based on chemical analysis, all the samples were identical, and when dissolved they measured strongly positive for digoxin by chemical assay. Additional analysis of the samples detected several compounds classed as bufadienolides as well as bufotenin (a hallucinogen). Chan Su is described in traditional Chinese medicine sources as a topical anesthetic and cardiac remedy, and is known to contain bufadienolides. Therefore, samples of Chan Su were obtained from an importing company in New York City for comparative analysis. Based on physical examination and chemical analysis, the Chan Su samples and the topical aphrodisiac samples were found to be identical.

Various other cardioactive compounds (steroids in their chemical nature) besides the bufadienolides have a very narrow margin of safety. Inadvertent intoxications in the course of therapy have been recorded repeatedly. These steroids adversely alter function of the heart muscle, with their most life-threatening toxic effects being several types of altered rhythms and hyperkalemia (excess potassium levels). Cardioactive steroids occur in several nontraditional therapies—Chan Su, teas made from oleander *(Nerium oleander),* and foxglove *(Digitalis purpurea).* In New York City this product marketed as an aphrodisiac was sold under names such as "Stone," "Love Stone," "Black Stone," and "Rock Hard," and was available through grocery stores, smoke shops, and even vendors on the streets. The record is unclear as to whether the purported aphrodisiac was distributed throughout the United States. However, similar products had been seized from suspected drug traffickers also in Miami, Philadelphia, and Tampa, and in North Carolina and Virginia. The gross misrepresentation of Chan Su, for which no rationale as an aphrodisiac exists, provoked a dangerous misuse. The pursuit of Eros claimed four more victims. (These cases were investigated by the New York City Department of Health and Mental Hygeine, New York City Department of Environmental Protection, and the FDA.) (Centers for Disease Control, 1995).

Toxic Encounters with the Spanish Fly

Cantharidin, an active chemical component of preparations long known popularly as Spanish fly, is derived from the dried and crushed bodies of blister beetles, of which various species occur widely on several continents. It purportedly has been used as a male sexual stimulant and for correction of erectile impotence since the time of the ancient Greeks. Unfortunately, it continues to be used despite a total lack of validation for its reputation. Because of its false reputation as an aphrodisiac, Spanish fly has at times been administered to women unwittingly with the misguided belief that it will aid in their being seduced.

This material is most noteworthy for its having vesicant or blistering properties when it contacts skin or especially mucous membranes internally. It is fortunate that many commonly available preparations labeled as Spanish fly may be found to contain only negligible amounts, if any, of cantharidin. However, from time to time it becomes available in concentrations that are able to cause severe toxicity. The literature indicates that manifestations of cantharidin poisoning range from local blister formation to gross hematuria (blood in the urine), damage to the heart muscle, severe injury to the lining of the gastrointestinal tract, and occasionally death. In mid-twentieth century this material was responsible for outbreaks of multiple injuries and fatalities, most notably in South Africa.

Symptoms of poisoning from swallowing of cantharidin include burning and severe reddening of the mouth, difficulty in swallowing, nausea, bloody vomiting, and blood in the urine plus pain and difficulty in urinating. Mucosal erosion and bleeding occur in the upper gastrointestinal tract. Renal failure is a common result of gross injury to kidney structures. Convulsive seizures and cardiac abnormalities occur rarely. Because of irritancy in the urethra, an effect on the male sexual organ known as priapism—an abnormal penile erection that is long-sustained and frequently painful—may occur, which doubtless is the origin for the mythology of Spanish fly. Women do not report sexual arousal, but may develop urethral, vaginal, and rectal bleeding.

Case Report 4

A fatal poisoning with cantharidin developed in a 38-year-old male in Pavia, Italy, after his voluntary drinking of a cup of tea that contained three teaspoonfuls of the powder for aphrodisiac purposes (Polettini et al., 1992). Nearly immediately he experienced a burning feeling of his tongue and mouth accompanied by an intense flow of saliva and difficulty in swallowing. A few minutes later he vomited after feeling a burning substernal pain suggesting a gastric spasm. When he was hospitalized about one hour after he drank the toxic tea, he was lucid, clearheaded, and cooperative. His breathing was regular and blood pressure was normal, and his heart rate was 100 beats per minute. Staff observed caustic lesions about and in his mouth and throat. He was able to void some urine that was clear, not bloody. However, laboratory measures already indicated that kidney injury was developing.

Attempts to aid the mucosal irritation with a soothing (demulcent) drink failed because of his inability to swallow. For two hours charcoal-hemoperfusion, which consists of running blood via an external circuit through a charcoal column hoping to remove a toxicant, was conducted without benefit. Continuous intravenous infusion of fluid to help maintain circulation against shock was not effective. No urine was being passed, and the man became comatose and showed a strong bleeding tendency. About 30 hours after the ingestion circulatory collapse occurred despite the intensive therapy and he died. Autopsy findings included severe necrotic and hemorrhagic lesions of the mucosa of the oral cavity, pharynx, esophagus, and to a lesser extent, the stomach and duodenum. Moreover, a severe state of kidney damage was evident (Polettini et al., 1992).

Party Pitcher Poisoning

Four associated cases of cantharidin poisoning were reported from the division of emergency medicine at the Temple University School of Medicine in Philadelphia, Pennsylvania (Karras et al., 1996). This episode resulted when a cantharidin-containing liquid was added to a pitcher of Kool-Aid drink, the perpetrator apparently intending to perform a test for aphrodisiac properties. Patients came for assistance with complaints of painful urination, urgency, and frequency, as well as a dark-colored urine. The symptoms developed two to four hours after drinking from the pitcher and noticing a peculiar taste. All admitted to marijuana use, but denied other recreational drug use. Patients presented with abdominal pain and/or blood in the urine, and two had rectal bleeding. One 18-year-old woman had similar signs in addition to a vaginal discharge that contained red blood cells. A low degree of the potentially very threatening condition, disseminated intravascular coagulation (multiple small clots within the blood vessels), was noted in two patients. Fortunately, all recovered and were able to leave the hospital on the third day. Medical management of cantharidin poisoning is merely supportive, consisting mainly of vigorous infusion of intravenous fluids to overcome dehydration and to hasten elimination of the toxic agent since no antidote is available. Karras et al. (1996) ventured that "given the widespread availability of Spanish fly, and the fact that ingestion is frequently unwitting, cantharidin poisoning may be a more common cause of morbidity than is generally recognized."

Products Having Androgenic Effects

Testosterone administration is not generally regarded by medical experts in the field to have activity against "true" erectile dysfunction (ED) or impotence. Therefore, CAM products that are claimed to act indirectly by amplifying testosterone secretion from the patient's gonads cannot be assumed to be effective (Reiter and Pycha, 1999). What they are more able to do is to supplement is the libido—the desire for sexual contact—when it has been impaired by an unusual falling off of testicular function because of disease, injury, or aging. Thus, the androgens are indeed able to serve as "libido hormones," but they will not reverse an organic problem of organic erectile deficit, e.g., from peripheral neuropathy in a chronic alcoholic male, from long-time occurrence of diabetes leading to peripheral neuropathy, or from surgical or traumatic nerve damage to the pathways regulating blood flow to the penis.

Moreover, the safety of using such supplements supposedly acting as precursors to promote testosterone secretion is in serious question if they are used for a prolonged duration. The androgens have a potential to favor growth of an unrecognized prostate tumor, and their use would be contraindicated (forbidden) if a prostate cancer were known to be present. Indeed, a major aspect of therapy for cancers having their origin in the prostate is the elimination or antagonism of all androgenic hormone sources in the patient. This formerly meant surgical removal of testes and adrenal glands. However, in recent times this has been circumvented by the use of a hormone therapy that instead can achieve a "chemical castration." Because this commonly is done via inhibition of all the secretions of the anterior pituitary gland, diverse adverse responses are possible. The therapy must also inhibit secretion of androgenic products of the adrenal cortex, from which arises androgenic hormones and the precursor molecule, dehydroepiandrosterone, or DHEA.

Thus, DHEA is joined by "andro," for example, androstenedione, the supplement product made famous by an exceptional Major League Baseball home run hitter Mark McGwire. He focused attention on andros by admitting to using androstenedione during his record-breaking 70-home-run year in 1998. The three andros besides DHEA are mainly used by bodybuilders, mostly male and under 50 years of age. All of these are agents that are unlikely to aid true ED. One can readily believe that not all use of either

Viagra or andros is by men actually qualifying for a diagnosis of ED, but rather are aiming to improve upon what is already within the normal range, making such agents into "recreational drugs." The andros are not known to be free from adverse effects on a long-term basis in older men who seek a restoration of more youthful sexuality. Even more of concern is whether they carry even greater potential risks from continuing usage by adolescents or young adults for athletic advantage or for bodybuilding. The answer to this question is totally unknown. (This topic is treated also in Chapter 13.)

Chapter 17

Good Fat and Bad Fat

For the past three decades or more dietary fat and cholesterol have been very negative phrases for a large proportion of the populace in the United States, as well as whipping boys for writers on health matters. They have consistently borne only undesirable connotations. However, viewpoints have begun to shift. It is now broadly recognized that our national epidemic of obesity cannot be laid entirely at the door of our intake of fats, and probably not to a primary degree, but rather to a habitual excess of carbohydrates in our food and drinks—too much sucrose or starch. Now our intake of saturated fats and cholesterol is no longer the scapegoat for causing the arterial disease of atherosclerosis.

Neuroscience researchers have recently emphasized the dangerous possibility that a chronic low-fat diet may endanger nervous system health by causing a damaging deficit of fat. Fat storage deposits generally are thought to be strictly nonfunctional, but this is not at all the whole truth. Their purpose can be easily understood as the body's means of preparation for not merely a "rainy day" but for a long period of food becoming scarce or unavailable. Although the problem of hunger still persists in the United States, a more common problem is being overweight.

Looking across the animal kingdom we find some other major biological reasons for storing of fat other than a hedge against a time of deprivation. One circumstance, most notably seen among birds, is to prepare females for egg-laying, incubation of the eggs, and tending to the offspring after hatching. If such females have inadequate fat stores their annual reproductive efforts will be greatly hindered or prevented. For women, a parallel may be seen in that without a minimal level of fat in the body a woman will no longer ovulate, and thus cannot begin to reproduce. This occurs in women who develop anorexia nervosa or in women athletes who train extremely, minimizing their body fat and resulting in amenorrhea. Clearly, the fat-free female body undergoes severe disruption of the normal hormonal balance. However, large initial fat deposits at conception are not required for the hu-

Consumer's Guide to Dietary Supplements and Alternative Medicines

doi:10.1300/5698_17

man species to have successful reproduction if food intake is adequate during the course of gestation.

Another major need of animals for fat deposits is for their being available as energy supplies during long-distance travels, as in annual migratory movements. Many species of birds but also some large mammal species illustrate this situation. But again this is not a real need for the human species. If it were true that we could explain our national obesity as "pre-migratory fat deposition" (as it is called by bird biologists), many in our population would be ready for a very long trip! More accurate would be to call it *premortality* fattening. In the current sociocultural milieu, even walking about the neighborhood is avoided in favor of driving to the sports club for exercise sessions. Only a minority of "fringe folks"—hobbyists (e.g., wilderness hikers), avid exercisers, the financially deprived, or the homeless—do serious traveling on foot.

Stored fat does serve a cushioning, protective agent, at least for infants. It has been noted that in some crashes, even of airplanes, the only survivor tends be a young child. This has recently been explained as owing to the protective value of their cuddly "baby fat." One might wonder whether reverse of this applies in old age when fat stores are largely lost and falls can be very threatening to survival. Most persons who have survived to old age are the thinner folks who outlived the overweight members of their age group. On the other hand, some observations suggest that extreme thinness can be risky also. Overweight persons, especially when their fat concentrates in the abdomen, are at heightened risk for cardiovascular disease and thus are likely to have succumbed to atherosclerotic vascular diseases and other conditions associated with type 2 diabetes. One clear advantage of being overweight is that it tends to protect heavier persons (especially well-documented in women) against osteoporosis, whereas the small-framed, thin woman (or man) is likely to suffer from low bone density and a significantly greater risk of bone fractures.

"Functional fat" is most clearly seen in the central nervous system (CNS), the brain, and spinal cord, as well as some peripheral nerves. Without their normal structural fatty coating (myelin), most neurons cannot retain their healthy function of nerve impulse transmission. For example, multiple sclerosis is a neurological disease that results from demyelination, a loss of the fatty myelin coating of neurons in the brain. However, this disease is not thought to be related to any dietary fat deficit.

Some readers will recall hearing the phrase *fatty liver* with respect to the effects of chronic alcohol abuse. The significance of fat accumulation in this case is that it reflects injury to the liver and failure of normal metabolic mobilization of fat from the liver.

Moreover, recent research suggests that the adipocytes (fat cells) may actually function as a part of the immune system. Pig fat cells were exposed to interferon-gamma, a small protein produced by infection fighting T-lymphocyte cells. This resulted in the production by the fat cells of hormonelike proteins, called cytokines, which react to fight off disease. (However, as fat cells accumulate too much fat, they secrete too much of certain biochemicals and too little others, causing abnormalities that researchers suggest might lead to diseases such as diabetes and cancer.) A cell's responding to lymphokines by secretion of cytokines has previously been a "badge" of a cell being part of the immune system. Who would have expected it to be shown by a lowly fat cell! Perhaps this could explain the survival disadvantage seen for extreme thinness. Hooray for fat—in the appropriate degree and in desirable places.

IMPORTANCE OF SERUM CHOLESTEROL LEVELS AND DIETARY FATS

For decades the American public has been taught to fear cholesterol and foods that may tend to elevate it. The evidence is overwhelming that lowering the total cholesterol level by diet and/or by means of pharmaceuticals of the statin class can decrease the serious complications of coronary artery disease. Although the overall cholesterol level has significance, the ratio of high-density lipoprotein (HDL) cholesterol (good) to low-density lipoprotein (LDL) cholesterol (bad) is more crucial. Simply put, the goal set before us in more recent times has been focused on improving the HDL-to-LDL ratio in order to maintain a healthy cardiovascular system and avoid atherosclerosis and its blocking of arterial blood flow.

The mainline viewpoint has been that a diet low in fats would best tend to achieve this goal, along with the important aim of moderating body weight (Steinberg and Witztum, 1990). This concept and various other factors led to a dietary pattern of lowered fats, but at the expense of a higher intake of carbohydrates. However, this concept was challenged some years ago by Robert C. Atkins, MD. For 35 years he stubbornly maintained that it was not a result of overconsumption of fats but rather an excess of the simple and complex carbohydrates, sugars and starches, that was the main reason for the accelerating epidemic of obesity and type 2 diabetes in the United States over recent decades. He advocated diets higher in fat and protein and low in carbohydrates. As many other diets came and went, the Atkins diet gradually rose to prominence as being successful for achieving good eight reduction. For his persistent nonconformity to the "truth" as preached by others, over decades Dr. Atkins was criticized (and even taken to court) by "experts" against whose practices Atkins' methods were arrayed. He was called erroneous and a failure, but he lived to see his position become most popular. Meanwhile other approaches that tended not to oppose the increase of the percentage of carbohydrate have been stuck with having fiddled while Rome burned because of the national epidemic of obesity. Broad agreement now exists that excessive carbohydrates are strongly associated with that epidemic. The public's adherence to that view may be seen in the producers of breads and pasta type foods in the early years of the new millennium having suffered a significant downtrend of their sales, notably by early 2004. Their response has been a rush by the food industry to modify their products so as to claim a "low carb" label.

Dr. Atkins's position rose in the long-term because medical research and practice came more nearly to agree with his anti-carbohydrate views. However, currently our society must confront a major public health problem, which represents at least in part the legacy of those who denounced Atkins's views. It is much a legacy also of the American food processing and marketing industry that has made great profits at the expense of our citizens' health by their choices of the composition of their products and by the strategy of escalating serving sizes for fast foods and beverages.

Along the way it was recognized that not all fats were equally to be avoided (Kris-Etherton et al., 2000). For some time we have heard that saturated fats were the "bad guys" by contrast with the "good guys" of unsaturated fats. More recently these distinctions have been refined to distinguish between trans and nontrans (i.e., cis) unsaturated fatty acids. According to the FDA, scientific evidence shows that it is largely the consumption of trans fats that raises "bad" cholesterol levels and thus increases the risk of coronary heart disease. Scientific reports have confirmed a relationship between trans fat and an increased risk of coronary heart disease. Food processors had already been required to list information revealing the overall fat and saturated fat content on the nutrition facts panel of foods, but on July 9, 2003, the FDA issued a regulation calling for food packaging to specify the content of trans fat for the sake of consumers who may wish to make more healthful ("heart healthy") choices by avoiding it. The FDA statement indicated, in part:

> Trans fat occurs in foods when manufacturers use hydrogenation, a process in which hydrogen is added to vegetable oil in order to turn the oil into a more solid fat. Trans fat is often but not always found in the same foods as saturated fat, such as vegetable shortening, some margarines, crackers, candies, cookies, snack foods, fried foods, baked goods, salad dressings, and other processed foods. (FDA, 2003b)

The FDA has estimated (a most remarkable feat) that in three years the new trans fat labeling will have prevented from 600 to 1,200 cases of coronary heart disease and 250 to 500 deaths per year. They further estimate that the change in labeling will save between $900 million and $1.8 billion each year in medical costs, lost productivity, and pain and suffering (FDA, 2003a).

ANTIOXIDANTS, FATS, AND HEART DISEASE

For some time there has been evidence pointing to a critical role for oxidative changes in LDL cholesterol for the pathology of atherosclerosis to proceed in arteries of the heart and brain. This has provided the theoretical basis for using antioxidant therapy to reduce one's risk for cardiovascular (CV) disease. This flows from the oxidative modification hypothesis of Steinberg and colleagues (1999). Their hypothesis assumes that unoxidized LDL is not particularly harmful, but once the LDL lipoprotein is altered by oxidation they cannot be recognized by the LDL receptors in the blood vessels and are instead taken up by scavenger receptors. The cells having scavenger receptors become overloaded with LDL cholesterol and are transformed into foam cells, which are the cellular hallmark of atherosclerosis. If the oxidative modification hypothesis were true, logically one would not have to worry about cholesterol intake or cholesterol levels if one had enough antioxidant molecules to prevent the oxidative changes. This leads to the current emphasis on supplemental antioxidant regimens. However, the hypothesis is contradicted by some data and still not fully confirmed.

Both alpha-tocopherol (vitamin E) and beta-carotene (vitamin A) have been studied in clinical trials for their ability to reduce the rate of CV events and of mortality. Neither one has given a clear-cut response. Vitamin E therapy decreased the incidence of heart attacks but not of mortality. A lower risk for cancer and heart disease has been shown both in observational studies of individuals with diets that contained more fruits and vegetables, but also in epidemiological studies of person with higher serum beta carotene levels. These findings suggested that beta carotene supplementation would be beneficial. However, a study of 29,000 Finnish male smokers supplementing with beta carotene showed no significant effect on coronary mortality or on the incidence of new angina pectoris, but was associated with an 8 percent *increase* in total mortality and an 18 percent *increase* in lung cancer. One commentator has suggested that the use of these agents cannot be expected to duplicate benefits seen for dietary intake of high amounts of the complex mixtures of vegetable antioxidants in the A and E families.

Key healthful nutrients and botanicals that can help to promote a healthy HDL-to-LDL ratio include, perhaps most important, the natural phytosterols. This term covers a group of "plant sterols and stanols." Especially high sterol levels are found in rice bran, wheat germ, corn oils, and soybeans. More than 40 phytosterols exist, but beta-sitosterol is the most abundant, comprising about 50 percent of dietary phytosterols. They have a chemical structure similar enough to that of cholesterol to enable them to oppose the uptake of dietary cholesterol, blocking it from being absorbed into the blood. Moreover, they can also block the reabsorption of endogenous cholesterol from the gastrointestinal tract where it appears in the bile secretions. Recently, functional foods containing phytosterols have become available in the form of margarines, spreads, and salad dressings. In most such products the phytosterols are found combined (esterified) with long-chain fatty acids. As "sitosterols complexe" or as beta-sitosterol they can be used as supplement capsules, which are derived from soybean oil and consist mainly of beta-sitosterol, campesterol, and stigmasterol. Adverse reactions to phytosterols are mainly mild gastrointestinal ones, including indigestion, feeling of fullness, gas, diarrhea, and constipation. However, phytosterol supplementation is generally well tolerated.

Three exceptional exogenous antioxidants exist that can oppose adverse effects of LDL-cholesterol. They are antioxidants that oppose the oxidation The LDL: grape seed extract, tocotrienols, and lutein. These protective antioxidants may be combined with phytosterols to provide optimal opposition to elevated cholesterol levels and their contribution to overall cardiovascular system poor health.

PHYSIOLOGICAL AND THERAPEUTIC ROLES OF OMEGA-3 FATTY ACIDS

Polyunsaturated fatty acids (PUFAs) can be divided between the "good guys" and the "not-so-good guys," represented, respectively, by the omega-3 and omega-6 fatty acids (FAs). Both of these include one important essential fatty acid (EFA) as well as others that also act as precursors of a number of regulatory agents known broadly as eicosanoids, more specifically as prostaglandins, thromboxanes, and leukotrienes (see Exhibit 17.1). The current U.S. diet generally contains such a great excess of omega-6 fats relative to the level of omega-3 fats that the omega-6 type becomes the "not-so-good guys." This ratio of omega-6–to–omega-3 fats is nearly the reverse of what seems to be desirable and optimal. A diet that has a high omega-6 to omega-3 ratio provokes a biochemical imbalance that favors inflammation and undesirable immune system actions.

EXHIBIT 17.1. Reported adverse effects of inadequate dietary Omega-3 FA intake.

Cardiovascular System

Higher degree of platelet aggregation
Higher risk for hypertension
Higher plasma levels of triglycerides
Greater blood vessel constriction
Higher risk of coronary artery disease
Increased risk for sudden cardiac death

Central Nervous System

Higher risk for major depression
Greater incidence of bipolar disorder
More episodes of mood instability
Higher risk for autistic disorder
Poor quality of sleep, daytime fatigue
Difficulty in concentration

Musculoskeletal System

Greater rate of rheumatoid arthritis
Higher risk for inflammatory disorders

Miscellaneous Symptoms

Weight gain
Dry hair
Brittle fingernails
Dry skin
Allergies

Source: Modified from Stoll (2001).

Experts studying the subject of dietary ratio of omega-6 to omega-3 FAs suggest that in ancient human history a dietary intake ratio of about one-to-one prevailed. The time of the industrial revolution showed a marked increase in this ratio of omega-6 to omega-3 fats in the diet. This probably reflected the advent of the modern vegetable oil industry as well as the increased use of cereal grains for fattening beef cattle. Unquestionably, many Americans currently eat a diet that produces a ratio of omega-6 to omega-3 rising to and even above 20 to 1. The optimal ratio presumably lies much closer to the supposedly "original" ratio, 1 to 1. For most persons resolving this problem calls for a great reduction in the omega-6 fatty acids eaten plus an increase of the amount of omega-3 fatty acids consumed. Sixty percent of the U.S. population eats fats at a ratio in the range from 8 to 1 to 12 to 1. However, the value may rise as high as 20 to 1 or 25 to 1 in some persons. The average ratio of omega-6 to omega-3 fat intake in the United States is said to be 9.8 to 1—much higher than recommended (2.3 to 1).

Therapeutic oils rich in omega-6 fats are derived from plants, include evening primrose oil (EPO), borage oil, black currant seed oil, and flaxseed oil. Omega-6 containing oils that are beneficial are those providing the essential linoleic acid. These are converted in the body to gamma-linoleic acid (GLA), arachidonic acid, and ultimately to certain of the prostaglandins, hormonelike molecules that affect the regulation of blood pressure and inflammation as well as the functions of the heart, gastrointestinal tract, and kidneys. More ordinary dietary sources of omega-6 fatty acids include cereals, eggs, poultry, most vegetable oils, whole-grain breads, baked goods, and margarine.

The healing powers of a number of therapeutic oils rich in omega-6 FAs—EPO, borage oil, black currant seed oil, and flaxseed oil among them—can be attributed to their high concentrations of GLA, which is converted into prostaglandins that can oppose inflammation. Supplements such as borage oil and evening primrose oil help to dampen inflammation because they are GLA rich. This can make them an attractive therapy for inflammatory conditions.

Specifically, omega-6 fatty acid sources with a high GLA content may help to the following:

- Reduce the discomfort of rheumatoid arthritis (Darlington and Stone, 2001). By promoting "good" prostaglandins, omega-6 FAs oppose the painful inflammation of joints in rheumatoid arthritis. By using a conventional prostaglandin-inhibiting anti-inflammatory drug (NSAIDs such as ibuprofen) simultaneously, the effects of both will be increased.
- Relieve the discomforts of premenstrual syndrome (PMS), endometriosis, and fibrocystic breasts. By their promoting "good" prostaglandins and blocking the "bad" variety released during the days before and during menstruation, omega-6 supplementation may be helpful in reducing uncomfortable menstruation-related symptoms such as breast tenderness, bloating, or cramps. Many PMS sufferers are found to have unusually low levels of GLA in their system, which may be why supplements rich in this omega-6 fatty acid seem to be helpful. Moreover, women with fibrocystic breasts frequently have low levels of iodine. GLA appears to enhance the absorption of iodine, which may help to explain its usefulness in fibrocystic breast syndrome.

- Reduce the symptoms of eczema and psoriasis. The essential fatty acids among both the omega-6 and omega-3 fats are important for healthy skin and hair; they are probably beneficial for virtually any chronic skin problem. For inflammatory skin conditions such as eczema and psoriasis, PUFAs may serve a dual purpose, serving as natural anti-inflammatories and as nutrients for healthy skin cells.
- Clear up acne and rosacea. GLA (as well as the omega-3s) in supplements such as borage oil may reduce the risk for pores being clogged and lesions developing. The essential fatty acid helps to treat rosacea by reducing inflammation, controlling the cells' use of nutrients, and by producing prostaglandins that stimulate the contraction of blood vessels.
- Prevent and improve diabetic neuropathy. People with diabetes cannot form GLA from the linoleic acid and as a result develop a deficiency of GLA. Research has shown that GLA supplementation in people with diabetes improves nerve function and may prevent painful neuropathy from occurring.

What might be the consequences of a dietary imbalance between the two groups of fatty acids? Scientific researchers are still in the process of establishing the answer to that question, not having reached a consensus viewpoint. However, more and more evidence is accumulating to suggest that a variety of modern human ills may result from this dietary imbalance. Examples suggested by some research are seen in Exhibit 17.1.

It is important to realize that the populace gets all the unsaturated omega-6 and omega-9 fats that we need from our present food intake. No supplements need to be taken to acquire these fats. Indeed, intake of some omega-6 fat supplements available in health food stores would serve to worsen health, not to improve it. This is because their intake raises the ratio of omega-6 fat to omega-3 fats. Thus, some authors recommend the reduction of usage for sunflower, corn, soy, safflower, and canola oils or products containing them. Hydrogenated or partially hydrogenated fats, margarines, vegetable oils, or shortening are not desirable because of their high content of omega-6 fats as well as their trans-FA content. Acceptable oil sources include high quality extra-virgin olive oil, coconut oil, avocados, and butter *if* it is made from milk supplied by grass-fed cows. Because nearly all beef cattle now are grain fed for weeks before slaughter, the benefits of earlier grass feeding will be lost. The beef resulting will typically supply predominantly omega-6 and very little omega-3 fatty acids and thus will of itself harm the dietary ratio. Fully grass-fed beef is available only through a limited number of special suppliers. Grass-fed bison meat is a healthful alternative that has a favorable fat chemistry and supposedly an added flavor bonus.

Dietary Recommendations for Omega-3 Fats

No "official" dietary recommendations have been made for omega-3 fats in the United States. However, Canada and the United Kingdom have such guidelines. Canada recommends a total omega-3 fat intake of 1.2 to 1.6 grams per day, which is similar to the recommendations of nutrition scientists in the United States, which do not distinguish between individual omega-3 fats. The United Kingdom does make a distinction among omega-3 fats, recommending that 1 percent of energy be obtained as ALA and 0.5 percent be from the combined levels of eicosapentaenoic acid (EPA) and docosahexaenoic acid (DHA).

Dietary Omega-3 Cardiovascular Health Claims Approved by FDA

On September 8, 2004, the FDA announced the approval of a qualified health claim for reducing the risk of coronary heart disease (CHD) by conventional foods that contain the omega-3 fatty acids EPA and DHA, which are contained in oily fish, such as salmon, lake trout, tuna, and herring. This will allow foods to bear a statement: "Supportive but not conclusive research shows that consumption of EPA and DHA omega-3 fatty acids may reduce the risk of coronary heart disease. One serving of [name of food] provides [x] grams of EPA and DHA omega-3 fatty acids" (FDA, 2004). In 2000, FDA announced a similar qualified health claim for dietary supplements containing EPA and DHA and the reduced risk of CHD. The FDA recommends that consumers not exceed more than a total of three grams per day of EPA and DHA omega-3 fatty acids, with no more than two grams per day from a dietary supplement. (For additional information, see FDA [2006].)

Researchers from Zurich, Switzerland, employed the phrase "Alpine paradox" as an analogy to the "French paradox" whereby a geographically-circumscribed human population shows the distinction of better-than-expected cardiovascular health, which is apparently because of a dietary factor. In this case Christa B. Hauswirth and co-authors (2004) provided evidence supporting their view that Alpine cheeses are the source of the Alpine paradox, the low cardiovascular disease rates among Swiss people. Alpine cheeses are those made from milk of cows feeding on grasses of Alpine meadows, which endows the resulting cheese with a more favorable FA profile, namely a high amount of alpha-linolenic acid (ALA), which serves the cow as precursor of the important omega-3 FAs, EPA and DHA.

Dietary Sources of Omega-3 Fats in the U.S. Diet

Not having ready access to Alpine cheeses, the sources of omega-3 fats in those eating the common U.S. diet are vegetable oils and, more important, fish oils that are the major source of EPA and DHA, and vegetable oils are the major source of ALA. Other sources include nuts and seeds, vegetables and some fruits, egg yolk, meat, and poultry. However, all of those dietary components together contribute only a small amount of omega-3 fats to the diet.

Of the commonly consumed oils in the United States, soybean and canola oil are the primary sources of ALA. The contents of ALA in soybean and canola oil are merely 7.8 percent and 9.2 percent, respectively. Flaxseed oil is a particularly rich source of omega-3 fats (ALA), but it is not yet a commonly used food oil. However, it is available as a dietary supplement product, which incorporates the oil into soft gelatin capsules or provides the oil in a dark bottle to oppose oxidation. Refrigeration is also desirable to ensure freshness, i.e., to prevent the oxidation that makes it rancid.

In October 2004 ConsumerLab reported on their analyses of 41 omega-3 oil products. Three of the products failed the tests, some did not contain their labeled amounts of omega-3 fatty acids, and one was rancid. The good news is that none of the products was contaminated with mercury or PCBs, unlike popular marine fishes that may be eaten for their omega-3 content (ConsumerLab.com, 2004).

For Future Reference, or for Now?

Common or green purslane, also called pigweed *(Portulaca oleracea),* is a succulent plant that is commonly regarded as a troublesome garden weed today but which has been used as a food and medicinal herb for more than 2,000 years (Phillips, 1995). Purslane is a uniquely rich source of alpha-linolenic acid (ALA), the richest among all known green leafy vegetables that have been examined, but it seems not to have been exploited as a supplement product source. Moreover, it is one of the few plant sources of EPA, and, besides the omega-3 components, it shows a good level of carotenoids. A PubMed search (1966 to June 2004) yielded nine papers relevant to the FA nutrient and antioxidant contents of purslane (for information on purslane see www.ipm.ucdavis.edu/PMG/WEEDS/purslane.html).

Tender young leaves and stems are eaten in soups and salads or are steamed, sauteed, or pickled by peoples around the Mediterranean basin and in the Middle East. It is also said to have been a part of the diet of the Australian aborigines. It is believed to be generally free of toxic effects, but the content of oxalate and nitrate could cause poisoning if used in excessive quantities. The plant is native to the region of southern Asia but has spread to Europe and even to the New World. Although not commonly consumed in the U.S. diet, purslane is found growing wild as a weed in all 50 states, and thus seemingly could be developed as an important source of dietary omega-3 fats. Jan Phillips (1995) in her *Wild Edibles of Missouri* presents tasty-sounding recipes for purslane use in salad or casserole forms.

Supplement Sources of Omega-3 Fats

A variety of omega-3 fat supplements are now made available to consumers. Most of these are derived from marine oils, usually containing 180 mg EPA and 120 mg DHA per capsule. Another source of omega-3 fats is cod-liver oil in soft gelatin capsules that may contain 173 mg EPA and 120 mg DHA. An industry source estimates that 300 tons of fish oil are used annually for fish-oil supplements in the United States. The average yearly intake of EPA and DHA from fish oil supplements in the U.S. diet is merely 0.6 to 0.9 mg per person. Thus, for most persons fish oil supplements are not now a significant source of omega-3 fats.

Fats for Cooking Oil

Olive oil is a monounsaturated oil, meaning that it has one carbon-to-carbon link that has not been saturated with hydrogen—the process that produces trans-fatty acids. Thus, olive oil would clearly be a more healthful choice of oil for use in deep-frying of fast foods, but it would be much too expensive, besides its having a distinctive taste that does not appeal to everyone. A study from the University of Barcelona reported that virgin olive oil also supplies high levels of vitamin E and flavonoids—biologically active compounds that are strong antioxidants. The study concluded that virgin olive oil might inhibit the oxidation of LDL cholesterol, suggested to reduce the risk of cancer.

An Omega-3 Marvel Source from Down Under?

Researchers in New Zealand and Australia have found that a marine bivalve mollusk, the green-lipped mussel *(Perna canaliculus)* harvested from New Zealand waters, has an analysis of fats and fatty acids more favorable than for vegetable oils and marine fish oil sources. Polyunsaturated fatty acids were the main group of fatty acids most of which were omega-3 fatty acids (40 to 41 percent). Saturated fatty acids comprised about 25 percent of total fatty acids. The major fatty acids were DHA (19 percent) and EPA and palmitic acid (15 percent).

A patented extract from *Perna canaliculus* (Lyprinol) has been produced and introduced into commerce as a therapeutic nutraceutical. A chemical analysis was run at RMIT University, Melbourne, Victoria, Australia, to provide a comparison between the composition of the oil derived from the New Zealand green-lipped mussel (Lyprinol) and two other oils rich in omega-3 fatty acids, flaxseed oil and tuna oil (Sinclair et al., 2000). The main lipid classes in Lyprinol were sterol esters, triglycerides, free fatty acids, sterols, and phospholipids, whereas the main lipids in the other two oils were triglycerides. The main omega-3 fatty acids in Lyprinol were EPA and DHA, whereas in flaxseed oil and tuna oil the main omega-3 fatty acids were ALA and DHA, respectively. The main sterols in Lyprinol were cholesterol and desmosterol (brassicasterol), and in flaxseed oil and tuna oil the main sterols were beta-sitosterol and cholesterol, respectively. According to current thinking, the profile of Lyprinol should be considered superior, although those of the others are surely favorable and healthful.

A nutrition researcher at the University of California–Davis (Halpern, 2000) reported that when two strains of rats were pretreated orally with Lyprinol they did not develop either of two types of experimentally induced arthritis. This was achieved with lower doses than for NSAIDs, and a dose 200 times less than is required for other seed or fish oils that supply PUFAs. Lyprinol inhibited activities of two types of white blood cells, neutrophils and macrophages. Much of its anti-inflammatory activity was associated with omega-3 and natural antioxidants. In contrast to NSAIDs, Lyprinol causes no gastric toxicity in stressed rats at a high dose (300 mg/kg), and does not alter platelet aggregation in rats or human subjects. The author's conclusion was that:

> clinical studies have shown very significant anti-inflammatory activity in patients with either osteoarthritis or rheumatoid arthritis, asthma, and other inflammatory conditions. Lyprinol is a reproducible, stable source of bioactive lipids with much greater potency than plant or marine oils currently used as nutritional supplements to ameliorate signs of inflammation. (Halpern, 2000, p. 272)

Lyprinol has been tested for therapeutic value mainly in osteoarthritis patients. In a small two-month trial in Seoul, South Korea, 60 patients with symptomatic osteoarthritis of the knee and hip received Lyprinol twice a day (Cho et al., 2003). The treatment led to a significant improvement of the signs and symptoms of osteoarthritis as determined by each of four efficacy measures, and without negative effects. The researchers concluded that

Lyprinol was very effective and that it constitutes a promising anti-inflammatory therapy relieving the signs and symptoms of osteoarthritis without adverse effects. Without any indication, we must wonder whether this study, reported in French allergy journal, was a nonrandomized, open trial lacking blinding and placebo control, which would weaken its impact.

An extensive review on antioxidants and fatty acids for the treatment of rheumatoid arthritis and osteoarthritis appeared in the *British Journal of Nutrition* (Darlington and Stone, 2001). The authors concluded that the "classical" dietary antioxidants—vitamin C, the tocopherols, beta-carotene, and selenium—are beneficial at high doses, especially in osteoarthritis. They indicate that PUFAs, including the omega-3s, some of which are precursors in eicosanoid synthesis, suppress cytokine formation so that the omega-3 FAs oppose the inflammatory effects of some omega-6 FAs, which increase the formation of two proinflammatory cytokines (TNF-alpha and interleukin-6) and of reactive oxygen species. That gamma-linolenic acid (GLA) is a precursor of prostaglandin E1 may explain its reported ability to improve arthritic symptoms. Fish oils rich in omega-3 FAs such as EPA also have been claimed to alleviate rheumatoid arthritis, possibly by suppression of the immune system and its role in the disease process. The marine oil from green-lipped mussels, and even from some vegetable oils (e.g., olive oil and evening primrose oil), appear to exert an indirect anti-inflammatory action, probably mediated via prostaglandin E1. Darlington and Stone (2001) voiced a conclusion on supplements and arthritis that is noteworthy: "overall, there is a growing scientific rationale for the use of dietary supplements as adjuncts in the treatment of inflammatory disorders such as rheumatoid arthritis and osteoarthritis" (p. 251).

Chapter 18

Cancer Cures: Are They Believable?

> The reason alternative cancer treatments are not yet mainstream has little to do with alleged therapeutic ineffectiveness and far more to do with political control over the therapy marketplace. Successful alternative approaches to cancer are a direct financial threat to this system. The politics of cancer have an overriding influence on the science of cancer and, ultimately, on what the public thinks about cancer treatment options.
>
> Burton Goldberg, MD (2000)

The one area of unconventional medicine that has provoked the most emotionally negative response and outright hostility from health care professionals is that of the purported unconventional "cancer cures."[1] People working in the realm of conventional medicine seem convinced that everything other than the conventional therapies is fraudulent and can only deceive and arouse false hope for those patients and their loved ones who might pursue them. Rightly enough they feel that persons who knowingly are deceiving people by offering invalid practices and promises are reprehensible in their behavior. However, the opinion that all of those providing such practices are knowingly misleading and offering false hope is very possibly untrue in some unknown proportion of cases. It is an extreme position replete with hubris to suppose that all who advocate alternative therapies are knowingly fraudulent—that none are genuinely believing in the therapy that they endorse and supply.

It may be anticipated that antiquackery forces will contend that persons who are unknowingly offering useless therapies are guilty of being willfully ignorant, and still are worthy of equal condemnation. True enough, physicians who use or promote unproven therapies may be sincere but self-deceived as to the validity of their practices. If current self-appointed "quack-busters" condemn all such physicians, very few of their esteemed predecessors would escape condemnation. Moreover, it is possible that

Consumer's Guide to Dietary Supplements and Alternative Medicines

doi:10.1300/5698_18

some unknown aspects of unconventional cancer therapies will eventually be validated by appropriate research not yet conducted. In the meantime, these treatments may enhance, interfere, or have no interactions with standard cancer therapy. Some of the CAM therapies are indeed said to improve symptom control with minimal or no side effects.

However, some CAM cancer approaches may have dangerous adverse effects or may potentially interfere with standard therapy, but it is of greatest concern that if used alone they may indirectly harm the patient by preventing or delaying the use of clinically validated standard treatments. This is not relevant to cancer sufferers for whom no conventional approach is deemed feasible for use—those for whom CAM offers a "last hope." Who is to say that should be denied to them?

A BRIEF VIEW OF CONVENTIONAL THERAPIES

Admittedly, medical research has not found a magical silver bullet to defeat all or most cancers as some might have anticipated from the "War on Cancer" of the past 40 or 50 years. But to minimize the great strides that have been made against cancer is also not realistic. Sixty years before this writing, as mid-twentieth century was approaching, *no* drugs proven to be anticancer agents existed. The only accepted, conventional therapies were surgery and radiation. By the outset of the new millennium at the turn of the twenty-first century about 75 such agents existed in about 15 subclasses as well as many more undergoing clinical trials.

Many of these individual chemicals and groups were indeed developed from natural sources—antibiotics from fungi, hormones from mammals, an enzyme derived from a bacterium, genetically engineered mammalian antibodies, and alkaloids or other classes of phytochemicals from herbaceous plants. The latter group includes the important agents vincristine and vinblastine, found in and developed from the periwinkle, *Vinca rosea* (now known as *Catharanthus roseus*). The mayapple *(Podophyllum peltatum)* yielded podophyllotoxin derivatives, and the Pacific yew tree *(Taxus brevifolia)* provided paclitaxel (Taxol). The group known collectively as camptothecins comprise a newer class of anticancer agents that originated from camptothecin, which was isolated from the bark of a Chinese tree. It was so poorly soluble and caused such significant toxicity that several more soluble and less toxic derivatives were developed. Such chemotherapeutic advances as these are in addition to significant advances toward a more effective use of surgery and radiation. Furthermore, new immunologic therapies are progressing toward becoming significant aspects of cancer therapy.

Today it is possible to list a number of cancers for which a significant chance of a curative outcome can be attained from antineoplastic drugs alone or in conjunction with surgery and/or irradiation. These are divided between the cancers of childhood and those typically occurring in adults (Calabresi and Parks, 1985):

Children: acute leukemias, Wilms' tumor, Ewing's sarcoma, retinoblastoma, and rhabdomyosarcoma.

Adults: Hodgkin's disease, diffuse histiocytic lymphoma, Burkitt's lymphoma, mycosis fungoides, testicular carcinoma, and choriocarcinoma in women.

These lists do not include the tumor types for which cures may occur, but quite rarely; those for which survival is significantly prolonged; or those in which palliation (symptomatic benefit) is known to be possible.

On the dark side, current chemotherapeutic drugs typically have a daunting number of severe adverse effects as shown in the following list.

Hematologic	***Epithelial***	***Central nervous system***
Bone marrow suppression that leads to deficiency of white blood cells and higher-than-normal susceptibility to infections	Loss of hair	Headache
	Lesions in the mouth	Dizziness
	Damage to the mucosal cells that line the digestive tract resulting in bloody diarrhea	Nausea
		Pain
		Fatigue
		Shivering

Most available anticancer agents are by definition cytotoxic, or oriented to killing cells. Their specificity is mainly based on their killing the more rapidly reproducing cells of cancers. However, the human body normally maintains a rather frequent replacement (high turnover rate) for certain cell types, which means that high turnover occurs not merely in cancerous growths but also in the healthy bone marrow, the skin (including the hair), mucosal cells of the digestive tract and genitourinary tract, and sex cells of the ovary or testis. Because of this, adverse effects are likely to occur through injury to those normal cells and tissues that show rapid cell turnover, as a parallel to the therapeutic action against cancer cells. New mechanisms for opposing cancer that avoid this catch-22 are needed. Some seemingly are now on the horizon.

However, for the individual patient diagnosed with cancer, these facts are not at all consoling, especially when an existing therapy is not available for them or if what is available has little chance for significant benefit. Early diagnosis is still the fundamental key to success in surviving cancer. The later the stage of progression of the disease at discovery, the worse is the outlook for effective surgery or eradication of the disease by radiation or chemotherapy. A bad prognosis is commonly seen, often correctly, as a death warrant. Seeking alternatives in the face of a hopeless prognosis is a natural reaction to an absence of hope from the viewpoint of conventional medical and surgical possibilities. People in this situation, or sometimes even more medically positive ones, decide to look beyond conventional therapies to unconventional ones. These provide offers of hope for benefits via alternative therapy when none is foreseen otherwise.

THE NATURE OF THE CHALLENGE

The reader doubtless realizes that cancer is very difficult to eradicate through chemotherapy, but may not have a full appreciation of the task, which is one of achieving selective toxicity to an extremely high degree. The therapeutic aim is to kill all the cancer cells while not killing the patient from lethal effects on the normal cells of vital organs. Examining some numbers will provide a better understanding of the magnitude of this problem. A patient with a widespread cancer such as leukemia, or a large solid-tumor growth such as a carcinoma, may have a staggering number of cancerous cells, any single one of which if surviving a therapy regimen would theoretically suffice to reestablish the cancer though all the others are killed. In short, the goal must be 100 percent eradication. That immense number of cells can reach one trillion.

Suppose that therapy kills 99.9 percent of the cells. It sounds very good doesn't it? But in fact it means that one cell out of each one thousand has survived, whereas the eradication of all except one cell would theoretically require a kill rate of 99.9999999999 percent. At a kill rate of 99.9 percent, a billion cells would still be alive, far from eradication, and more than plenty to keep the cancer going and growing. This daunting numbers game emphasizes how wondrous it is when a cancer patient shows five-year survival, the rule-of-thumb criterion for "cure" achieved by means of an eradication. Moreover, it places a great question mark on the risk level of depending upon an unproven remedy, especially when the conventional approaches offer some hope. When the situation is too grave, and no hope is offered other than easing pain and other symptoms, it is more understandable that people will grasp at any offer of hope. Seeking an alternative in the face of a very negative prognosis is a natural response to a lack of hope for recovery from the conventional surgical, radiological, and medical possibilities.

The elusive and challenging goal of beating cancer has attracted the attention of many biomedical scientists and physicians. The result is the pursuit of every conceivable approach that might be proposed as a means to the end of killing cancer cells while not killing too many normal cells for the patient to survive. Some of the methods of therapy devised stretch the capacity for scientific acceptance because of a far out, implausible underlying theory. Skepticism is the natural, ingrained response of scientists in such cases, and generally in situations new and incompletely explained. (Be aware however that merely completing a medical curriculum does not typically produce a scientist.) Most new methods are based on laboratory data from animal models of cancer, although they still undergo formal clinical evaluation. In such cases a medical scientist is more optimistic because of *plausibility* lent by the animal research, but he or she still must withhold a conclusion until clinical validation of the experimental therapy is received. In the more implausible examples from unconventional cancer therapy no supportive animal research exists. However, hope for overcoming one's cancer is hard to turn down. We will shortly examine some old and new examples of unconventional therapies that have been used by cancer patients despite the scientific criteria for their acceptance having not been met.

CURRENT STATUS OF UNCONVENTIONAL THERAPIES

Complementary cancer therapies do not propose to substitute for the conventional ones but propose to serve as adjuncts to improve outcomes. These are currently receiving more consideration by the scientific and medical communities. NCCAM at the NIH is devoted to research concerning both alternative and complementary therapies. Although some CAM therapies have been in use for many years, few well-designed, properly conducted clinical studies have investigated their efficacy and their adverse effects. Great ethical difficulty exists in proposing to evaluate an unconventional cancer therapy used alone, as this might involve abstaining from use of a conventional therapy. Although the latter might indeed not have a high expectancy of long-term benefit, withholding whatever level of life-prolonging effect it would provide in favor of a therapy of unknown capacity to prolong life constitutes an unethical choice for a physician by today's standards. Thus, an institutional human research committee would not likely give approval for such a design. For this reason, new pharmaceutical candidates for anticancer action generally will first be evaluated as an adjunct to established therapy, while the control group receives the "standard" therapy and a placebo.

Many doctors treating cancer patients seemingly have not been concerned with gaining knowledge of alternative therapies and typically dismiss talk of them out of hand.[2] Surely they frequently are prone to discourage a discussion of their use with patients (Boon et al., 2000). According to Boon et al. (2000), data from an ongoing five-year study at the University of California–San Francisco showed that only one-third of women with breast cancer disclosed their using alternative treatments to their physicians, whereas almost all women discussed their medical treatment with any alternative practitioner that they consulted. The three main reasons why women failed to discuss such alternative therapies stemmed from their perceptions of, and attitudes toward, their physicians. They are (1) an impression that the physician was disinterested; (2) expectation of a negative response, being condemned, embarrassed, or reproached; and (3) the belief that their physician had inadequate training in and/or a negative bias against alternative approaches.

Such feelings deterred most women from discussing their alternative medicine usage. Even in the instances when a patient attempted to initiate discussion of CAM remedies, their efforts were often not reciprocated, and unresponsiveness was taken as a sign that the physician did not want to hear about the patient's practices. Other reasons included the perception that disclosing CAM use to physicians was not relevant to or within the realm of the doctor-patient relationship. Indeed, it seems very likely that the perception of "inadequate training" would be true as often as not.[3]

However, this situation is showing signs of change as medical school curriculum planners and major cancer centers are embracing integrative medicine, by which is meant a combining of the conventional therapies with some aspects of the unconventional or CAM therapies. This trend seeks to allow patients and physicians to consider together the possible adjunctive use of CAM approaches. More recently, clinical reports on CAM therapies have begun to appear in mainline medical journals, and research programs for CAM have been developed by several comprehensive cancer centers. The Memorial Sloan-Kettering Cancer Center in New York City established an Integrative Medicine Service in 1999 including inpatient and outpatient clinical care, research, and education, and provides information about over-the-counter products.

Similarly, the M. D. Anderson Cancer Center in Houston, Texas, has launched a Complementary/Integrative Medicine Education Resources Web site that supplies evidence-based reviews of complementary or alternative cancer therapies as well as links to other authoritative resources. These reviews evaluate the designs and the results of published research on herbal, nutrition, mind-body, energy, and other biological-pharmacological-organic therapies. Detailed scientific reviews are provided to assist health care workers in guiding patients who would like to integrate these therapies with conventional treatments. Patients who have a leaning toward CAM methods will supposedly be welcomed in sharing that outlook with their oncology physician, which was seldom true for medical practice broadly in the 1990s.

M. A. Richardson and colleagues (2000) at the University of Texas M. D. Anderson Cancer Center assessed the prevalence and predictors for the use of CAM by cancer patients attending the outpatient clinic. Of 453 participants, 99 percent had heard of CAM practices. Of those, 83 percent had used at least one CAM approach. Such use was greatest for spiritual practices (80.5 percent), dietary supplements (vitamins and herbs, 63 percent), and movement and physical therapies (59 percent). The researchers found that the use of alternative treatments was more common among women, younger patients, those who had undergone cancer surgery, or those who were poor. Most of these participants expected CAM to improve their quality of life (77 percent), boost their immune system (71 percent), prolong their life (63 percent), or reduce their symptoms (44 percent). Moreover, about 38 percent hoped that CAM therapies would cure their disease. Despite high hope for CAM, about 60 percent of participants said that they had not discussed alternative and complementary therapies with a physician. The authors concluded that "given the number of patients combining vitamins and herbs with conventional treatments, the oncology community must improve patient-provider communication, offer reliable information to patients, and initiate research to determine possible drug-herb-vitamin interactions." Evidently this research was persuasive to the center's administration in view of the integrative medicine (Richardson et al., 2000) program.

R. K. Nam and colleagues (1999) determined the prevalence and patterns of the use of complementary therapies in men diagnosed as having prostate cancer as well as among those at high risk for the disease. Of men attending a prostate cancer support group, 80 percent of those seen as being at high risk for prostate cancer used some form of CAM. Because some CAM therapies used by prostate cancer patients include botanicals (for example, PC-SPES) and phytochemicals (such as lycopene and soy isoflavones), which exert significant biological effects, these authors emphasized the importance of physicians obtaining accurate data from their patients on their use of CAM materials.

NCCAM Supports Research on CAM for Cancer

To promote high-quality research the National Center for CAM, the National Cancer Institute (NCI), and the National Heart, Lung, and Blood Institute (NHLBI) in 2000 funded 11 centers for CAM research. Such centers are aimed at providing resources needed for a rigorous scientific investigation of CAM materials and methods. Research conducted at these centers is expected to examine the potential efficacy, safety, and validity of CAM practices as well as the physiological or psychological mechanisms underlying or contributing to the effects of such practices.

Examples of natural products used in unconventional approaches to cancer therapy (not for prevention) under study in 2003, funded by federal grants through NCCAM, included the following:

- *Flaxseed,* being assessed as an alternative high-phytoestrogen dietary intervention for possible favorable effects in hormone-dependent prostate cancers
- *L-carnitine,* being tested for a capacity to oppose fatigue in terminal cancer patients who show a deficiency of the amino acid
- *Mistletoe,* being tested for antineoplastic activity in persons with inoperable or metastatic breast, pancreatic, colorectal, or lung cancer
- *Noni,* being tested to determine the maximum tolerated dose of freeze-dried fruit extract, to define toxicities resulting from its ingestion, and to obtain preliminary data on its efficacy for anti-tumor and symptom-control capabilities in cancer patients
- *Pancreatic enzyme therapy,* undergoing a Phase III trial comparing the efficacy of gemcitabine, a conventional therapy, with that of combined pancreatic enzyme therapy plus a specialized diet (Gonzalez regimen) in treating patients who have stage II, stage III, or stage IV pancreatic cancer
- *Shark cartilage,* being tested in a Phase III study of the efficacy of a combination of chemotherapy and radiation, with or without a shark cartilage preparation, for treating patients with inoperable, stage III, non-small-cell lung cancer as well as in a randomized phase III trial is testing the efficacy of shark cartilage in treating patients who have advanced colorectal cancer or advanced breast cancer (NCCAM, 2006).

EXAMPLES OF UNCONVENTIONAL THERAPIES

Metabolic therapies and supposedly immunoaugmentative therapies used by CAM practitioners, or even at times by patients independently of any practitioner, have been many and varied. We will consider a broad sample of them here. Some are touted as the cure that the pharmaceutical companies and the American Medical Association have blacklisted for the sake of their greater economic gain. A tendency to believe in conspiracy theories or urban legends may make one a better prospect for believing in such "cancer cures." Although one of the notorious classics of the 1950s and 1960s, laetrile, might have been thought to be dead and gone, apparently someone failed to drive a stake into the heart and it seems yet to be alive and well at clinics of Baja California, Mexico, and elsewhere.

Chaparral Tea for Cancer

Chaparral tea is a long-standing Native American remedy that originated among the tribes of the American Southwest desert, where other names such as creosote bush or greasewood are applied to the woody shrub *Larrea tridentata.* It has long been used in the form of the dried leaves, green stems, and fine twig tips for tea making by Native American traditional healers there and by residents of northern Mexico. However, it has been regarded by medical authorities as an ineffective and dangerous potion since it came into wider use since 1969 as a cancer remedy and antiviral agent. In 2002 the FDA declared a supplier to be in violation for a Web site making such therapeutic claims as:

> A potent and stable concentrate from the leaf resin of the Creosote bush (Chaparral) which has broad spectrum anti-viral . . . anti-inflammatory, . . . , anti-microbial, anti-tumerogenic properties. Useful as a natural alternative for Chronic Fatigue Syndrome, Herpes Simplex 1 & 2, Atherosclerosis, Chicken Pox and Shingles, Roseolovirus, Kaposi's Sarcoma, AIDS, HIV 1 & 2, Human Leukemia Virus 1 & 2, and Hepatitis B Virus. Also useful for all inflammatory conditions . . . (CDER, 2002)

Meanwhile, an Internet search will lead a seeker to sources of supply and to product "information" that support use of the botanical forms of chaparral. Promotional sources suggest that chaparral acts against various accumulative toxicants, such as metallic poisons, environmental pollutants such as pesticides, and drugs, to "detoxify" and thus permit the restoration of vital organs such as liver and kidneys and of the immune functions so as to once more be capable of "fighting off cancer." These unsupported claims are essentially those shared by various "cancer cures," botanicals or otherwise, having scientifically unproven status and consequently rightly evoking a negative response of a skeptical mind.

However, chaparral is the source for a compound now seemingly being scientifically validated to a degree as an anticancer agent. In October 2004 Ralph Moss of "The Moss Reports" described a resurrection of interest in chaparral as a source for cancer therapy despite that it had been severely damaged by previous reports of users experiencing serious liver injuries (Sheikh et al., 1997) amid concern for its potential cancer induction. Moss reported that the derivative of chaparral known as M4N is undergoing trials for the treatment of head and neck cancers, a type of neoplasm that is notoriously difficult to treat. According to a press release (Anonymous, 2004) research physicians at the Medical University of South Carolina announced that the component derived from chaparral called M4N shrinks inoperable tumors of the head and neck region. The researchers injected M4N directly into tumors of eight patients who were ineligible for surgery because they had advanced intractable (untreatable) forms of cancer. They observed that the agent shrank the tumor growths in these patients, apparently by killing cells. Lead investigator Terry A. Day, MD, reported to the 6th International Conference on Head and Neck Cancer in Washington, DC, on August 10, 2004, that the study not only revealed efficacy, but also showed that M4N was tolerated well without direct toxicity.

A few months earlier Frank R. Dunphy, MD, and colleagues (2004) from the Duke Comprehensive Cancer Center, Durham, North Carolina, presented results of their Phase I study, in which M4N also was injected directly into tumors of patients with relapsed or refractory (i.e., treatment-resistant) head and neck cancer. This mode of administration was used in the two trials because M4N had shown activity in animals when injected directly into tumors. Again their observations showed that therapeutic results were dramatic; in three patients injected, the tumors responded by crusting within a week of the first injection, followed within two weeks by necrosis and ulceration. The patients treated at Duke were not free of side effects—one had an episode of heart block requiring hospitalization, and another developed a fistula from the trachea to the skin, which required withdrawal from the study. All patients had pain at the injection site severe enough to require their receiving intravenous morphine. The authors drew the conclusion that intratumor injection of MN4 was feasible and displayed promising antitumor activity against relapsed or refractory squamous cell cancer.

Both of these groups were participating in an NCI-sponsored clinical trial with material supplied by a small drug company, BioCure Medical. M4N was first investigated as an antiviral agent, being tested as an anti-HIV treatment in China. Later it was found to halt the growth of cancer cells as well. A sequence of misadventures concerning overseas clinical trials that brought M4N under a cloud is described by Moss (1994) (cancerdecisions .com/102404_page.html).

Essiac Tea

Essiac is a herbal mixture that has been widely used in Canada for more than 70 years. The original recipe was a combination of four herbs said to have been devised by a Native American (Ojibwa) healer with the intent "to purify the body and put it back in balance with the great spirit." It was popularized, beginning in the 1920s, by a nurse in Ontario named Rene Caisse, whose name spelled backward is Essiac. Nurse Caisse obtained the formula to treat a cancer-stricken family member, which reportedly was successful. The original four plants were burdock root *(Arctium lappa),* Indian rhubarb *(Rheum palmatum),* sheep sorrel *(Rumex acetosella),* and the inner bark of slippery elm (*Ulmus fulva* or *U. rubra*). Advocates claim that Essiac acts to strengthen the immune system, improve appetite, relieve pain, and improve overall quality of life, while also often reducing tumor size and prolonging the life of people with many types of cancer (Medline Plus, 2005).

In 1938 members of a Royal Cancer Commission of Canada visited Miss Caisse's clinic and heard testimonials from patients she had treated, but were concerned by her reluctance to provide the formula to them for further analysis. Their report concluded little evidence existed for an anticancer efficacy of Essiac. Nevertheless, between 1959 and 1978 Caisse worked with a prominent American physician, Dr. Charles Brusch, to modify the recipe and promote its use. As a result of their clinical and laboratory work, four more ingredients were added to the original recipe—watercress, blessed thistle, red clover, and kelp. These were claimed to strengthen its action and improve its taste.

Before her death in 1978, Caisse gave her formulas for Essiac to a company in Toronto intending that they would test it and make it available at a reasonable cost. The Department of National Health and Welfare gave permission to conduct human studies of its safety and effectiveness, but later withdrew its permission in 1982 because the research was not proceeding as planned. Restrictions were placed on promotion of Essiac for use in treating cancer. However, the formula continues to be manufactured in New Brunswick (Canada) and is still available in health food stores. Another Canadian product patterned after the one developed by Caisse and Brusch is produced in British Columbia and is widely available in health food stores but is openly promoted as merely a health-enhancing herbal tea. Most people trying Essiac today use it as an adjunct to more conventional therapies or as a component of palliative care for terminal stages of cancer. This example from our North American neighbors set the stage for twentieth century developments in the United States such as laetrile.

Green Tea: The Safest Tea for Cancer Benefits

In Chapter 24 the role of antioxidant components of green tea is discussed from the viewpoint of cancer chemoprevention. However, some animal studies have also found that injections of extracts of tea catechins cause implanted breast and prostatic tumors to decrease in size (Kaegi, 1998b). Thus, these findings support the need for further research on the value of green tea components in cancer therapy as well as prevention. Preparations of green tea in the form of capsules or tablets are now widely available, having been developed for the market with a significant background of laboratory and epidemiologic research. Unfortunately, the difficult aim of confirming their clinical effectiveness to lower cancer risk or overcome established human cancers has not yet been achieved.

Amygdalin (Laetrile, "Vitamin B-17")

A notorious example of a controversial "cancer cure" is that of amygdalin or laetrile. Amygdalin is a plant component that occurs in the pits of many fruits—raw nuts, lima beans, clover, and sorghum, but especially in apricot pits. It is a cyanogenic glycoside, i.e., it contains a sugar, but when metabolized it releases toxic hydrogen cyanide (the chemical used for executions in "the gas chamber"). The latter is the hypothetical basis for the supposed cancer-killing activity of amygdalin products. The names laetrile and amygdalin have often been used as if there were synonymous, but in fact they are not identical materials. The laetrile/amygdalin that was and is manufactured in Mexico and made available through cancer clinics there, and by mail to the United States, reportedly is produced from crushed apricot pits. However, the chemical makeup of the laetrile patented in the United States was different in being a semisynthetic form of amygdalin. Neither material was ever approved by the FDA.

Amygdalin was first isolated in 1830, and it was used as an anticancer agent in Russia as early as 1845. In the 1950s, laetrile, the supposedly nontoxic and curative form of semisynthetic amygdalin, was developed and patented in the United States as an anticancer agent employed as part of a "metabolic therapy" program that included a special diet, high-dose vitamins, and pancreatic enzymes. Whatever the source, amygdalin is commonly given by intravenous injection over a period of days to weeks, and then by mouth for maintenance therapy. Laboratory animal studies were conducted with laetrile, but they were said to show little evidence for efficacy against cancer. But "believers" claimed that bias negated the "true" outcome. By 1978 it was claimed that more than 70,000 people in the United

States had been treated with laetrile, but none was claimed to yet be living. Did they survive longer, the same duration, or a shorter time than they would have without laetrile? Were their final weeks better or worse for having taken it? No answers seem to be at hand for even such basic questions.

Many anecdotal reports, lacking a complete description of the diagnostic and therapeutic history of patients, and case reports were published in 1953 and 1962, but they failed to confirm a significant lasting benefit. The case reports provided some details of the diagnosis, treatment and follow-up of patients, but they failed to provide acceptable scientific evidence to support the use of laetrile for cancer. A politically charged atmosphere was created by accusations that "the medical establishment" was attempting to block a useful anticancer drug from the public marketplace for nefarious reasons.[4] In 1978, the NCI requested case reports from physicians who believed their patients had benefited from laetrile therapy. Ninety-three cases were received, 67 of which were complete enough to be evaluated. An expert panel concluded that two of them had complete responses and four experienced a reduction in tumor size. Based on these six out of 67 cases, NCI sponsored clinical studies of laetrile, as had been demanded by its proponents.

The first trial of laetrile was a Phase I study in six cancer patients to establish the dosage, mode of administration and schedule of treatment. The researchers found that amygdalin caused minimal adverse side effects. In 1982, a Phase II study with 175 patients probed what types of cancers might respond to amygdalin. Most patients in this study had breast, colon, or lung cancer. Amygdalin was injected for 21 days, followed by oral maintenance therapy using doses and procedures similar to those devised in the Phase I study. Vitamins and pancreatic enzymes were given as part of a metabolic therapy program that also included dietary changes. One stomach cancer patient showed a decrease in tumor size, which was maintained for ten weeks while the patient was on therapy. However, in 54 percent of the patients a measurable added growth of their cancer occurred by the end of treatment. All of the patients showed progression of their cancers seven months after completing therapy; i.e., none went into remission. Some patients reported an improvement in their ability to work or do other activities, and other patients said their symptoms reduced. However, improvements did not last after therapy stopped. (The same commonly would be said for conventional therapies.) Based on this, the NCI concluded that no further clinical testing of laetrile was warranted (NCI, 2005).

Although laetrile is not legal in interstate commerce, it apparently has been produced and distributed on an intrastate basis, as well as being imported from Mexico. In July 2003 a federal jury in Brooklyn convicted a New Yorker of three counts of criminal contempt after he continued to sell laetrile despite a court injunction in 2000 ordering him to stop (Anonymous, 2003). He had used an Internet site and a massive e-mail marketing campaign guaranteeing a cancer-free life to those who used his products. He was charged with having promoted and dispensed these products with false promises that they could prevent or cure cancer. When a search warrant was executed at the defendant's house during the undercover investigation after the preliminary injunction it was found that he had on hand in his basement ready for shipping to customers around the world enough laetrile to supply a single person for more than 242 years. From somewhere in the never-never land of cyberspace one can order laetrile to one's hearts content!

Dr. Burzynski's Many "Antineoplastons"

If it were possible to be more controversial than the laetrile "cancer cure," it would likely be the "antineoplaston therapy" of Stanislaw Burzynski that has achieved that honor. He is a physician born and educated in Poland, where he received an MD degree in 1967 and a DMsc degree in 1968. He did not undergo specialty training in cancer nor did he complete any other residency program. His bibliography shows no clinical research on cancer, on urinary biochemistry, or on "antineoplastons" during his early career. The term *antineoplaston* is evidently one he coined for the supposed biochemical agents he extracted from human urine that he described as peptides capable of exerting an anticancer action.

Dr. Burzynski for more than a decade has been operating a cancer therapy practice in north Texas where he apparently has administered his experimental therapy to hundreds of patients annually. He is subjected to "star status" by the medical scientists operating Quackwatch.org. That Web site is devoted to exposing the unconventional therapies that are deemed unsafe and/or unproven to be useful for medical treatment of the diseases claimed by their sponsors. Although Burzynski has submitted to the FDA requirements for clinical trials on a new therapeutic agent—when ordered to do so by a court—his reports to the FDA are said not to have provided suitable data from which any conclusion can be drawn regarding either safety or efficacy against any cancer.

One particularly strong critic of Burzynski and antineoplastons is Saul Green, PhD, a retired biochemist, who formerly did cancer-related research at the prestigious Memorial Sloan-Kettering Cancer Center for 23 years. He attacks the chemistry on which Burzynski bases his supposed discovery (Green, 1993). Green also accuses him of lying about having a PhD (www.quackwatch.org/01QuackeryRelatedTopics/Cancer/burzynski2.html).

Green further asserts that the extraction methods described would lead to simpler types of chemicals rather than the supposed peptide composition claimed for materials he obtained from human urine and named "antineoplastons." The plural is used because Burzynski's work has gone through multiple phases over time, resulting in differently numbered versions of "antineoplaston." His recent publication of clinical data was on two of them, "A10" and "AS2-1" (Burzynski et al., 2006).

Green states that by 1985, when Burzynski received a U.S. patent he claimed to be using eight antineoplastons to treat cancer patients, whereas merely two fractions were being used by 2001. Much of the clinical research conducted by S. Burzynski continues to be questioned. In short, a considerable basis exists for questioning whether *any real evidence* exists in support of antineoplastons for efficacy up to the present. If it exists, it has not been well displayed either to the FDA or to the medical community (The Cancer Letter, 1998).

Dr. Burton's Immunoaugmentative Therapy (IAT)

Another "cancer cure" seemingly akin to that of Burzinsky was developed by Lawrence Burton, PhD (zoology), in the 1960s and 1970s. Burton died in 1993 but his "therapeutic system" may be still be carried on. It consisted of a complicated concept of a protein acting as a tumor-inducing factor (TIF), an inhibitory protein toward that factor, plus more two proteins that "block" and "deblock" the receptors to the TIF. In a thorough critique of this subject published in *JAMA*, biochemist Saul Green (1993), came to a conclusion that the patented procedures for isolation of these components did not suffice to support the proposition of their actual existence or their supposed biological activities. Neither did chemical analyses of samples by independent laboratories detect the sort of proteins supposedly contained in injectable solutions brought from Burton's Bahamian clinic to the United States by outpatients.

However, such analyses did serve to indicate that those solutions were neither sterile nor free from pyrogenic (fever-inducing) components. Evidence of viral DNA indicated that the putative therapeutic materials might instead provoke disease, viral infections, in the unsuspecting recipient. More trappings of pseudoscience were Burton's claimed "secret formulas" for producing a therapeutic combination individualized for each patient as determined by his (also secret) computer-based diagnosis of their particular state of imbalance. Give the proper formula to overcome the imbalance, and the ability of the immune system to overcome and destroy the cancer is restored. *Presto, chango!* The patient's cancer is destroyed and he or she is cured!

This "house of cards" theory depends upon the basic premise that the healthy, normal immune system has a capacity to seek out and destroy any cancerous cells. Dr. Green declared that, sad to say, the mystique of omnipotence imparted to the mysterious immune system is not sufficient to make it happen that way. He declares that this beautiful but false hypothesis that a healthy or a "boosted" immune system can overcome all cancers is spoiled by the ugly facts. At Green's writing more than a decade ago, various evidence indicated that even an optimally functioning immune system is not always able to control the onset of the most common, major types of cancer. Thus, he dismissed many seemingly scientific therapies that hinge upon the same hypothesis so as not to be relied upon. Even so, it should be acknowledged that some current anticancer approaches employing natural agents that are supposed to provide immunoenhancement may exert other biological effects (such as inducing apoptosis) that might indeed be a plausible basis for efficacy against cancer. An incorrect initial premise may occasionally lead to a successful outcome; this was true relative to a major pharmaceutical antineoplastic agent, Cytoxan, or cyclophosphamide.

However, a thorough consideration of Green's critique of immunosurveillance as a normal defense against cancer must look to an update of immunologists' current views on this controversial topic. One finds that although the initial launching with a good early acceptance of the concept of "immunosurveillance against cancer" was followed by a later rejection, the pendulum has swung back toward its favor. A review by Dunn et al. (2004a,b) states that

> after a century of controversy, the notion that the immune system regulates cancer development is experiencing a new resurgence. An overwhelming amount of data from animal models—together with compelling data from human patients—indicate that a functional cancer immunosurveillance process indeed exists that acts as an extrinsic tumor suppressor. (2004a)

Another states

> The last fifteen years have seen a re-emergence of interest in cancer immunosurveillance and a broadening of this concept into one termed cancer immunoediting . . . The latter . . . holds that the immune system not only protects the host against development of primary nonviral cancers but also sculpts tumor immunogenicity. (2004c)

Similarly, a German writer (Atanackovic, 2004) stated that, "Recent studies clearly prove the existence of cancer immunosurveillance and justify renewed hope for the development of effective vaccination therapies for solid tumors." In short, the current view acknowledges that the immune-system response is effective but not so almighty as earlier pictured against cancer, that it even may at times facilitate a cancer. Whether this new concept still justifies any major hope for achieving a significant anticancer benefit from dietary supplements through immunoenhancment must still remain an unanswered question.

Shark Cartilage

This material has been in use by cancer patients for a number of years on an uncertain premise that sharks *never* get cancer; thus, it is deduced that their tissues must contain a cancer-inhibiting agent. Some investigations have suggested that even bovine cartilage has similar anticancer activity, which undermines the hypothesis of shark cartilage being unique. We must acknowledge that research arising from a false hypothesis can lead to the discovery of a truly active biomaterial. A shark cartilage preparation is being tested with federal funding from NCCAM as previously described.

Hydrazine Sulfate

In the 1980s and early 1990s, the National Cancer Institute sponsored research to determine if hydrazine had metabolic actions that might improve cancer patients' survival or help reverse cancer-induced cachexia, a wasting syndrome characterized by extreme weight loss in advanced cancer. Despite an early favorable response in a small number of cases, three larger clinical trials did not detect any improvement in cancer patients' survival, weight loss, or quality of life from taking hydrazine sulfate. The FDA never approved the chemical for use in cancer therapy. The use of hydrazine sulfate as an alternative, unregulated remedy against cancer is made possible via direct-to-consumer marketing on the Internet. It was linked to the death of a patient from toxic liver and kidney failure by a report from Hainer et al. (2000) in *Annals of Internal Medicine*.

Case Report 1

A 55-year-old man with sinus cancer, when first seen had a two-week history of rash, itching, worsening malaise, and jaundice. He had previously refused surgery, radiation, or chemotherapy, choosing to obtain hydrazine sulfate through an alternative medicine Internet site. He had used it for four months when he developed a troublesome rash. Liver and kidney function tests were done, and tissue biopsy samples from his liver and kidneys were examined. The patient was admitted to the hospital with a diagnosis of kidney failure, hepatic encephalopathy (brain dysfunction related to liver failure), and severely impaired clotting ability of his blood, owing to the liver ceasing to produce the proteins essential to coagulation. Despite aggressive treatment, the patient died after developing gastrointestinal hemorrhage. Autopsy revealed a breakdown of the kidneys and a near-massive liver necrosis, which were attributed to the hydrazine. The physicians reporting this case (Hainer et al., 2000) stated that "this case graphically illustrates the potential danger of therapies purchased online. Furthermore, it illustrates the importance of reporting adverse events resulting from the use of medications, medical devices, or even special nutritional products" (p. 879). Authors of an accompanying editorial (Black and Hussain, 2000) concluded that little evidence supports an ability of hydrazine sulfate to shrink or cure cancers. Even though a few cases of serious adverse effects have been previously reported, the chemical is still easily available for dangerous, unsupervised self-medication.

Iscador/European Mistletoe Extracts

European mistletoe *(Viscum album)* is a parasitic plant that has been used in the treatment of many diseases for thousands of years (it is a different species from the familiar North American mistletoe). It appears in legend and folklore as a panacea. Use of mistletoe as a cancer therapy was promoted early in the twentieth century by Rudolf Steiner, PhD (1861-1925), who was founder of "anthroposophy," a therapeutic concept that blended spiritual and scientific principles to apply them to healing, especially focused on cancer. Steiner's proposal was that the prevailing balance between "lower organizing forces" (which control and organize cell growth to form tissues and organs) and his so-called "higher organizing forces" is what determines a person's susceptibility to cancer. An imbalance between these opposing forces promotes the onset of cancer (Kaegi, 1998b).

Steiner somehow (perhaps from knowing of folklore claims for its supposedly extraordinary powers) came to view mistletoe as having a number of features that suggested it could stimulate the "higher organizing forces" to restore a healthy balance in cancer patients. Mistletoe liquid extracts containing key medicinal components of this plant are marketed under several trade names, such as Iscador, Helixor, Eurixor, and Isorel, most of which are available in Europe. These Iscador products have been used for decades to treat cancer, mainly in Europe and parts of Asia. To this day anthroposophic medical clinics are said to exist in Switzerland and Germany that promote the use of Iscador products! Not only in several European countries, but also in South Africa, Iscador is commercially available and legally prescribed. The proposal of Steiner is not deserving to be dignified by calling it a hypothesis. It was never subjected to a scientific test because it was too nebulous and vague to it permit to be tested and proved or disproved scientifically. This is an example of a crackpot or crackbrained basis for claims of a cancer cure. "Cures" such as this so taint the perceptions of all unusual approaches to cancer as to deny an open-minded hearing to ones that might offer a more reasonable basis for application.

Mistaken concepts do at times lead to important scientific discoveries. The question remains as whether Steiner, despite his unscientific approach, might have stumbled upon something valuable in mistletoe thanks to the insight of the folklorists. Extracts of the mistletoe plant have been shown in recent years to kill cancer cells and to stimulate immune cells in vitro. Several chemical components of mistletoe have been suggested to be responsible for these effects—alkaloids, viscotoxins (small proteins that have cell-killing activity and possible immune system stimulating activity), and lectins (complex molecules combining protein and sugars). However, the question remains as to whether these findings can be extended from in vitro to the in vivo situation of human patients. Unfortunately, acceptable data from well-designed clinical trials to verify that mistletoe or its components are an effective therapy against human cancer are lacking.

The available literature on mistletoe has been published primarily in non-English journals and consists mainly of anecdotal reports, small case series, and a few clinical trials that provide only inconclusive outcomes. In 1998 a Task Force on Alternative Therapies of the Canadian Breast Cancer Research Initiative examining this literature found that "most of the studies had significant design limitations, making it difficult to interpret their results and seriously limiting the value of their findings." Their report did indicate that multicenter clinical trials were ongoing in Europe and were being planned in the United States and Canada (Gorter et al., 1999).

However, a study of considerable interest on research involving 10,226 cancer patients in a prospective long-term study was published in Germany (Grossarth-Maticek et al., 2001). The matched-pairs, nonrandomized study (subjects are first matched in pairs, and then assigned to the two groups) found that the survival time of patients treated with Iscador was longer for all types of cancer studied. Among 396 matched pairs, mean survival time in the Iscador groups (4.23 years) was nearly 40 percent longer than for the control groups receiving no mistletoe product (3.05 years). Results of two randomized, matched-pair studies largely confirmed the results of the nonrandomized research. The authors concluded that therapy achieved a clinically relevant prolongation of survival time of cancer patients.

Still, pharmaceutical mistletoe preparations are not marketed in the United States as they are in Germany. The National Cancer Institute has an online information source on mistletoe extracts: www.cancer.gov/cancer topics/pdq/cam/mistletoe. Apparently, no research group has applied for an Investigational New Drug (IND) application from the FDA to evaluate mistletoe as a treatment for cancer. Here again we find people who are determined to obtain and use therapies not available in the United States. In 2001 movie/television star Suzanne Somers revealed that she had tested positive for breast cancer and had undergone a lumpectomy. She chose to use a combination of conventional and complementary treatments for cancer aftercare—radiation plus the Iscador product that she described as "homeopathic" (incorrect, but probably because it was obtained through a homeopathic practitioner) on her Web site, which related her experience (suzannesomers.com/products/tapes/Health.asp).

A company in Germany produces Iscador, the oldest and most widely used among the various preparation of mistletoe available in Europe. It has gained wide acceptance in Europe and Asia for use mainly as a *complementary* therapy before and after surgery and/or radiation for solid-tissue cancers. The entire plant is ground to make a water extract, which is a conventional approach. However, after this step an unusual process begins—the extract is fermented by means of a bacterium, *Lactobacillus plantarum.* (Perhaps not entirely unusual considering that we obtain both tabasco sauce and soy sauce after a process of fermentation.) The resulting broth is filtered, and the aqueous product is administered by subcutaneous injection near or into the tumor, or sometimes systemically by intramuscular or intravenous routes. Among the varieties of the product is an oral form, which is especially used in the case of brain and spinal cord tumors, being claimed to oppose dangerous elevation of intracranial pressure.

In Europe, Iscador products are now being tested with some reports of positive results for treating HIV disease (AIDS), chronic hepatitis C, and immune deficiency related to childhood exposure to post-Chernobyl radioactive fallout (Chernyshov et al., 2000). A study of Iscador in 16 HIV-positive patients and eight healthy persons (van Wely et al., 1999) analyzed drug-related adverse effects and found flulike symptoms, gingivitis, fever, local reddening of the skin, and eosinophilia (elevation of the white blood cells known as eosinophils). The adverse effects were not severe, and local inflammation at sites of injection is an accepted aspect of injected therapy using biological products. The rate of systemic adverse events was higher in the HIV-positive patients. In addition, changes in laboratory values were an increased blood urea level and a slight decrease of total plasma protein caused by a minor decrease in albumin. These findings suggest that Iscador may be justified for use because of its low risk-to-(possible)-benefit ratio.

However, overdosage may occur from oral intake or intravenous mistletoe doses. The toxic risk for mistletoe products may include a slow heart rate, seizures, or death. Clearly, the last chapter of The Mistletoe Story has yet to be written.

Modified Citrus Pectin

Pectin is a natural product long known in a food context as the gel component of ripe fruits such as apple, orange, grapefruit, and lemon that allows them to be used in making jellies. It is a complex carbohydrate that is classified as a soluble fiber. In a medical context, preparations of pectin are being used as bulking agents for relief of constipation and have been promoted as a source of fiber that may be protective against colon cancer by favoring the more rapid removal of possibly harmful chemicals through avoidance of constipation.

However, a newer concept of medical value is associated with the supposed capacity of citrus pectin to oppose cancer, especially prostate cancer. Citrus pectin is claimed to exert superior binding properties enabling it to promote the excretion of toxic heavy metals. Modified citrus pectin (MCP) has been reduced to a smaller-sized molecule that enables its absorption and a systemic action, whereas pectin in unmodified state is confined to acting within the intestinal tract. It is thought that MCP in the circulation is able to bind and inactivate a molecule that seems to be a key one for the cancers' metastatic behavior—setting up distant secondary growth sites of prostate cancer cells. Aggressive cases of prostate cancer are prone to metastasize to distant structures such as the lungs or the spine. The major concept of metastasis by cancers views the adhesion of cancer cells to endothelial cells and to one another (cancer cell aggregation) as being equally key components in the process of metastasis. If it were not for metastasis, many more cancers could be successfully treated by surgical removal of the original growth. Thus, a means of opposing metastasis would be highly valuable in improving the chances for surviving cancer.

Galectin-3 is a mammalian protein that researchers have implicated in a variety of biological functions including cell proliferation and differentiation, tumor cell adhesion, angiogenesis, apoptosis ("cell suicide"), tumor progression, and metastasis (Fuchs, 2003). Recent research indicates that both forms of cell adhesion in metastasis—that to the vascular endothelium and that of cell aggregation—are mediated by galectin-3, and that both are required for metastasis to occur. This molecule lodges on the cell membrane of prostate cancer cells, where it supports both the formation of the original tumor and its spread to new sites via metastasis. MCP is said to bind by "molecular hooks" on galectin-3, but in doing so MCP interferes with the adhesion process and thus with both tumor formation and metastasis. It also is proposed that galectin-3 is necessary to the process of angiogenesis—formation of new capillaries to feed the tumor. Thus, interference with this action of galectin-3 would provide yet another anticancer mechanism for MCP.

Cancer of the prostate is a very common type of neoplasm. Statistics indicate that about 70 percent of men over the age of 70 years have it. Fortunately, most will not die from it. An important fact regarding prostate cancer is that the tumor causing death usually is not the original tumor in the prostate but rather the growths that occur in other organs after metastasis. More critical is the occurrence of prostate cancer in too many men younger than 70 years who have a higher chance of dying from it. MCP has been studied most in persons having prostate cancer. Prostate-specific antigen (PSA) in the blood is used as a test for cancer. In a small-scale study by Stephen Strum, MD, on seven men with prostate cancer, a dose of 15 grams per day of oral MCP treatment for at least six months was seen to slow the time for doubling of the values of PSA in the blood, which serves as an index for the rate of growth of the cancer. Another ten patients, who similar to the first group had failed other therapy or relapsed, took MCP for a year and in seven of the ten the PSA doubling time was significantly extended. This is interesting, but we would wish for data on longer-term measures of outcome for this therapeutic approach (Guess et al., 2003).

Direct testing for opposition to metastasis has been conducted in a rat model of prostate cancer. For rats receiving oral doses of MCP the level of metastasis was reduced from that seen in a control group. Rat and human studies cited here were published only in a pamphlet form; they are quite intriguing, but not so convincing as if they were found in a medical journal for which they would have undergone peer review. The mode of action that is proposed for MCP is clear and plausible in this case, in contrast to some modes discussed previously. Much more definitive data from tests in cancer models and patients are greatly needed before MCP can be regarded with confidence.

Noni Juice

As is befitting for a reputed panacea, preparations from the tree (or trees) known as noni are said to exert an anticancer action. Noni *(Morinda citrifolia)* is a fruit tree native to the southeast Asia region and distributed widely throughout the Pacific islands (as far east as Hawaii) that seems to have been extensively used in folk medicine by people of Polynesia for more than 2,000 years. This plant is suspected by some to occur in three subtypes or closely related species. Moreover, it continues in a medicinal role following the path of an indigenous remedy while also being brought to the wider world as a dietary supplement product, mainly in an oral liquid form, e.g., the brand Tahitian Noni Juice (McClatchey, 2002). Its qualities are extolled in not only English, but also French, "Les incomparables qualités du fruit du noni!" However, a concern has been expressed for an adverse response to develop hyperkalemia if it is taken to excess (Mueller et al., 2000).

Noni supposedly has shown a broad range of health benefits, the most remarkable claims being for anticancer activity in both laboratory animal models and clinical practice (Solomon, 1998; Wang and Su, 2001). The mechanism for these reputed effects remains unknown, but the plant's antioxidant action is implicated. The concept that *Morinda citrifolia* possesses an anticancer action at the initiation stage of carcinogenesis was studied (Hirazumi and Furusawa, 1999). This research consisted of testing for a suppressive activity of 10 percent Tahiti Noni Juice (TNJ) in the drinking water of rats that were then exposed to a chemical carcinogen, DMBA (7,12-dimethylbenzanthracene). Later the researchers measured the levels of DMBA-to-DNA adducts, which are the products of chemical interaction between molecules of the carcinogen and the DNA in animal cells. Formation of such adducts is an index of a cancer-provoking action by the chemical. The rats given treatment with noni for a week prior to DMBA when compared with untreated controls showed that levels of the adducts were reduced by 30 percent in the heart, 41 percent in the lung, 42 percent in the liver, and 80 percent in the kidney. Mice showed an even stronger positive effect. In 1995 evidence was found of an anticancer action for noni in mice that were injected with a human lung cancer cell line. Also, researchers have reported (1999) identifying an immunomodulating component of noni juice in a polysaccharide-rich fraction.

These appear to be promising animal results. The NCCAM has supported an early stage human trial of noni with respect to its claimed value (see Chapter 32). In order to explore the mechanism of the supposed anticancer effect, the antioxidant activity of the noni juice was examined by a standard in vitro test. TNJ manifested a dose-dependent antioxidant activity, which was then compared to the effects of vitamin C, grape seed powder, and pycnogenol with the recommended daily serving size being the RDA of each in the United States, or by their manufacturers recommendation. Data suggest that some hindering of carcinogen-DNA adduct formation may be related to antioxidant or radical scavenging activity of TNJ, and may be a basis for the supposed human cancer-opposing action of *Morinda citrifolia,* for which no published studies were retrievable.

The beneficial actions of noni juice, according to the hypothesis of a researcher in Hawaii, Dr. Ralph M. Heinicke, are said to be derived from its content of proxeronine, which is said to enter body cells where it is converted to an alkaloid, xeronine. This compound, it is alleged, then "combines with biochemicals such as hormones, enzymes, serotonin, antioxidants, vitamins, minerals, and other elements. The combination of Proxeronine and the other biochemicals are in specific and varied combinations depending on how the body's homeostasis is out of alignment" (Solomon, 2006).

Unfortunately, this purported scientific background for noni juice has not appeared in published scientific or medical literature, discounting a writing on the pharmacologic activities of noni components that was published in an obscure and inappropriate outlet, *Pacific Tropical Botanical Garden Bulletin* (1985; 15: 10-14), which was referred to by Will McClatchey, PhD (2002) as "an outrageous publication," unreferenced and written too authoritatively, and lacking adequate data. Indeed, the very existence of Heinicke's (postulated) proxeronine and xeronine is not recognized in the general biomedical literature or by a specialized source on plant chemistry, as noted in the very useful review of the noni literature by McClatchey (2002), who indicates that the chemical nature and structures for these molecules have never been supplied.[5]

However, these concepts were presented to the world in a small paperback format by Dr. Neil Solomon (1988). Moreover a brief description of Heinicke's work and theory is available on the Web site of the only commercial noni source, the TNJ, that receives his personal endorsement (www.iwr.com/noni-juice/xeronine.htm). One literature item of interest is a positive test of a noni preparation for antidiabetic activity in diabetic rats (Olajide et al., 1999).

In summary, the supposed basic chemical research on noni is not available for others to evaluate. This smacks of a classical scientific "scam." However, as indicated elsewhere, a deluded hypothesis may at times point the way to a true discovery concerning a natural product having medical value. In time a full judgment on noni may become possible. Meanwhile, advertisements for products based on the xeronine concept of noni are prevalent, although printed material studiously avoids reference thereto.

Pawpaw

The abundant plant chemistry foundation for the pawpaw plant regarding medical applications stands in stark contrast to the situation of noni fruit and juice previously described. Pawpaw is a small deciduous tree that recently has been growing in popularity as an ornamental because of the edible fruit it produces—oval fruits three to six inches long that weigh five to 16 ounces and turn from black to yellow-orange as they ripen. They have a taste similar to banana or pear with a custard consistency, features that caused the plant to be named alternatively as American custard apple, the West Virginia banana, the Indiana/Hoosier banana, and poor man's banana. The fruit is said to be an excellent source of the vitamins A and C, and is described as a tropical fruit for the temperate regions. An extensive site for links concerning the pawpaw is found on the Internet at www.fred.net/kathy/pawpaws.html.

A former professor of pharmacognosy at Purdue University's School of Pharmacy and Pharmacal Sciences, Jerry McLaughlin, PhD, was lead researcher for many years of extensive laboratory research on the North American pawpaw tree *(Asimina triloba).* He retired from academia to enter a new role as chief scientist for a botanical supplement company focusing on products based on the active constituents of this species. Under Dr. McLaughlin's direction an oral product known as Paw Paw Cell-Reg has been made available as a treatment "Selective for Abnormal Cells." The carefully couched description avoids admitting that the product is made available to help rid the body of cancer, as a complementary therapy, by its selective cytotoxicity toward neoplastic cells. The laboratory researches on components extracted from pawpaw (primarily from the bark of twigs and small branches) demonstrated that animal tumor cells are indeed targeted selectively for a cell-killing action. The group identified more than 40 related pawpaw compounds having similar anticancer properties in experimental test systems.

Not only were the pawpaw compounds effective in killing human mammary cancer cells that had become resistant to other anticancer agents, but also they seemed to show a special affinity for such resistant cells. The research group's findings were detailed in 1992 by papers in *Cancer Letters* and the *Journal of Pharmacy and Pharmacology* (Oberlies et al., 1997a,b). Further research indicated that these substances act to "pull the plug on the energy-producing mechanisms in the cell." Thus, their use as a complementary approach in conjunction with conventional therapy seemingly has plausibility and promise. Presumably, development of pharmaceutical agent(s) based on pawpaw was inhibited by the difficulties related to nonpatentability of plant substances. Clinical studies on Paw Paw Cell-Reg have been reported to complementary and alternative medical meetings.[6]

Antioxidant Vitamins A, C, and E

The proponents of using antioxidant supplements often recommend combining three vitamins—A, C, and E—claiming that these three can improve one's general well-being while strengthening one's immune system, and that these effects may oppose not only the development but also the progression of serious diseases, including cancer. The daily doses they advocate typically exceed those accepted by nutritional authorities (the recommended daily allowances) as appropriate and necessary for maintaining health.

Some animal studies have shown an ability of vitamin A, beta-carotene, and other retinoids to enhance immune responses, to retard tumor growth, and to diminish the size of experimental animal tumors. For instance, beta-carotene increased the production and tumoricidal activity of white blood cells—monocytes, lymphocytes, and macrophages. More recently, an animal study found that fenretinide, a synthetic vitamin A analogue, inhibited cell growth in human mammary cancer cell lines. In rats it inhibited mammary gland development, suppressed carcinogen-induced mammary cancer, and caused shrinkage of invasive mammary cancer.

Still no direct evidence supports a benefit of vitamin A versus cancer in a human patient. When high doses of vitamin A were given to lung cancer patients the results of the study showed no benefit. Moreover, a 1994 report of a large study involving smokers who received supplemental beta-carotene and vitamin A gave quite unexpected results—an increased risk of lung cancer! As a result of this outcome, researchers are proceeding much more cautiously in examining the proposed value of vitamin A and/or its precursor, beta-carotene, in the prevention or treatment of cancer. However, the validity of this study has been challenged by Dr. Abram Hoffer with regard to bias in the experimental groups' preliminary levels of smoking, and with respect to the results showing a statistical significance, but likely not a real clinical significance (www.doctoryourself.com/news/v3n15.txt).

What of the combination of these three? Can it provide a "triple play" against cancers? Proponents of megadose vitamin therapy for cancer who usually recommend combinations of vitamins A (or beta-carotene), C, and E believe that this combination therapy is likely to have a synergistic beneficial effect greater than the sum of all the individual parts acting alone. The Canadian Breast Cancer Research Alliance published a review by a committee to study the role of unconventional, alternative therapies for cancer (Kaegi, 1998a,b,c). These three vitamins were one focus of a study on antioxidants. It's rationale and limitation were described as follows:

> There is clear evidence that a diet rich in fresh fruits and vegetables reduces the risk of many diseases, including some types of cancer. The specific factors responsible for this protective effect are not completely understood. However, it seems likely that it is related to complex interactions between constituent phyto-chemicals that have not yet been completely identified, let alone incorporated into supplements. There is therefore concern that the administration of food

extracts or supplements in any form may not confer the benefits of fresh foods. (Kaegi, 1998a)

The analysis by the Canadian Breast Cancer Research Alliance found several studies that reported on the effects of combined vitamins in therapy for patients (usually) with advanced cancer. Some of these provide minimal evidence for increased benefit. However, methodologic weaknesses undermined the possible acceptance of data from the studies. Proponents claimed to find that only certain patients are "good-responders" to the vitamin regimen, but no means has been identified for predicting those who would be good responders before beginning the treatment. Thus, it is statistically invalid to focus on those and to disregard the "nonresponders." Unfortunately, at this time insufficient evidence exists to believe in A-C-E therapy of cancer and to warrant a person having confidence in its use.

However, a favorable outcome was reported from a multiple, low-dose antioxidant treatment in Paris, France (Hercberg et al., 2004). The researchers noted a reduction of the rate of occurrence, i.e., on the risk for cancer, among men but not in women. The antioxidant supplements used included beta carotene, ascorbic acid, vitamin E, and selenium, and also zinc, which is not commonly so classified. The study involved 5,141 men aged 45 to 60 years and 7,876 women aged 35 to 60 years old. They were randomly assigned to take a daily capsule containing either 120 mg of ascorbic acid, 30 mg of vitamin E, six mg of beta carotene, 100 micrograms of selenium, and 20 mg of zinc, or a placebo capsule. The participants were followed for a median of 7.5 years to record occurrence of cancers. When the researchers determined cancer incidence according to sex, they found a significant protective effect of the antioxidants in men, who were 31 percent less likely to develop cancer than were women. A similar trend was found in men for death rates; after 7.5 years the low-dose antioxidant supplementation lowered the total cancer incidence and the all-cause mortality rate for men but not in women. Hercberg and colleagues (2004) speculated that the difference might reflect men having a lower baseline intake level than women for certain antioxidants, especially beta-carotene. The levels of supplementation were not as high as those commonly endorsed by "nutritional doctors."

Megadose Vitamin C (Sodium Ascorbate) Therapy

The researchers who drew great attention to using megadose vitamin combinations as a therapy for cancer were Linus Pauling, PhD (a Nobel Prize winner for chemistry and for peace), Ewan Cameron, MD, and Abram Hoffer, MD. Dr. Hoffer entered this arena from his specialty of psychiatry because of his successful use of high-dosage niacin (vitamin B3) plus vitamin C against psychosis. He chanced to be called upon for his nutritional therapy experience in treating a cancer patient who subsequently had a quite remarkable recovery. The advocates of vitamin C against cancer were further influenced by animal laboratory data indicating that vitamins, both alone and in combinations, exert positive effects in whole animals or in vitro cell systems. They caused a reduction of tumor growth, immunomodulation, and enhancement of a highly vital function lost by cancer cells—cell differentiation (progressive development of more specialized features). All of these actions seem potentially beneficial to cancer patients.

The hypothesis in favor of vitamin C was tested by Cameron with encouragement from Pauling in patients with advanced cancer. A positive effect of apparently extended survival was seen according to initial clinical reports. He and others following this approach usually use injections of a solution of the more soluble and nonacidic salt of ascorbic acid, sodium ascorbate. However, the findings of those early trials were only able to be presented as anecdotal reports, being an uncontrolled series of cases. Therefore, the results could merely be called suggestive rather than conclusive. Some have protested that limiting such studies to only advanced-stage cancer patients disadvantaged ascorbate therapy from showing its full potential. Unfortunately, no randomized, controlled tests using sodium ascorbate on the progression of either early or less advanced cancer have been reported, so the therapy remains unvalidated, though it may be questioned whether adequately tested or not. (Extensive coverage of this topic will be found Chapter 25.)

Vitamin E Therapy

Some correlative, descriptive studies have indicated that low serum levels of vitamin E (often known alpha-tocopherol) are associated with a slight increase in the risk of cancer for some populations studied. Because vitamin E exerts antioxidant properties and is alleged to have immunostimulant effects, some observers infer that it should be protective against cancer. However, the epidemiologic data are too limited and inconsistent to provide definitive support for the conclusion that a higher intake of vitamin E will reduce one's risk for cancer.

SPES and PC-SPES for Prostate Cancer

Prostate cancer (PC) is the second most common cause of cancer death among men in the United States. PC-SPES was marketed in the United

States (DiPaola et al., 1998) specifically as a remedy for patients diagnosed with prostate cancer. Case reports were published of biopsy-conformed cancers being greatly reduced under PC-SPES therapy. However, in early February 2002 FDA's Safety Information and Adverse Event Reporting Program issued a notice warning consumers to stop using the herbal supplements PC SPES and SPES. The basis for this was that both products were found to contain undeclared prescription drugs that could cause serious health effects if not taken with medical supervision. Laboratory analysis of the products by the California Department of Health Services revealed that samples of PC SPES contained warfarin and SPES contained alprazolam, both of which are legally available only by prescription. The illegal presence of these agents is puzzling because neither is appropriate for the claimed purposes of the products—PC SPES and SPES were marketed for "maintaining prostate health and strengthening the immune system." BotanicLab, the manufacturer of the products, immediately issued a nationwide recall. Subsequently, on June 1, 2002, BotanicLab officially closed down the business. Detailed data from NCCAM concerning possible further research can be found at www.nccam.nih.gov/health/alerts/spes/, and a safety notice from the FDA can be found at www.fda.gov/medwatch/SAFETY/2002/safety02.htm#spes.

An Unconventional-Type Enzyme Therapy "Crosses Over"

European medicine, especially in Germany, has accepted the idea that orally administered enzymes can exert a systemic action of therapeutic value. This goes against a perhaps overly simplistic "scientific" concept that enzyme molecules are too large to be absorbed from the intestine, and moreover, that being proteins they would be thoroughly digested before they could be absorbed. However, a small number of mainline U.S. medical researchers undermined this prevalent outlook by showing that orally dosed protein molecules can provoke the production of useful, therapeutic antibodies, which means the protein had to be absorbed. This finding arose in the course of efforts to overcome certain autoimmune diseases. Immune cells associated with the intestinal lining are thought to provide access for undigested proteins; uptake by other cells lining the intestinal tract through endocytosis (a cell engulfing the molecule) is also a possibility.

One natural and unconventional enzyme therapy for cancer, Wobe-Mugos, has made a successful crossover by becoming FDA-approved in 2000 as an orphan drug on application from Marlyn Nutraceuticals of Scottsdale, Arizona. The approval calls for its use only in treating one specific cancer, multiple myeloma, which has long been known as incurable, and for its being used as an adjunct to other therapies. It consists of a mixture made from an extract of the calf thymus gland combined with enzymes from the papaya fruit, the pancreas of cows, and the pancreas of pigs, and is administered as an enteric-coated tablet. It had been successfully used in Europe for clinical trials in conjunction with chemotherapy since 1977. Numerous European reports claim that it reduced the severity of symptoms, extended life, and improved the quality of life of multiple myeloma patients. However, a proposed Phase III multicenter clinical trial of its use as sole therapy was stopped and canceled (www.annieappleseedproject.org/mulmyelwobe.html).

The component enzymes of Wobe-Mugos are pancreatin, papain, bromelain, trypsin, chymotrypsin, lipase, and amylase. The ways in which they are proposed to act are multiple, including (1) stimulation of immune functions through activation of the T-lymphocytes and natural killer cells and the secretion of tumor necrosis factor, (2) destruction of circulating antibody-antigen complexes provoked by the cancer cells, and (3) "unmasking" of cancer cells by removing their "protective guise" behind normal components of the patient's cellular chemistry, such as fibrin or fats that attach to the surface of cancer cells. This would better permit identification of the target and would facilitate immune system attacks on the cancer. A division of Marlyn Nutraceuticals has marketed a very similar product under the name of Wobenzym as a dietary supplement, nominally for its use as a digestive aid (www.thewayup.com/products/0221.htm).

THE TOXICITY FACTOR IN CONVENTIONAL THERAPY

A major factor causing people to consider unconventional, natural remedies is the severe adverse effects that are associated with use of contemporary cancer chemotherapy and radiation. Proponents of CAM therapies tend to use quite pejorative language against conventional therapies—"cutting, burning, and poisoning"—while promoting their particular alternative cancer remedies as being free of any damaging side effects. Some breast cancer patients express the view that they had nothing to lose because CAM was not harmful (Boon et al., 2000). Therapies considered by the women interviewed were mostly those involving orally ingested substances, such as herbs and other supplements. Although those might have not been totally free of potential risks, they are unlikely to cause anything akin to the level of toxic effects on noncancerous tissues that is likely when using conventional chemotherapy, but neither are they sure to kill enough cancer cells.

That the mode of action for chemotherapy is to kill cells, and that the discrimination between cancerous and noncancerous cells is far less than perfect also turns away some patients who hope and believe that a less drastic mode of attack against the problem may be available. Gotay and Dumitriu (2000) told how a researcher from Hawaii posed as a shopper looking for alternative treatments for a person with cancer. Clerks in the local health food shops were happy to give advice and information, describing many of their natural products as "cleansing," "balancing," or "immune boosting." Doctors should try using such descriptions/explanations for chemotherapy. Indeed, it is a fact that a great variety of conventional anticancer drugs originated from plant materials, but that did not avoid their being highly toxic.

PERSONAL CHOICES

Many cancer patients search Internet sources for information on complementary and alternative medicine. Schmidt and Ernst (2004) conducted a study to evaluate the quality of the information so obtained and to identify the treatments most frequently described. Thirty-two Web sites were included in their analysis. The quality of the sites was scored on a point system, and results varied between 8 and 14 points with a maximum of 14. Most sites issued recommendations for numerous treatments, which typically were judged to lack support by sound scientific evidence. The most frequently discussed therapies were herbal medicines, diets, and mind-body therapies. Three sites were judged to hold the potential for harming patients through the advice offered. The most popular Web sites on CAM approaches to cancer offer information of "extremely variable quality," and many endorse unproven therapies, some of which were judged to be "outright dangerous."

Another viewpoint is expressed by the person behind one of the Web sites very likely included in the Schmidt and Ernst (2004) analysis—Dr. Ralph Moss and "The Moss Reports: The World's Leading Cancer Treatment Information and Referral Service":

> I don't think the answer is to become a hardened cynic with regard to new or alternative cancer treatments. In many ways that is even worse than being too trusting, for it prejudges and effectively rejects potentially beneficial new treatments when they do come along. What is needed is an open-minded attitude towards new treatments combined with a searching attempt to get at the bedrock truth concerning any proposed treatment for this intractable disease. In other words, the approach that I characterize as "friendly skepticism." (Moss, 1994)

Chapter 19

Immunoenhancing Supplements: Are They Effective?

It is bad not to do any research, but badly done research is even worse.

Bernardo Houssay (1956),
1947 Nobel Prize winner

INTRODUCTION

A rudimentary understanding of the following basic terms in immunology will be required to deal with this subject: antibodies, complement, cytokines, leukocytes, lymphocytes, natural killer cells, and phagocytes. Please refer to the Glossary at the end of this book if you are uncertain about the definitions of these terms. Be forewarned that immunology is a very complex science, the technical literature of which is more incomprehensible than other science if one has not studied it thoroughly.

In the realm of immunonutrition, as in many other biological research areas, much scientific understanding of normal physiological relationships has been gained through observations of abnormal conditions. Cases of persons experiencing starvation reveal that severe protein-energy malnutrition is associated with a significant impairment of various aspects of immunity, sush as cell-mediated immunity, phagocyte function, complement system activity, secretory immunoglobulin A antibody levels, and cytokine production. However, overnutrition and obesity also are said to reduce immunity according to a distinguished nutrition researcher, Dr. R. K. Chandra (2002), who emphasized that deficiencies of single nutrients also can result in an impaired immune response, which may occur even when the deficiency state is relatively mild. He also observed that the micronutrients zinc, selenium, iron, copper, and vitamins A, C, E, B_6, and folic acid all have important influences on immune responses (see also Erickson et al., 2000; Grimm and Calder, 2002). Another commentator on nutrients as modulators of im-

doi:10.1300/5698_19

mune function (Hinds, 1991) emphasized L-arginine as an enhancer of lymphocyte reactivity, and the omega-3 fatty acids of fish oils as antagonists of autoimmune-type inflammation. Both may have useful clinical significance.

The capacity to modify the activity of the immune system by supplementation that involves specific nutrients is termed *immunonutrition* (Grimm and Calder, 2002). Therefore, immunonutrients are those compounds that are ordinary dietary components that are influential toward the immune system's response mechanisms. These agents include substances such as certain amino acids, fatty acids, nucleic acids, and trace elements (Rivera et al., 2003). In particular, the amino acids glutamine and arginine, the omega-3 fatty acids, and ribonucleic acids (RNAs) are now being added to standard nutritional-support solutions for hospitalized patients to provide formulations called immunonutrition. Although some authors use the terms *immunoenhancement* or *immunostimulation,* more likely one will encounter the use of *immunomodulation* to describe agents' producing unspecified effects on immune system activities. In medical practice such solutions are administered enterally (via a nasogastric tube, that delivers into the upper intestine) or parenterally (a line to deliver intravenously).

Randomized, controlled trials have shown that recipients of immunonutrition have outcomes superior to those found in control subjects who receive only the standard nutritional support. However, conceivably the standard parenteral or enteral solutions may actually have an adverse effect that is canceled by the additional nutrients, but this is unknown because data are lacking from randomized trials to test the standard nutritional solutions versus no such nutritional support. Moreover, because nutritive agents may either up- or down-regulate the immune response, their effects may vary and be specific for certain diseases.

Many therapeutic advances during the past quarter-century have arisen from better understanding of the intricacies of our defense mechanisms encompassed by the term *immune system.* Indeed, enough mainline studies of parenteral or enteral nutritional therapy have been done for three meta-analyses to have been reported concerning nutrient components on immune functions. Most such trials used a combination of arginine and omega-3 fatty acids, or arginine and omega-3 fatty acids and nucleotides. Others combined these types of nutrients with glutamine or branched-chain amino acids.

Those researches were briefly reviewed in an editorial of April 2003 in the *BMJ* by a professor of nutritional immunology of the Institute of Human Nutrition at the University of Southampton School of Medicine in the United Kingdom. Dr. P. C. Calder (2003) pointed out that three potential targets exist for immunonutrition: the mucosal barriers of our body, the cellular defenses, and local or systemic inflammatory reactions. He stated that the nutrients most studied for intravenous use to gain immunonutritional benefit are arginine, glutamine, branched-chain amino acids (all in the L-form), omega-3 fatty acids, and nucleotides. These specific nutrients have been shown to improve the immune system function after surgery. Such experimental feeding formulas also contained large doses of antioxidant vitamins and minerals, e.g., vitamins A and E and selenium. Mixtures of some or all of these five key nutrients are present in commercially available enteral products.

Parenteral formulas containing glutamine or omega-3 fatty acids are also available commercially (de Pablo and Alvarez de Cienfuegos, 2000). The picture was described thus by Calder (2003):

> Major surgery is followed by a period of immunosuppression that increases the risk of morbidity and mortality due to infection. Improving immune function during this period may reduce complications due to infection. Critically ill patients are at greater risk of adverse outcomes than surgical patients. In these patients complex variable immune and inflammatory changes occur that are only now being well defined. (p. 117)

Thus, we find mainline medical practice acknowledging the role of critical nutrients for maintenance or restoration of healthy immunologic activity. Moreover, knowledge in this area is beginning to progress not only for hospitalized postsurgery patients but also for all the rest of us who live in a world of continually new strains of influenza as well as a new coronavirus causing SARS (severe acute respiratory syndrome). Concerning methodology, it is becoming possible to detect and/or confirm that certain supplements, both nutrients and botanicals, can alter immune functions in ways that are beneficial.

However, large, interindividual variations exist in many immune functions even among healthy persons. Genetics, age, sex, smoking, habitual levels of exercise, alcohol consumption, diet, stage in the menstrual cycle, physical or mental stresses, history of infections, and vaccinations are believed to be the important contributors to observed interpersonal variation (Calder and Kew, 2002). Nutritional status is accepted as being an important factor in immune competence knowing that undernutrition impairs immune system activities, leading to a suppression of immunity. Although it is clear that some persons whose immune responses fall significantly below normal are more susceptible to infectious agents and have more illness or death from infections, it has not been clearly shown that variations in immune function among healthy persons determines their susceptibility to infection.

BOTANICAL SUPPLEMENTS AND IMMUNONUTRITION

Operating on a parallel but independent track from conventional medical therapy via immunonutrition, unconventional practitioners have made the immune system a very major target for nutritional supplements (especially for the antioxidants), with aims and claims for their helping to prevent diseases of various types. This is in addition to the general claim for many botanical/herbal agents that they can help to improve ("boost") immune system activities to oppose serious diseases, especially of latter life. The 2003 SARS epidemic is a case in which attention was focused on claimed immunoenhancing effects of dietary supplements. Clearly this may recur if further serious outbreaks of this new viral disease occur, or when older ones such as regular influenza or the threatening avian flu reemerge.

A paper by Wilasrusmee and colleagues (2002) reported investigations of in vitro immunomodulatory effects of ten commonly used botanical supplement products on immune function relevant to transplantation procedures. Dong quai, ginseng, and milk thistle all showed nonspecific immunostimulatory effects in terms of lymphocyte proliferation, whereas ginger and green tea had immunosuppressive effects. Dong quai and milk thistle both increased responsiveness also in a second test, whereas ginger and green tea once more decreased the responses. The immunostimulatory effects of dong quai and milk thistle were consistently seen in both cell-mediated immune response and antibody-related nonspecific lymphocyte proliferation. The authors concluded that green tea, dong quai, ginseng, milk thistle, and ginger all have effects on in vitro immune assays that may be relevant to human transplantation patients. Their direct actions on the immune system might serve either to enhance or to oppose the immunosuppressive agents routinely required by organ transplant recipients. The adverse influence of one botanical, St. John's wort, on the immunosuppressive action of a transplantation medicine, which was exerted indirectly by accelerating its metabolism, is described in Chapter 9.

Nonetheless, many claims for the nutritional supplements regarding immune system activity are still overly simplified. In addition, too few instances of a claimed anti-infective benefit have been confirmed by clinical research. Printed materials promoting supplements as clinically effective immunoenhancing agents should be considered with a goodly dose of cautious skepticism. The scope of illnesses that are related to immunity functions is broad, ranging from those stemming from a deficiency or inadequacy of immune system actions to those that stem from an overactivity or misdirection of the immune system's actions.

In the latter case we refer to illnesses arising from what we call either autoimmunity or allergy, or even less well defined illnesses that seem to stem from unfavorable immune system activity. One could say that these may not be examples of overactivity so much as cases of misdirected actions. Thus, the question exists of whether autoimmune and allergic diseases can be improved by opposing or reducing immune functions without causing other serious problems, i.e., producing a dangerous immunosuppression that may interfere with our intrinsic defenses against cancers or infections. That is one of the hazards of several 1990s Rx therapies for autoimmune diseases such as rheumatoid arthritis and Crohn's disease. One of them in October 2004 was the subject of an FDA Warning Letter that the risk for lymphoma is increased several-fold for persons treated with Remicade (infliximab) and possibly also other TNF-alpha (tumor necrosis factor-alpha) blocking agents (www.fda.gov/medwatch/SAFETY/2004/remicade _dearhcp.pdf).

This is a new area that mainline medicine has begun exploiting to advantage, but one with considerable inherent difficulties and dangers. Thus, reason for concern exists regarding whether supplements that exert an immunity-enhancing action also might aggravate those disease states having an autoimmune foundation.

OVERVIEW OF CONFERENCE ON IMMUNONUTRITION (1999)

In September 1999 the National Institute of Allergy and Infectious Diseases held a two-day conference, cosponsored by the Office of Dietary Supplements of the National Institutes of Health, on immunonutrition that is very relevant for our consideration. The workshop provided information on the effects of micronutrients on innate and adaptive immunity, mucosal immunity, cytokine production, gene expression, and intracellular signaling pathways. One session focused on the implications of basic research findings for treatment of disease. An initial overview on how dietary characteristics modulate immune responses concluded that the field is in its infancy. Areas in particular need of research include the role of micronutrients in innate and mucosal immunity as well as the early phases of development of immune cells. Cases of direct interactions between micronutrients and pathogens were described; for example, a benign strain of infectious agent becoming virulent by passing through micronutrient-deficient mice was described.

At the conclusion of the workshop, a panel of experts (CDC, 1999) composed of basic scientists, infectious disease specialists, and clinical epidemiologists submitted an array of topics needing future research that included the following:

- The development of a panel of assays that could be used for general screening for any impact of nutrients on immunocompetence (the ability to mount a normal response)
- The need to define reproducible molecular and immunologic markers that can be used in both human and animal researches
- The need for continued basic mechanism studies on both the role of micronutrients as antioxidants or as regulatory molecules within the immune system, and the effects of micronutrient status on the decline of immune function in the elderly
- The need for investigators to link basic molecular mechanistic studies to fieldwork in areas of endemic infectious diseases of the greatest public health importance
- The need for innovative approaches for combining nutritional supplementation and conventional immunotherapy in new forms of intervention
- The need to recruit young investigators with state-of-the-art skills in immunology and to promote their collaborative research with nutrition or infectious disease experts

These recommendations indicate that this field is still rather immature, and it thus is to be expected that an inadequate scientific foundation exists for drawing many conclusions on the role of dietary deficiencies, and of dietary supplementation, in healthy functioning of our immune system.

CAN NUTRIENT SUPPLEMENTS AID THE IMMUNE SYSTEM?

Whether the competence of the immune system to mount a normal immune response when needed can be improved for apparently healthy persons by botanicals or through nutritional supplementation is still open to scientific question. Although many animal or in vitro studies have been done, the question of the results carrying over to the human situation has seldom been satisfied. However, this is hardly the conclusion one would reach from reading promotional materials about many nutrients, much less the botanical products touted as enhancers of immune function. In this instance again we find that the information provided to consumers tends to mislead rather than inform by suggesting that much more knowledge is available than actually exists. Many supplements have been found in laboratory animal tests to have significant and seemingly desirable effects on immune system functions. Of these are very few for which human confirmation of the laboratory data are available. Exhibit 19.1 gives a sample of the dietary supplements that are commonly endorsed as "immune boosters."

EXHIBIT 19.1. Selections of a major "nutritional doctor" for "immunity boosters."

Nutrients or Metabolites

Vitamin C: Recommends 2.5 grams per day; aids immune cells to attack bacteria.

Vitamin A: Recommends 5,000 IU up to 50,000 IU for viral upper respiratory problems.

Alpha-lipoic acid: A dual-function antioxidant—water and fat soluble.

N-Acetylcysteine: Antioxidant/radical scavenger; favors glutathione and opposes homocysteine (a risk factor for cardiovascular disease).

Lycopene: Protective antioxidant to aid maintenance of immune system activities.

Zinc: Recommends as gluconate (12 mg) lozenges for use at the onset of cold to shorten its duration, which is supported by published clinical findings.

Botanicals

Echinacea (Echinacea purpurea *or* angustifolia): Enhanced number and activity of WBCs, popular for opposing colds, *not* recommended for continuous use.

Elderberry (Sambucus nigra): May shorten duration of flu symptoms, said to directly inhibit the virus, used as syrup or lozenges.

Ginkgo biloba: Flavonoids and ginkgolides act as antioxidants and benefit circulation.

Cranberry: Shown active against urinary tract infections by stopping bacterial adhesion on the bladder mucosal surfaces.

To these might be added (among others):

Blueberry: Mechanism believed as for cranberry, an excellent source for antioxidants.

Goldenseal (Hydrastis canadensis): Similar to echinacea and elderberry, no more than three weeks continuous use, liquid form has a strong taste, best with a fruit juice.

Astragalus (Astragalus membranaceus): Similar to echinacea and elderberry.

Unfortunately, few of these claims are yet supported by substantial clinical trials.

Echinacea is the most popular among various botanical remedies claimed to have value for preventing or overcoming infections. Traditionally, it has been used both by topical and systemic routes, but is supplied most commonly as an oral dosage form. The best-researched usage is for treatment and prevention of upper respiratory tract infections, especially colds. Although echinacea may be helpful in this manner, the human trial data, though more often than not positive, are not fully convincing to those who pursue an evidence-based standard.

MICRONUTRIENTS AND THE IMMUNE SYSTEM

Although the major emphasis in medical immunonutrition currently is upon the amino acids, fatty acids, and ribonucleic acids, roles also exist for the vitamins, minerals, and metabolites. This is discussed also in Chapters 21 to 23, but we will consider it in broad terms here. The first anti-infective defenses are physical barriers—the skin and mucous membrane surfaces of the body. In ascorbic-acid deficiency the integrity of these tissue barriers may be subverted because a sufficiency of ascorbate is essential for the integrity of the connective tissues. A severe deficiency state (scurvy) is characterized by a generalized structural breakdown (Cameron and Pauling, 1973). Vitamins A, C, and E as antioxidants may support a reduction of oxidative injury occurring during a bacterial infection because the body's own leukocytes secrete prooxidant radicals important to their defensive actions. Avoiding injury to and deterioration of healthy tissues may be a significant role of both vitamin and nonvitamin antioxidants.

A recent review by Bhaskaram (2002) found that micronutrient deficiencies and infectious diseases often coexist and show complex interactions that lead to a vicious cycle of malnutrition plus infections. Such a combination is mainly observed in underprivileged people of developing countries, particularly in rural regions and especially in young preschool children. He says that the micronutrients vitamin A, beta-carotene, folic acid, vitamin B12, vitamin C, riboflavin, iron, zinc, and selenium all have immunomodulating functions, and thus they influence the susceptibility of humans to infectious diseases and the course and outcome of such diseases. Practically all forms of immunity may be adversely affected by deficiencies of one or more of these nutrients. Animal and human studies have shown that adding the deficient nutrient to the diet can restore a deficient immune function and resistance to infection. This does not mean that an above-normal nutrient level will elevate immune function to a supranormal level, as many dietary supplement promotions might seem to suggest.

Another review (Bogden, 2004) declares that compelling evidence confirms that severe zinc deficiency can cause a substantial impairment of cellular immunity which can favor an infection and even death. The effects on immunity of mild to moderate zinc deficiency are much less severe and more subtle. Bogden says that zinc supplementation in combination with other micronutrients can enhance immunity when an immune deficit arises from an underlying deficiency. Calder (2003) emphasized that copper, iron, and selenium as trace mineral elements are needed for optimal activity of the immune system. Deficiencies of zinc and vitamins A and D are thought to reduce the functions of natural killer cells, but supplementation with zinc or vitamin C may enhance their functions.

Beta-Carotene, precursor of vitamin A, has been found by Herraiz et al. (1998) to protect against a natural type of immunosuppression—that resulting from skin exposure to ultraviolet (UV) light. That vitamin's protective action seemed to be less for a sample of healthy older men (average age 65.5 years) than for younger ones, which may point to another age-related decline.

Calder and Kew (2002) conclude that higher intake of some nutrients above normal levels can enhance immune function. However, they also warn that excess amounts of some nutrients may impair immune function. Finally, they conclude that growing evidence suggests that probiotic bacteria can improve host immune function. However, whether such an effect is observed in healthy individuals is not clear.

However, indications exist that apparently healthy elders may be more at risk for nutrient deficiencies that may impair immunity. Dr. R. K. Chandra (1997), in his commentary piece, concluded that overwhelming evidence of immunological enhancement exists following nutrient supplementation in the elderly. He especially endorsed vitamin E at a dose of 200 mg per day.

PREBIOTICS AND PROBIOTICS FOR IMMUNE SYSTEM BENEFITS

Probiotics are living, nonpathogenic microorganisms that can affect the host in a beneficial manner by their presence among the gastrointestinal (GI) microflora—bacteria living harmlessly in the colon (Hamilton-Miller, 2004; Manning and Gibson, 2004). *Prebiotics* are nondigestible food ingredients that stimulate the growth and activity of probiotic bacteria already established in the colon. These topics are increasingly seen as clinically significant. Animal research indicates that having an optimal gut microflora can raise an animal's resistance to pathogenic bacteria, lower their blood level of ammonia, increase stimulation of immune responses, and reduce the risk of cancer. However, rather few reports of human intervention studies on probiotics exist. Multiple mechanisms of action have been postulated—improved lactose digestion, microbial competition for space or nutrients, immunomodulation, and a production of antimicrobial agents. (Some writers postulate that excessive immune stimulation may occur as an adverse response.)

Probiotic preparations, for example, have been shown effective in opposing a wide range of GI diseases (Erickson and Hubbard, 2000). Either *Lactobacillus rhamnosus* GG alone or a combination of *Bifidobacterium bifidum* and *Streptococcus thermophilus* have shown efficacy for treatment of *Clostridium difficile* infection as well as for reducing the frequency and severity of infectious acute diarrheas in children. Prevention of antibiotic-induced diarrhea has been demonstrated by a concurrent administration of either *Lactobacillus* GG or *Saccharomyces boulardii.* Data to support probiotic efficacy in prevention of traveler's diarrhea are less adequate. It is believed that selected probiotic preparations can prevent relapse of ulcerative colitis when it is quiescent. One review concludes that additional studies are needed to take full advantage of this traditional approach to human GI diseases.

A form of probiotic therapy known as Primal Defense claims on its label to employ distinctive "Specially cultured probiotic strains designed to be resistant to Heat, Cold, Stomach Acids, Chlorine, Fluorine and Ascorbic Acid" and to be "the only probiotic that contains HSOs (Homeostatic Soil Organisms)." No research articles were found by a PubMed search using such phrases. These friendly organisms are said to "keep the human GI tract in a state of homeostasis by increasing intestinal absorption and keeping it free of parasites, yeasts, molds, other fungi, harmful bacteria, viruses, and additional pathogens such as spirochetes, rickettsiae, chlamydiae, protozoa, and helminths." (Walker, 2001).

The prebiotics concept, which was launched as recently as 1995, is concerned with these nondigestible but selectively fermented food ingredients and their effects in the colon that could reduce the risk for GI diseases (Van Loo, 2004). Nondigestible prebiotics are the oligosaccharides, comprising a shorter chain of sugar molecules than is found in a polysaccharide. Prebiotic laboratory feeding studies that examined lactosucrose and fructo-oligosaccharides in both cats and dogs have shown positive effects on their microflora balance. Prebiotics exert an osmotic effect in the intestinal lumen and are fermented by bacterial action in the colon. Their array of effects are relevant to the fields of intestinal function, lipid metabolism, absorption of minerals, bone formation, and immunology. Some emphasis is also given to an importance of prebiotics in the management of osteoporosis, alleviation of menopausal symptoms, and opposing an onset of cancer. It will be of interest, looking forward, to see how many of these "areas of promise" eventually are supported by adequate evidence.

Modification of intestinal flora because of the presence of selectively fermented prebiotics has been observed to be a central factor in determining probiotic properties. The probiotics can interact positively with varied intestinal physiologic processes by means of the large intestinal surface contact, including their improvement of health via a reduction of disease risks (Marteau et al., 2001; Marteau and Seksik, 2004). On the down side, prebiotics may induce gaseousness and bloating, but abdominal pain and diarrhea only occur with large doses. An increase in gastroesophageal reflux also has been associated with excessive daily doses. Individual intolerance factors probably include the prior presence of irritable bowel syndrome or gastroesophageal reflux.

POLYSACCHARIDE PRODUCTS FOR IMMUNOENHANCEMENT

Carbohydrates are biomolecules found abundantly in nature in highly diverse forms and types, ranging from simple sugars, the monosaccharides (such as glucose and fructose), to oligosaccharides and polysaccharides, to the glyco conjugates of many glycoproteins. Supposedly immune-response-stimulating plant components are found among various polysaccharides from several sources. One is larch arabinogalactan, a polysaccharide powder derived from wood of larch trees, primarily *Larix occidentalis* (western larch), which consists of about 98 percent arabinogalactan (containing arabinose and galactose sugars). Arabinogalactans are found in a variety of plants but have high abundance in the *Larix* genus (Anonymous, 2000). Western larch is also known as mountain larch or western tamarack and is native to the Pacific and the inland northwestern United States as well as parts of British Columbia. In plant tissues, the arabinogalactans are implicated in such diverse functions as cell-to-cell adhesion, nutrition of growing pollen tubes, responsiveness to microbial infections, and as markers of identity. Larch arabinogalactan is approved by the FDA as a source of dietary fiber, but it also is being used as a dietary supplement for supposed therapeutic benefit as an immunostimulant that has been considered as a cancer protocol adjunct.

Arabinogalactans, pectin, and other saccharide-related polymers have also been obtained from aerial parts of sage *(Salvia officinalis)* and are being evaluated for value in medicinal use (Capek et al., 2003). Glucomannons and galactomannans are among the soluble fibers that are considered to exert a blood-cholesterol-lowering action. They share a common base component of the sugar mannose, as well as glucose and galactose, respectively. Some galactomannans and arabinogalactans are prominent components of the polysaccharide fraction of roasted coffee. Highly branched arabinans, xyloglucans, and arabinogalactans are polysaccharide components from apples that doubtless have antiadhesion properties that likely help to keep apple eaters and their doctors apart. A review by nutritionist R. N. Tharanathan (2002) gives a broad view of the often bewildering diversity of carbohydrates. Jenkins and co-authors (2000) considered the relationships of polysaccharides to metabolism of simple sugars and lipids as determinants of a person's risk for coronary heart disease.

DIETARY SOURCES FOR CRITICAL IMMUNONUTRIENT FACTORS

Dietary sources for L-arginine include dairy products, meat, poultry, and fish, as well as nuts, rice, whole wheat, soy, and raisins. It can also be taken in supplement form as capsules. Intravenous L-glutamine therapy aims to repair and maintain the mucosa of the intestinal tract as well as to stimulate the immune system. Moreover, the amino acid is valuable as an indirect source of energy for brain cells after its metabolic conversion to glutamate. The brain uses glutamic acid for energy almost as well as it does glucose, and with less biochemical stress in doing so. The problem is that glutamate does not readily cross the blood-brain barrier. However, glutamine is freely able to cross, and then the brain cells can convert it to the glutamate for their energy needs. Moreover, L-glutamine is one of the important precursors of the vital radical scavenger and antioxidant glutathione. Fortunately numerous good dietary sources of L-glutamine are available, including meats, fresh fruits, and vegetables; moreover, L-glutamine supplements are widely available.

The branched-chain amino acids (BCAAs)—leucine, valine, and isoleucine—are reputedly the easiest for the body to use in repair, which has made them very popular with many bodybuilders. BCAAs also are useable for incorporation into new proteins, both structural and enzymatic. The three BCAAs are all essential amino acids and are also precursors of glutamine. They are easily obtained from meat, whey protein, egg protein, and other dairy products, and they also are available in supplement form.

Nucleotides are the basic units of nucleic acids, which are the building blocks for not only DNA but also RNA. They must be available to make cell division possible. When the immune system is under stress, new cells are needed to help fight infection. White blood cells, bone marrow cells, and the mucosal cells of the intestine all show a high rate of turnover, which requires plentiful sources of the necessary nucleotides. The organ meats such as liver and kidney are rich in nucleotides, as are legumes and seafoods. Breast milk is perhaps the richest source of nucleotides. It is recognized that formula-fed infants are generally more prone to infection than those who are breast-fed. Some researchers believe that the ready accessibility of such nucleotides is primarily responsible for the difference.

Chapter 20

What Is the Price of Globalism? Heavy Metals, Heavy Risks

Imported ethnic-traditional remedies may carry a health risk from their content of toxic metals such as lead, mercury, arsenic, or cadmium.

Many people are able to recognize names of certain dangerous heavy metals such as the metallic elements lead, arsenic, and mercury. However, the occurrence of such elements in some ethnic remedies is not reference to name of the element but rather to the name of its mineral salt, which goes by another and more innocent name. *Cinnabar* is a name that sounds downright appetizing until one learns that it is a name for mercuric sulfide, a quite toxic compound. Likewise, *realgar* is the term for arsenic sulfide, and *litharge* is really lead oxide.

All of these are known to occur in mixtures comprising Indian or Chinese "herbal" medicines, supplied in the form of capsules, pills, or balls. They also are well known to occur in remedies from the Mideast, Asia, and from "Latin and South America. Chapter 1 told of a misadventure involving a heavy metal, lead, that occurred in the early 1970s. Examples in this chapter show that the problem continues to the present day. Besides the four metals previously named, one case report found the element thallium, used formerly in rat-killer formulations, to be present in and responsible for poisonings from a Chinese remedy called Nutrien. Two women were poisoned, but not fatally, by use of contents of a single package that showed analyses of 3.05 percent thallium and 2.88 percent lead (Schaumburg and Berger, 1992). As analyses of other samples did not detect their being similarly adulterated; the basis for the situation was not discovered.

One relevant research, from the University of Mississippi School of Pharmacy and the National Center for Natural Products Research (Huggett et al., 2001), analyzed samples of four significant botanical products for five metal elements—arsenic, cadmium, chromium, lead, and nickel. The

Consumer's Guide to Dietary Supplements and Alternative Medicines

doi:10.1300/5698_20

botanicals were echinacea, passion flower, St. John's wort, and valerian. The arsenic, chromium, nickel, and lead were detected in all species at quite low levels compared to cadmium, which had levels nearly 40 times as high. The concentrations all were explainable as plant uptake from the soils. The amounts of organochlorine agents detected in all samples must be attributed to anthropogenic (human-induced) causes, i.e., use of pesticides on croplands. However, the authors' conclusion was that levels were not high enough to constitute a health hazard. Thus, metals from the soil are not likely to be a problem, whereas purposeful addition of metals to botanical material as an active component of the remedy does comprise a serious problem, as examples will indicate.

CHUIFONG TOUKUWAN

Supposed herbal remedies from Asia have been found repeatedly to also contain high levels of heavy metals; consequently, their use may result in toxicity. Chuifong toukuwan appeared as early as 1974 in the United States for use as an arthritis remedy, and it was banned by the FDA in 1978 when it was found to contain both toxic heavy metals and Rx drugs. By "banned" is meant that the FDA declared the product to be mislabeled, illegal to import, and subject to seizure if found by customs inspectors. However, via an Internet site (www.envirodocs.com/chinese_herbs.htm) that promises access to "rare healing treasures" are offered, including (surprise!) chuifong toukuwan, with only botanical components being listed. Is it really as represented, and not lead-laden as in the 1970s?

Use of the 1970s' version chuifong toukuwan would also increase the body burden of a less familiar toxic element, cadmium, and could possibly contribute to kidney damage and malfunction in persons exposed to this substance. Upon chronic exposure cadmium accumulates in certain organs, most particularly the kidneys. Not only cadmium but also several analgesic drugs contained in chuifong toukuwan can cause cellular injury to the kidney tubules enabling the loss of lower-molecular-weight proteins into the urine. Cadmium is a cumulative toxicant, with a biological half-life (the time for body levels to decrease by one-half) of greater than ten years in humans. In short, if you take it in, you are stuck with it—it essentially won't leave you!

The FDA declares by a 2004 revision of earlier bulletins that "Chinese herbal medications have a history, dating back to 1974, of containing strong prescription drugs." Certain unapproved foreign digestive remedies containing lead are cited on the same FDA Web page, including "Alarcon,

Azarcon, Coral, Greta, Liga, Maria Luisa, or Rueda." Greta, for example, is 99 percent lead oxide! Azarcon was associated with lead poisoning by Bose et al. (1983).

Lead Poisoning from a Chinese Herbal

Case Report 1

A 59-year-old woman was admitted to Stanford University Hospital in January 1977 with complaints of diffuse pain and anemia (Lightfoot et al., 1977). She had used the services of an herbalist-acupuncturist for the sake of her post-traumatic joint pains. In September she had received and had taken as instructed ten red "herbal pills" three times a day. In November, she developed knee- and hip-joint pains, and in December, pains in her breasts and abdomen plus insomnia. Moreover, she noticed constipation and difficulty in using her hands. At admission she was found to be a pale woman with mild distress from widespread body aches. Her mood was rather unsettled with weepy and irritable spells. A neurological examination showed no sensory or motor defects. Two of her teeth had a small visible "lead line," indicative of an accumulation of elemental lead. Some of her red blood cells showed "basophilic stipling," which also is an indicator of a high lead accumulation. Her whole-blood level of lead was 90 mcg/dL (normal, 10 to 60 mcg/dL). The 24-hour excretion of lead was 281 mcg/day versus a normal level of 0-80 mcg/day. Blood samples from the patient's husband were normal for lead, which tended to exclude some source of household or environmental exposure.

An analysis conducted on the red herbal pills revealed an average lead content of 0.5 mg each. The woman's daily intake of 30 pills would provide a daily lead intake of up to 15 mg of elemental lead per day. This level is well within the recognized toxic range. A constant intravenous infusion was initiated consisting of 2 mg/day of edetate calcium disodium, a chelating agent that ties up the lead in a nonionic form and facilitates its urinary excretion from the body. Intravenous fluid also was given to encourage a liberal urine output. The patient noticed rapid and dramatic relief from her abdominal, joint and muscle pains, as well as from her depression and irritability, within 24 hours. By the second day of therapy her blood levels of lead had fallen and her urinary levels had risen. Investigators from FDA and the Public Health Service discovered that the herbalist-acupuncturist had received the pills from Hong Kong and did not know of their lead content (Lightfoot et al., 1997).

Indian Herbal Diabetes Remedies As Source of Lead Poisoning

Case Report 2

A 39-year-old Indian man with a ten-year history of type 2 (non-insulin-dependent) diabetes, being controlled by the antidiabetic drug glibenclamide, came to a clinic in England with the complaint of a ten-day history of feeling ill (malaise). His accompanying loss of appetite and upper abdominal pain clearly suggested a liver problem. Liver function tests were performed, and elevated levels of liver enzymes were found. Tests were negative for hepatitis viruses A, B, and C; Epstein-Barr virus;

or cytomegalovirus. A urine test indicating a probable excess of lead was confirmed by a whole-blood analysis for lead. This measurement gave a blood lead level value of 5.3 units versus normal values of less than 0.7 units for men not exposed to lead sources.

The patient was treated for five days with a lead-binding chelating agent, and he showed significant improvement. Analysis of an Indian "diabetes medicine" he had been taking disclosed that it had an inorganic lead content of 19 percent by weight, which was the only factor of exposure discovered. Comparative isotopic ratios for the Indian remedy and the patient's blood confirmed that the remedy was the likely source. The authors concluded that this case of hepatitis was the result of lead poisoning arising from an ethnic remedy he had taken for diabetes in addition to a Western antidiabetic medicine (Keen et al., 1994).

Case Report 3

Another Indian male, 35 years old, came to a U.K. clinic with complaints of weakness, malaise, nausea, and abdominal pain six weeks after a three-month visit to India during which he obtained and began to take a nonprescription traditional diabetes medicine. A coarse stippling of his red cells pointed to an overexposure to lead, tests for which confirmed an elevation of nearly four times the normal value. Analysis of the remedy confirmed that lead was present to a degree sufficient to explain the patient's blood level. Treatment with the chelating agent penicillamine restored him to the normal, subtoxic range for lead and reversed his symptoms of poisoning (Pontifex and Garg, 1985).

Crema de Belleza Manning

Although it does not qualify as a dietary supplement but rather as a cosmetic product, it is of concern that a beauty cream manufactured in Tampico, Tamaulipas (Mexico), caused mercury poisoning in consumers and their family members in Texas and Arizona (McRill et al., 2000; Weldon et al., 2000). The findings, involving a mercury-contaminated cream called Crema de Belleza Manning, triggered a statewide health investigation in Arizona. This is another incident that highlights the potential hazard of purchasing certain products produced outside the United States and imported for or by the target ethnic population.

Analysis showed that the cream contained 6 to 10 percent calomel, or mercurous chloride. Although the skin does not easily absorb this form of mercury, sunlight and heat can cause mercurous chloride to break down into forms that are readily absorbed, the authors explained. Mercury levels began to decrease after the patients stopped using the cream, but average levels remained high even months after they stopped.

Case Report 4

Another report suggests that mercury poisoning from beauty creams containing calomel (mercurous chloride) occurs regularly (Weldon et al., 2000). This case involved a 15-year-old boy who resided in Texas near the border with Mexico. In September 1995 he developed weakness, fatigue, insomnia, muscle pain, severe headache, cough, sore throat, constipation, and abnormal sensations (paresthesias) of the hands and feet. Added problems that followed were loss of taste sense, loss of weight (15 pounds), and an increasing weakness of his limbs. His neurologic symptoms were diagnosed as arising from severe demyelinating polyneuropathy, a serious pathology.

In a hospital in November an MRI scan of his brain was normal, but a heavy-metal test of the urine demonstrated an elevated mercury level—nine times the upper limit of the normal range! A chelating agent was administered to facilitate removal of mercury. Investigations seeking to identify the source of exposure failed to find mercury in the soil, paint, or indoor air at his residence, school, or work. It was found that he had used the Crema de Beleza-Manning to treat acne for five months in 1995. Analysis of the product showed again a 6 to 10 percent mercury content by weight. Later surveys found that the cream was present in many homes in the six most populous Texas counties along the Mexican border with the United States. Most users had high urinary levels of mercury (Weldon et al., 2000).

METROPOLITAN MARKET FOR DANGEROUS ETHNIC REMEDIES

New York City is commonly regarded to be a crossroad of the whole world. Because of its population from scores of far-flung countries, it becomes a locale for toxicity problems that formerly were thought of as occurring only in peoples of the Third World. One of the areas of concern is for ethnic remedies from diverse regions having in common their use of lead-containing concoctions (Pérez-Peña, 2003). In early November 2003 the New York City Department of Health and Mental Hygiene sounded a warning and performed searches concerning one such remedy, Litargirio. This product has been marketed in the Dominican Republic for years as a remedy for every sort of malady from body odor to foot fungus. Reportedly, Litargirio has been widely used by Dominicans as a burn remedy and as a tonic for sore feet, but no one could say how widely because of its being unregulated.

The city health officials warned on November 5 that the substance was poisonous. The city began trying to persuade those operating herbal medicine shops that cater mainly to Hispanic communities to stop offering it for sale. Litargirio contains high levels of lead, which can cause brain damage if too much enters the bloodstream. Several Dominican companies make it, distributing it as a yellow or orange powder in cellophane packets. It has been exported to the United States in years past. Health officials said the powder was also sold at bodegas (bars or wine shops), pharmacies, and beauty supply stores.

Litargirio powder usually is sprinkled on the skin, where it is not readily absorbable into the systemic circulation. However, if it gets on the hands of the user, it can be ingested unintentionally. The City Health Commissioner warned "there is absolutely no health benefit from using it, only danger. If you're using it, stop right away, and go to a doctor to get a blood test for lead" (Pérez-Peña, 2003, p. 1). The hazard is especially critical for children who are at risk for impaired development of higher mental functions. The FDA is considering a ban on any further importation of the material.

Litargirio is just a small part of a vast array of traditional ethnic remedies sold in little shops around New York City and other major metropolitan areas of North America. This trade is often conducted in various languages besides English, and it has been going on without much official oversight. According to *The New York Times* (Pérez-Peña, 2003) in early 2003 among Chinese neighborhoods across the country, stores supplying folk remedies did a brisk business in herbal concoctions intended to ward off the SARS infection, even though Toronto, Canada, was the only site for its occurrence in North America. This unregulated trade in dangerous products conducted in immigrant communities is not limited to remedies. New York City health officials found unsafe levels of lead in imported cosmetics and in ceramic pots sold in some areas of the metropolis. Physicians have been alerted repeatedly to the problem (Chan et al, 1977; Pontifex and Garg, 1985; Kew et al., 1993; Espinoza et al., 1985; Elden and Torre, 1997).

CONCLUSION

Because of the increasing ethnic diversity of the United States with new immigration sources over recent decades, numerous ethnic communities have not forgotten their remedies used in "the old country." These are less familiar to workers in health-related capacities than in a former age when the "old country" was western Europe. Thus, state and federal public health agencies have added another item on their plate. However, it is generally not so pressing as are more acute problems—SARS, HIV, West Nile virus, STDs (sexually transmitted diseases), and thoughts of bioterrorism. A public awareness that ethnic remedies may be a bane rather than a boon becomes quite important. People should not become adventuresome in seeking health benefits by using imported products from Asia and the Third World in general because toxic agents have been employed as ingredients in their traditional remedies.

PART IV: More Certain Supplement Marvels

Medical doctors claim that their discipline is founded on scientific knowledge. Yet, although the ideas of evidence based medicine are widely accepted, clinical decisions and methods of patient care are based on much more than just the results of controlled experiments.

Kirsti Malterud (2001)

Chapter 21

Marvelous Micronutrients: The Vitamins

> . . . suboptimal intake of some vitamins, above levels causing classical vitamin deficiency, is a risk factor for chronic diseases and common in the general population, especially in the elderly.
>
> Fletcher and Fairfield (2002)

BASIC FOUNDATIONS

By definition, vitamins are vital biochemicals that our bodies are unable to produce in adequate amounts, if at all; thus through human history they have been obtained from foods in our diet. Furthermore, a severe enough and prolonged enough deficiency of vitamin intake in the diet will result in one or more specific metabolic malfunctions leading to the development of a specific deficiency disease having a set of distinctive signs and symptoms. When a supplemental supply of a vitamin is provided, persons will be protected from developing the deficiency disease despite being on a diet that would otherwise elicit one.

This describes the classical physiological nutritional usage of vitamins. However, the use of supplemental amounts that go well past supplying the physiologic need can comprise a pharmacologic application of a vitamin. Indeed, for a minority of vitamins an elevated level of intake/supplementation may constitute a toxicologic dose.

In marginal instances a chemical is listed on a roll call of vitamins even though it does not meet the criteria to the fullest degree. For example, our supply of vitamin K would not be obtained from our food intake except for the action of certain species of bacteria that inhabit our intestinal tract. These helpful microbes do us no harm while benefiting from our food intake. At the same time, we receive the important benefit of their producing an excess of vitamin K, which we then can absorb along with the materials

Consumer's Guide to Dietary Supplements and Alternative Medicines

doi:10.1300/5698_21

resulting from the digestion of our food. Also, vitamin D is not fully qualified as a vitamin because it can be synthesized only if we obtain the necessary precursor molecule in our diet and we have sufficient skin exposure to sunlight, which is required to drive the synthetic reaction. Thus, it is better called a *conditional* vitamin.

Moreover, deficits of a few members of the vitamin class do not readily manifest a clear-cut human deficiency disease despite one having been produced experimentally in laboratory rodents or chickens. We generally share with such species the same list of demonstrated vitamins, with the major exception of ascorbic acid. Whereas rats and mice do not develop scurvy on a vitamin C-deficient diet as humans do, the nonrodent laboratory and pet species the South American cavy (better known as guinea pig) does indeed require vitamin C in its diet. This discovery in 1907 of the one laboratory species that can serve as an experimental model of scurvy made it possible later for the discovery of the cure or prevention of scurvy.

This is a classical story of the earliest beginning of knowledge concerning vitamins, with respect to vitamin C. It is known chemically as ascorbic acid but may be employed also as the mineral ascorbates—the sodium, magnesium, or calcium ascorbate salts that are more soluble and less acidic than the acid. In the navies of European countries of the sixteenth and seventeenth centuries it was recognized that after many months at sea sailors were prone to develop a disease known as scurvy. This was characterized by weakness, pain, bleeding in the skin and gums, loosening of the teeth, and at times illness ending in death.

A British Navy surgeon, James Lind, in 1747 developed a hypothesis and tested it in a model fashion for his era, namely, that scurvy was a consequence of a limited selection of foods available to the common sailors (probably not so much so for the officers) during long ocean voyages. A shortage of fresh fruits would have been a conspicuous feature of their larder. The doctor set up a groundbreaking human trial in which he tested fruits for content of a preventive dietary factor against scurvy. Having made the dietary alteration the toll of illness and death from scurvy was clearly reduced from the usual. Because of a subsequent use of limes to supply the factor responsible for avoiding the deficiency disease, British navy members by the nineteenth century became known to others as "limeys."

It was more than a century and a half later before the identity of this antiscorbutic (against scurvy) factor was isolated and identified by a Hungarian chemist, Albert Szent-Gyorgyi who held both a medical degree and a doctorate in chemistry. During his research on cellular respiration mechanisms he succeeded in isolating a reducing agent from plants such as oranges and lemons, which blocked the effect of the oxidase enzymes. He found it not merely difficult but impossible to obtain enough of the target factor using expensive oranges and lemons. However, he was successful in extracting and isolating large quantities of it from a more available, rather inexpensive source, paprika, a common food item grown in plentiful supply around his home region.

Not only the importance of his discoveries but also the wide metabolic importance of ascorbic acid were recognized when in 1937 Szent-Gyorgyi received the Nobel Prize in physiology and medicine. His research eminence was amplified during the nearly 40 years of his later life spent after World War II in the United States. During that period his still quite significant research concerned the contractile mechanism of muscle cells and cellular metabolic regulations relevant to cancer.

Before Szent-Gyorgyi, a Polish biochemist named Casimir Funk, who moved to the United States in 1915, was the pioneer who originated the vitamin concept. After his discovery in 1911 of the amine comprising vitamin B1 (thiamine), in 1912 Funk coined the term *vitamine* (from vital + amine). A deficiency disease that is cured by thiamine had long been known as beriberi, a form of neuritis. Funk was able to make his discovery only after an animal model of human thiamine deficiency disease was developed in chickens by a Nobel laureate Dutch researcher, Christiaan Eijkman, in 1897.

However, when subsequent research showed that not all essential food factors are amines in their chemistry, Funk's term was shortened to *vitamins.* He is credited with stirring public interest in vitamins with publicity given to his book *The Vitamines* as well as his 1912 research paper that attributed several diseases, such as scurvy, beriberi, rickets, and pellagra, to vitamin deficiencies. In later researches Funk contributed to knowledge of the hormones of the pituitary gland and the sex glands, and he emphasized the vital importance of a proper balance between the actions of hormones and vitamins.

THE TWO SUBGROUPS OF VITAMINS

Vitamins are subdivided into two groups by virtue of their solubility characteristics: the water-soluble and the fat-soluble classes. The smaller number are the fat-soluble ones that can be remembered by the term ADEK. All the others are water soluble. Thus, vitamins A, D, E, and K all are associated with poor water solubility—the tendency to be associated with oils in foods we eat. If persons lacks fat-emulsifying secretions in their bile they will not absorb well either the fatty acids in the oil or the ADEK vitamins.

HOW MUCH IS ENOUGH?

Panels of nutritional scientists have for years struggled with the daunting challenge of providing answers to the question of how much is a sufficient quantity of each of the vitamins. Formerly their answers were broadcast in terms of MDRs, or minimal daily requirement levels for each vitamin. Controversial aspects of this led to a change to "recommended daily allowance" levels (RDAs) being promulgated. This was the basis for the phrase on vitamin products showing "% RDA" for each component that has had such a value assigned. Currently, the phraseology has changed again to RDI, meaning recommended daily intake for vitamins and minerals. However useful these various guides may be to the consumer, they are perpetuating misconceptions. An MDR was conditioned by the amount of a vitamin required to avoid an overt deficiency disease such as those mentioned previously, but it does not deal with the possibility, or probability, that milder, subclinical deficiencies that are not easily recognized may also occur.

The higher, more adequate levels of the RDAs and RDIs still are misleading by suggesting a "one-size-fits-all" concept of needed levels of vitamins for many different individuals. Some persons at an extreme of the distribution of biological variability may require a significantly higher amount than the RDI level of intake. Clearly, different individuals are not identical in their body size, shape, composition, and metabolic rate. This prevents a perfect estimate of the required level being made for each member of a large population of persons. Thus, if one looks at these values correctly, they should be seen as approximations, not necessarily as an amount that will be optimal for everyone. Nutritional physicians are inclined to endorse vitamin intakes clearly above the RDIs rather than possibly to err on the side of an inadequate intake.

Indeed, it is important to recognize that the amount needed will vary over time in a single person with changes related to aging or to disease states that reduce the efficiency or capacity of dietary nutrients being absorbed. The malabsorption stemming from a chronic high ingestion of alcoholic beverages would be a very significant illustration of this principle. An inadequate diet often aggravates the alcohol problem, making alcoholism the most severe cause of overt malnutrition in the United States. Illness or other stresses may also elevate the tissue needs, most notably for vitamin C. Here again we encounter the uncertainty principle; we cannot know with certainty the precise, optimal vitamin level for each person.

Moreover, another fallacy promoted by MDRs, RDAs, and RDIs is that we *must* have our quantity of vitamins every day because our bodies cannot store a surplus today for a future "rainy day." Although this generalization has some basis in truth, it is indeed a general principle that does not fit all the vitamins equally well. The most extreme case of an exception to this generality is the case of vitamin B_{12}, for which normal stores would generally not be fully depleted before many months of total deprivation.

WHO NEEDS TO SUPPLEMENT VITAMIN INTAKE?

Everyone needs an adequate level of vitamin intake because they are vital! This doesn't mean that everyone needs a supplemental amount beyond what they obtain in their food, or at least not at all times. Reasons and times exist for a greater need by certain individuals than may be the general case. Growing infants and children have an especially critical need. Women during and after pregnancy, especially if they are breast-feeding, and at times between multiple pregnancies are clearly in a special class. In old age persons may have less appetite for the amount of good nutritional foods that they once ingested, so they do not eat adequately. As the quote at the outset of this chapter indicates, many persons in the U.S. population, especially the elderly, are at risk of chronic illness for lack of a fully adequate vitamin intake.

Alcoholism leads to a lifestyle in which an individual neglects healthful eating, and consequently alcoholic persons as a group are the most prone to significant nutritional deficiencies of any subgroup in the U.S. population. In the case of thiamine deficiency states sometimes become severe enough to be life threatening. Both heavy drinking and heavy smoking, which tend to go together, put a person at risk from excess oxidative stress. This will be aggravated by an inadequate supply (needing to be greater than normal to be adequate) of the antioxidant vitamins A, C, and E. One of several views on the causes for premenstrual syndrome (PMS) suggests a role for deficient dietary factors, and implicates vitamins B_6 and E as well as magnesium.

VITAMINS FOR PREVENTION OF CHRONIC DISEASES

The prevention of deficiency diseases is a relatively short-term prophylaxis. Values for prophylaxis of chronic diseases in adults are now recognized on a long-term basis. These concern coronary heart disease, cancer, and osteoporosis, with all vitamins except thiamine and riboflavin providing actions of this sort. The coronary connection involves a state of elevated levels of the amino acid homocysteine being a contributing factor in promoting atherogenic changes in the coronary arteries (hardening of the arteries). People having the highest plasma total homocysteine measures are at twice the risk for coronary disease as those showing the lowest homocysteine levels. The risk elevation is similar to that seen with cigarette smoking or having elevated cholesterol levels. Three vitamins are able to oppose this risk factor by normalizing the blood levels of homocysteine—folate, vitamin B_6, and vitamin B_{12}.

IMPORTANT FEATURES OF INDIVIDUAL VITAMINS

Vitamin A (Carotenes)

Vitamin A (chemically, *all-trans* retinol) shows the most promise of any of the three important antioxidant vitamins for a growth-regulatory action, which might influence the process of cancer development. This is because it belongs to a chemical group called retinoids, which are known to exert biological growth-influencing activities. Indeed, both vitamin A and several provitamin forms (carotenoids and beta-carotene) have been proposed as chemopreventive agents for cancer because some epidemiologic studies have shown that the risk of certain types of cancer is higher for people having low dietary intakes of the foods rich in vitamin A and beta-carotene, as well as among those with low measures for serum levels of vitamin A and beta-carotene. Beta-carotene has two major advantages over vitamin A: it is much less toxic because of intrinsic mechanisms limiting the amount of beta-carotene transformed into vitamin A, and it also appears to have some immunostimulant effects that can be exerted independently of its conversion to vitamin A.

However, the growth regulatory actions of the retinoids make them a potential risk if consumed by a pregnant woman in quantities able to influence adversely the embryonic-fetal development process. This has been of most concern with respect to systemic use of the retinoid Accutane for dermatologic benefits to the extent of a contraindication to such usage. This issue also concerns the possible teratogenicity of high-dose vitamin A intake during pregnancy. Health care practitioners should be familiar with the possible hazard of excessive dosages of vitamin A and its analogues. Vitamin A daily doses of more than 8,000 IU (international units) are not recommended for pregnant woman as they are not necessary for good health. Foods high in beta-carotene can provide the necessary amounts of vitamin A and, in contrast to the synthetic analogues, their use has not been associated with vitamin A toxicity or teratogenicity in humans or animals.

Vitamin B_1 (Thiamine)

The discovery of thiamine was associated with a recognition that people could develop a deficiency disease (beriberi) by eating an excessive amount of *polished* rice, whereas rice not so processed was quite healthful. The discovery of a nutrient factor in the hull of the rice that later proved to be thiamine was made on the basis of this clue. Beriberi occurs when a high intake of carbohydrates or alcohol exists along with a low thiamine intake. Stores of thiamine also can fall to a dangerous degree during severe or total fasting, when the person's energy metabolism is confined to storage molecules from organs (e.g., liver glycogen) or fatty tissues, and B-complex vitamins are not being taken. Persons who undertake a lengthy voluntary fast should be taking a thiamine supplement to avoid the serious potential consequence, the deficiency disease known as beriberi, one form of which endangers the health of the heart muscle. The nervous system is also very much at risk as thiamine is intimately associated with energy metabolism of nerve cells.

This is the reason that thiamine, along with the rest of the B-complex, rightly compose the heart of multivitamin supplements. The usage of carbohydrates to generate energy is especially dependent upon vitamin B_1. This is so critical that for a person whose thiamine stores are depleted, as in a severe alcoholic crisis, administration of a glucose infusion is contraindicated (not to be conducted) before the person is given injections of B_1 to rapidly raise its level in the cells. Brain pathology occurring acutely in alcoholism is known as Wernicke-Korsakoff syndrome. If a person with this state is not diagnosed and promptly treated by injections of thiamine, a high probability of a fatal outcome exists. It is difficult to discriminate the role of malnutrition from that of direct alcohol toxicity to the brain in the long-term development of alcoholic dementia, which can appear within the first decade of a person's alcohol abuse.

Vitamin B2 (Riboflavin)

In the body, riboflavin is mainly found as an integral part of two "flavin" coenzymes, flavin adenine dinucleotide (FAD) and flavin mononucleotide. Those enzymes that need a flavin coenzyme (called flavoproteins) are critical for the metabolism of carbohydrates, fats, and proteins. FAD is a vital link in the electron transport (respiratory) chain, which is central to cellular energy production. Flavins also are necessary to the metabolism of drugs and toxins in conjunction with cytochrome P-450. Riboflavin is indirectly needed for the antioxidant function of glutathione. The enzyme glutathione reductase is an FAD-dependent enzyme that participates in the regeneration of active glutathione after it has been reduced in its scavenging reactive oxygen species. Riboflavin deficiency has been associated with signs of increased oxidative stress. A second mechanism for this outcome is that riboflavin deficiency can decrease xanthine oxidase activity and result in a reduced blood uric acid level. While it is regarded mostly as an undesirable waste product, uric acid in the blood is one of the most active water-soluble antioxidants.

Because flavoproteins are involved in the metabolism of other vitamins (vitamin B_6, niacin, and folic acid), severe riboflavin deficiency may impact many enzyme systems in addition to those previously described. Along with other B vitamins, increased riboflavin intake has been associated with a desirable lowering of plasma homocysteine levels. Research in animals suggests that riboflavin deficiency may impede absorption of iron, increase intestinal loss of iron, and/or impair iron utilization in synthesis of hemoglobin. Humans findings show that improving riboflavin supplies will increase circulating levels of hemoglobin when they are deficient.

Riboflavin deficiency rarely occurs alone; it frequently is found in combination with deficiencies of the other water-soluble vitamins. Symptoms of riboflavin deficiency include sore throat, redness and swelling of the lining of the mouth and throat, cracks or sores on the outsides of the lips and at the corners of the mouth, inflammation and redness of the tongue (magenta tongue), a moist and scaly skin inflammation (seborrheic dermatitis), the abnormal formation of blood vessels in the clear front of the eyeball (corneal vascularization), and a decreased red blood cell count in which the remaining red cells contain normal levels of hemoglobin while being of normal size (normochromic normocytic anemia). Severe riboflavin deficiency may result in decreased conversion of vitamin B_6 to its active coenzyme form and a decreased conversion of tryptophan to niacin. Alcoholics are at increased risk for riboflavin deficiency because of decreased intake, decreased absorption, and impaired utilization of the vitamin. Persons having anorexia nervosa rarely consume adequate riboflavin. Lactose intolerance may prevent people from consuming adequate milk or dairy products as good sources of riboflavin. People who are very active physically (athletes and laborers) may show slightly increased riboflavin requirements, but supplementation has not been found to elevate their exercise tolerance or athletic performance.

Two case-control studies found a lower risk (33 percent to 51 percent) of age-related cataract in men and women of the highest quintile (fifth) of dietary riboflavin intakes compared with those in the lowest quintile. Similarly, a recent cross-sectional study of 2,900 Australian men and women, 49 years of age and older, found that those in the highest quintile of intake for riboflavin were merely 50 percent as likely to have cataracts as those in the lowest quintile. Although these observational studies suggest a role for riboflavin in preventing cataracts, placebo-controlled intervention trials are needed to confirm this apparent relationship.

Most plant and animal foods contain at least small quantities of riboflavin. Because wheat flour and breads since 1943 in the United States have been enriched with riboflavin (as well as thiamin, niacin, and iron), the average intake of riboflavin for men is about 2 mg/day and for women is about 1.5 mg/day, well above the RDI. Similar intake levels have been found for a population of elderly men and women. However, riboflavin is easily destroyed by exposure to light—up to one-half of the riboflavin in milk can be destroyed after two hours of exposure to bright sunlight. Nevertheless, a serious deficiency of riboflavin is not likely to occur in the United States without major malnourishment.

Vitamin B3 (Niacin/Niacinamide)

Despite much research and development of synthetic drugs for improving the blood-fat picture for diabetics and others, the natural substance niacin continues to be of some value in this realm. *Atherogenic dyslipidemias* is the technical phrase for an abnormal blood-lipid/fat profile that is associated with a heightened risk for the development of arterial atherosclerosis, which predisposes to heart attack and stroke. Niacin has been an effective therapy for treating a broad range of dyslipidemias. However, a view worthy of respect is that of a distinguished clinician, Lewis Lasagna (1994), who has declared that niacin still has a place in the management of dyslipidemia, "but not on the basis of self-diagnosis and self-treatment" because of its potential for causing hepatitis. This is seen in some cases within as little as one week after starting usage, but in some as late as 48 months.

A randomized, double-blind, parallel clinical trial reported in 1994 compared doses of immediate-release (IR) and sustained-release (SR) niacin for effectiveness in reducing levels of LDL cholesterol and triglycerides and increasing levels of HDL cholesterol and for the occurrence of adverse reactions, especially hepatotoxicity. The SR niacin was seen to lower LDL cholesterol levels significantly more than did IR niacin at doses of 1500 mg/day and higher, whereas IR niacin increased HDL cholesterol levels significantly more than SR niacin did at all dosages. The reduction in triglyceride levels was similar with IR and SR niacin. However, 39 percent of the patients on the IR dosage form withdrew before completing the 3,000-mg daily dose. The most common reasons for withdrawal were fatigue and/or vasodilator symptoms. However, 78 percent of those taking the SR dosage form withdrew before completing the 3,000-mg daily dose.

At that daily dose the most common reasons for withdrawal were gastrointestinal tract symptoms, fatigue, and increases in levels of liver aminotransferases, often with symptoms of hepatic dysfunction. Although none of the patients taking IR niacin showed hepatotoxic effects, 52 percent of those taking SR niacin did. The authors concluded that an SR form of niacin is hepatotoxic and should be restricted from use. IR niacin is preferred for management of hypercholesterolemia, but it can also cause significant adverse effects and should be taken only by patients who are carefully monitored by experienced health professionals, as indicated by Lasagna (1994). Niacin is among the drugs that appear to have an increased likelihood of causing hepatotoxicity in patients having a preexisting liver disease. Such persons with any sort of liver disease are warned against the use of niacin in doses high enough for lowering LDL levels.

Another instance of a pharmacologic application for niacin is its mostly former role in orthomolecular psychiatry to control major psychoses. Prior to the era of antipsychotic drugs for treating schizophrenia began in the 1950s, large doses of niacin, along with other members of the B complex, were found by Abram Hoffer, MD, to show success in reducing symptoms of psychosis. Considering this background, it is interesting that a recent report suggests that the risk for the brain degeneration of Alzheimer's disease (AD) is lowered by a high B_3 content of one's diet. The study was published in July 2004, and was conducted at the Rush Institute for Healthy Aging in Chicago. The lead author, Martha C. Morris, MD, noted that high therapeutic doses of niacin have been credited with a reduced risk of cognitive decline, as in Alzheimer's disease, but no prior studies had tested for an association between AD risk and the dietary intake of niacin (Morris et al., 2004).

Morris and colleagues (2004) studied more than 3,700 subjects from a Chicago community all of whom were over the age of 65. The subjects filled out detailed food frequency questionnaires, and over an interval of more than five years took a series of cognitive tests. The researchers randomly selected 815 subjects for closer analysis. All persons in this group were free of AD at the outset, but by the end of the study 131 of them were diagnosed with AD. After analyzing the data, the Rush Institute team found a clear association between niacin intake and reduced cognitive decline and AD risk. Morris stated that when subjects with the highest niacin intake were compared to those with the lowest intake, the high niacin group had an 80 percent reduction in risk. The reduced risk was primarily related to dietary intake, and the protective action of niacin ingested in the form of supplements was less strong.

Vitamin B_{12} (Cyanocobalamin and Hydroxocobalamin)

One of the major "miracle drug" discoveries of the mid-twentieth century was indeed that of vitamin B_{12}, the cure for pernicious anemia. First described in 1855, pernicious anemia was usually a fatal affliction until 1926, when it was found that a heavy intake of slightly cooked liver for six months could reverse pernicious anemia for persons with the disease. The role in this anemia of the cobalamins—the collective term for different chemicals having B_{12} activity—was not established until the vitamin was first isolated in 1948 in the form known as cyanocobalamin. It was named for two very unique features of the molecule—the presence of an atom of cobalt and of a cyanide group. Liver proved to be a rich source of cyanocobalamin. Hydroxocobalamin, another active form, which has a hydroxyl rather than a cyano group, later became available as an effective alternative for therapy. Moreover, a third therapeutic molecule known as methylcobalamin is widely available in Europe and used more there than in the United States. These three molecules are why the plural, cobalamins, or at times the generic singular, cobalamin, are used to represent all, which are unlikely to show qualitative differences.

The most obvious need of human beings for vitamin B_{12} is for support of the maturation of red blood cell (RBC) precursors in the bone marrow, which requires also adequate amounts of folic acid (also called folate). Lacking adequate intake of either of these vitamins, the result is a state of macrocytosis or macrocytic anemia, which alludes to the abnormally large size of the immature red cells (macrocytes) being released from the bone marrow. Thus, the disease actually consists more of a qualitative deviation than a quantitative one, i.e., not simply a deficit of RBCs. Those cells that are released from the bone marrow into the circulation, the immature macrocytes, also are called megaloblasts, so pernicious anemia is also known as megaloblastic anemia. This occurs because the megaloblasts fail to undergo the full maturation, which involves shrinkage to the more compact size of a mature RBC.

The oxygen-carrying capacity of such macrocytes is greatly reduced from that of the normal mature RBC. For a person who suffers from extreme macrocytic anemias, many tissues are deprived of their normal oxygen supplies. Not only will the vigor and energy level of the person's muscles be reduced but also the function of their nervous system will be impaired by a state of hypoxia (oxygen deficiency). Moreover, other vital metabolic functions of nerve cells are also served by cobalamins. Thus, a B_{12} deficiency may be manifested in terms of reduced cognitive, sensory, or motor capacities. Qualitative changes may extend to alterations in personality or even a diagnosis of a psychotic condition.

Vitamin B_{12} is unique among the vitamins in that it includes both a complex organic portion and an inorganic portion, an essential atom of the trace element cobalt. It is synthesized only by some bacteria, not by animals and plants, but it occurs naturally in small amounts in animal foods including fish, milk and milk products, eggs, meat, and poultry. To find it in plant sources is exceptional. Fortunately, a healthy person need ingest only about 3 to 5 micrograms (one-thousandth of a milligram, one-millionth of a gram) of vitamin B_{12} per day. This tiny amount usually can be obtained from a normal diet, mainly from animal foods. However, for strict vegetarians, vegans (who consume no animal-derived products, including milk and eggs), necessary alternative sources are blue-green algae products and bean sprouts. The whole adult human body normally contains about 5,000 to 10,000 micrograms (5 to 10 mg) of vitamin B_{12}, equally distributed between the liver and the nervous system. To deplete the body starting from this normal level requires a total loss of intake that lasts not days or weeks but many months or a year. Barring starvation, a total cutoff of B_{12} is more likely to occur because of a failed absorption than from a total lack in the diet. Diminished serum B_{12} levels have also been found to be associated with the onset of atrophy of the gastric mucosa along with gastritis, and in the course of omeprazole therapy in GERD (gastroesophageal reflux disease) patients who are positive for the bacterium *Helicobacter pylori.*

Assuming an adequate supply in one's diet, a deficiency of cobalamins generally is the result of insufficient intestinal uptake of the vitamin from the food as a result of the following:

- Gastric abnormalities—atrophic gastritis of old age, or partial gastrectomy
- Bariatric (stomach-stapling) surgery for treating morbid obesity
- Intestinal dysfunction from partial surgical removal or bypass of the duodenum
- Severe diseases of broadly deficient absorption—malabsorption syndromes
- Insufficient release of intrinsic factor (the protein secreted by gastric glands that is essential for the intestinal absorption of B_{12}), which is more likely to occur in upper age groups
- Deficiency of hydrochloric acid (HCl) in the gastric juice, which is more likely with old age, regular use of laxatives, excessive use of antacids, or with an antisecretory agent, especially proton pump inhibitors such as omeprazole (Prilosec) and the newer, closely similar

esomaprazole (Nexium) and others acting alike for the treatment of peptic ulcer or GERD.

Clearly, this list shows a greater risk for B_{12} deficiency with advanced age. A recent review in the *Canadian Medical Association Journal* (Andres et al., 2004) stated that such deficiency is found in 20 percent of elderly persons in the general population of industrialized countries. Of these persons, a food-cobalamin malabsorption syndrome was indicated as being responsible for more than 60 percent of all cases, and failure of uptake owing to lack of intrinsic factor, i.e., pernicious anemia, was responsible for 15 to 20 percent of all cases. Thus, only a small proportion of cases are attributed to inadequate dietary intake. Food-cobalamin malabsorption, which has been recognized only recently as a significant cause of cobalamin deficiency among elderly people, is characterized by the inability to release cobalamins from food.

Older people showing malabsorption of protein-bound B_{12} from foods may produce enough intrinsic factor and yet have an inadequate ability to absorb B_{12} taken in food. Malabsorption of protein-bound cobalamins by the elderly may instead result from their having a reduced secretion of pepsin and gastric acid, and a consequent hindrance to the cleavage of cobalamin from its tie with proteins in the diet. This cleavage is essential for the cobalamin to join with intrinsic factor to complete B_{12} absorption. Because of this, in 1999 the Institute of Medicine of the U.S. National Academy of Sciences recommended that older people should receive the majority of their B_{12} intake, the RDI of 4 micrograms per day, in the synthetic form from supplements rather than relying on natural sources from foods.

Younger persons prone to substance abuse behaviors may develop a toxicity called myeloneuropathy (spinal cord injury), which has been observed following excessive inhalation ("huffing") of nitrous oxide (an analgesic gas for dentistry) as a euphoriant abuse agent. Toxicity occurs because nitrous oxide can chemically inactivate most of the cobalamin molecules present. The resulting toxic response to B_{12} deprivation can also be a risk for patients having low body stores of vitamin B_{12} , if they are treated with nitrous oxide for analgesia rather than being exposed in its "recreational" use.

Vitamin B_{12} and HIV Infection?

Researchers at the Department of Epidemiology of Johns Hopkins School of Hygiene and Public Health (Tang et al., 1997) conducted a study to examine a possible associations between serum levels vitamin B_6, vitamin B_{12}, and folate with the risk and rate of progression from "infected with

HIV" to time of first diagnosis of AIDS. The follow-up period was approximately 9 years. A time-course analysis (Kaplan-Meier) found that participants initially having a low serum vitamin B_{12} level had a shorter AIDS-free interval than did those with adequate vitamin B_{12} levels ($P = 0.004$, a highly significant difference). The median AIDS-free times for the two groups were four years versus eight years, respectively. No such association was found with low serum levels of vitamin B_6 and folate. Intervention studies are needed to test whether correcting a low serum vitamin B_{12} level early in HIV-1 infection will alter the course of the disease.

Folic Acid/Folate and Homocysteine

Folate serves as a cell growth regulatory factor without which anemia occurs. It is necessary for maturation of cells in the bone marrow, megaloblasts, which are precursors of the red blood cells (RBCs). When they mature normally, a progressive shrinkage of the cell size occurs. With a deficiency of folate the cells are released from the bone marrow in an immature state as macrocytes, meaning that they are larger than normal, as well as not functioning normally. Thus, folate-related anemia is called macrocytic anemia or megaloblastic anemia. The biochemical failure and structural abnormality are functionally equivalent to the anemia of a B_{12} deficit called pernicious anemia.

Both folate and B_{12} have important nervous system roles, as well as complementary roles in the bone marrow cells, but the neural effect of B_{12} is more prominent. Indeed, an excess of folate for a person deficient in B_{12} will mask the signs of B_{12} deficit related to the bone marrow. However, this may allow a B_{12} deficit affecting the brain to progress further than it would otherwise; such a happening may leave the person with irreversible injury to the motor functions of the nervous system. Brantigan (1997) described in *JAMA* how this happened to his wife who had taken folate supplements. She developed quite advanced neurologic problems from B_{12} deficiency before a correct diagnosis was reached, since no sign of anemia existed. He opined that vitamin B_{12} deficiency is neither a benign condition nor one easily diagnosed in all cases by general physicians. (Patients, beware!)

It is because of such situations that the FDA several decades ago put an upper limit on the amount of folate to be permitted for nonprescription products so as to reduce the probability of injurious events from such masking. Supplemental folate in flour was introduced in 1974 to avoid damage to an infant's nervous system development (neural tube defects, most commonly spina bifida) as a result of folate deficit during the early weeks of pregnancy. This was followed by a significant rise in the average folate level for the U.S. population. Such an action was still being debated in Australia as of 2004, whereas another even wider action by the FDA requiring folate fortification was placed on U.S. food processors as of 1998 despite a dissent from Brantigan.

Evidence continues to accrue supporting the proposition that an adequate folate level is protective against heart disease. Canadian researchers found in a 15-year study of 5,000 men and women that those with the highest folate levels were nearly 70 percent less likely to die from a heart attack with coronary disease than were the persons having the lowest folate levels. Raising folate blood level lowers the level of homocysteine, an amino acid indicator for vascular disease. It seems that homocysteine contributes to the narrowing of the arterial vessels, thus reducing the availability of blood and oxygen to the heart muscle. Moreover, the effect on cerebral vessels brings an even higher risk for stroke. It is now realized that it is of equal (some say even greater) importance to achieve a lower homocysteine level as it is a lower cholesterol level. Yet measurement of homocysteine has not become a universal clinical chemistry measure and therapeutic target, as is true of cholesterol. Thus, medical practice lags significantly behind expert knowledge because of the economics (HMOs [health maintenance organizations] haven't agreed to pay for homocysteine assays on top of the LDL and HDL cholesterol measures!). The solution for consumers is to start eating plenty of good folate sources regardless of what one's homocysteine reading may be, and thus to make it fall. Orange juice, lentils/beans, and green leafy vegetables—broccoli, asparagus, and spinach—are the dietary pathway to a safer level of homocysteine.

New research data presented at the American Heart Association's Council for High Blood Pressure Research annual conference in October 2004 showed that young women who consume more than 800 micrograms (μg) of folate per day can reduce their risk of developing high blood pressure by almost a third compared to those who consume less than 200 μg/day (Rim et al., 2004). Folate also reduced the risk in older women to a lesser degree. The researchers studied more than 150,000 women to test if a link existed between risk of high blood pressure and their level of folate intake, including supplements. Folate intake was ranked in quintiles (fifths) for the analysis. Two age groups were studied, women of ages 26 to 46 years old and those aged 43 to 70 years. Researchers found the greatest effect was among the younger group. Younger women in the highest folate intake quintile, consuming more than 800 μg/day (micrograms per day) of total folate, dietary intake plus supplements, had a 29 percent lower risk for high blood pressure than did those in the lowest quintile, consuming less than 200 μg/day of folate. Older women who had total folate intake of 800 μg/day had a 13 percent lower risk versus the lowest quintile. The benefit of folate was independent of other factors such as exercise, salt intake, and diet, which are known to influence the risk of high blood pressure.

One final reason for taking steps to lower one's homocysteine level pertains to bone health past midlife. Two papers appeared simultaneously in the *New England Journal of Medicine* in May 2004 on this topic (van Meurs et al., 2004, McLean et al., 2004). Both one from Europe and one from the United States found that in older persons high homocysteine levels were a predictor for bone fractures. A study from the Netherlands found an association between circulating homocysteine levels and the risk of osteoporotic fracture in 2,406 subjects 55 years of age or older. The risk was similar in all three subgroups studied, and was also similar in women and men. A homocysteine level in the highest quartile was significantly correlated with an increase by a factor of 1.9 in the risk for fracture. The U.S. research studied 825 men and 1,174 women ranging in age from 59 to 91 years from whom blood samples had been obtained to measure plasma total homocysteine. The participants were followed for 16 to 19 years and rates of hip fracture were calculated for quartiles of total homocysteine blood levels. Men and women in the highest quartile had a greater risk of hip fracture than those in the lowest quartile; the risk was nearly four times as high for men and 1.9 times as high for women. The authors concluded, "These findings suggest that the homocysteine concentration, which is easily modifiable by means of dietary intervention, is an important risk factor for hip fracture in older persons" (McLean et al., 2004).

Vitamin C (Ascorbic Acid/Ascorbate)

At the beginning of the chapter we have already described the vitamin deficiency state for ascorbate and the discovery of its physiological role, which has fundamental importance to the integrity of all tissues, but it also has life as a pharmacologic agent beyond that of a vitamin, which is quite interesting. This has warranted a more complete coverage in Chapter 25.

Vitamin D

Natural vitamin D can be produced in the human body from its common dietary precursor, but only when the skin is adequately exposed to sunlight. Such exposure drives a chemical reaction to produce what was long thought to be the essential "active vitamin D," but that product actually turned out to also be a precursor that is finally activated in the liver and kidneys. Thus, production may be impaired also by liver or kidney disease. However, essential sunlight exposure often cannot be easily achieved, especially in the winter months, so a deficiency disease will occur unless the diet is well supplemented by a fish liver oil (e.g., cod). The classical manifestation of deficiency disease is caused by inadequate absorption of calcium as well as its metabolism and deposition in the bones, resulting in a bone pathology known as rickets.

People living at higher latitudes are more at risk because of longer, darker winters during which they can get no sunlight exposure, even if it were not too cold to leave skin exposed. Some authorities believe that people whose skin is highly pigmented because of their ethnicity are at particular risk for insufficient sunlight exposure when they reside outside the tropical or subtropical zones of the earth. This puts them at higher risk for deficient levels of vitamin D.

Elderly persons among the U.S. population seem to be at greater risk for being deficient in vitamin D than are younger persons. Vitamin D is essential not only to assist in the maintenance of healthy bones but also in normal muscle and nerve functions. A deficit of vitamin D leading to adverse changes in any of those systems could cause an elderly person to be more prone to experience a fall and also a bone fracture. Because vitamin D production depends on the skin being exposed to sunlight, this may be the missing factor for such elderly persons, for whom intake via supplements becomes more critical than for younger persons. It also may be that metabolic formation of the active molecule in the kidney and liver occurs less efficiently in elderly persons.

Besides the classical action to promote calcium uptake from the diet and to regulate its availability to the bones, nerves, and muscles, some researchers have in recent years discovered that an inadequate level of vitamin D is a risk factor for certain cancers. Presently, the evidence points to a higher rate of death from cancer of the skin, colon, prostate, ovary, and breast for persons living in low-sun areas versus those in more sunny regions of the United States. (This should not be seen to contradict the evidence that overexposure, e.g., sunburn in early life, may be a risk factor for skin cancers.)

Vitamin D deficiency is currently becoming recognized as a growing public health problem in the U.S. population segment at higher risk for osteoporosis, the elderly. As the population ages, osteoporosis is becoming even more common. More than 60 million Americans, 41 million of them women, will be at risk of either osteoporosis or low bone mass by the year 2020 according to the National Osteoporosis Foundation.

Older men have a risk for osteoporosis as well as women. This may be greater if their habitual midlife diet did not supply an adequate intake of calcium and vitamin D. Their risk level also becomes greater with habitual exposure to smoking (2.3 times higher) and alcoholic beverages (2.4 times higher). Obesity was protective (relative risk was 0.3) as it also is for women.

Vitamin E

The tocopherols (especially alpha- and beta-tocopherol) are among a group of chemically related substances comprising vitamin E that are outstanding for their biological antioxidant capacities. A great deal of evidence has accumulated that oxidation of the serum LDL (low-density lipoprotein cholesterol) is of major importance to the disease process of atherogenesis (calcified and fatty deposits in the walls of major arteries). This would suggest that the level of vitamin E available may be an important influence on one's risk for developing atherosclerosis.

In fact, some sources suggest that remarkably little evidence shows that vitamin E supplements can significantly reduce lipid peroxidation in *healthy* humans. Evidence of increased oxidative stress was not a criterion for subjects to be included in the trials. If only some participants had an excess of reactive oxygen species, then the extra vitamin E may have benefited too few persons to change the overall outcome values. Such uncertainty exists about the ability of vitamin E to enhance antioxidant defense mechanisms to a degree that is clinically significant, that much more substantial data regarding LDL oxidation and atherosclerosis are needed.

Some correlative, descriptive studies have indicated that low serum levels of vitamin E are associated with a slight increase in the risk of cancer for some human populations. Because vitamin E exerts antioxidant properties and is alleged to have immunostimulant effects, many observers deduce that it should be protective against cancer. However, it is possible to believe that antioxidants reduce the risk for initiation of cancer while still not finding grounds to believe that they are significantly helpful once cancer has begun. In addition, much controversy exists over the possibility that antioxidants may interfere with the killing of cancer cells by certain anticancer drugs. Vitamin E is regarded by some as especially effective in opposing prostate cancer, if used along with other dietary supplements such as selenium and vitamin D. Other possible prostate cancer preventives include whole flaxseed or its oil, milk thistle, and the spice curcumin (turmeric).

In recent times it has been discovered that another chemical group besides the tocopherols contributes to the total vitamin E benefits received from one's intake of oils known for supplying that vitamin. These are known as tocotrienols, and they have a slightly different molecular structure from the alpha-tocopherol form of vitamin E. This difference was found to make them far more potent as antioxidants, up to 60 times more effective in protecting cells from oxidative damage than was alpha-tocopherol. More significantly, the tocotrienols are similar to alpha-tocopherol in that they also reduce platelet clumping and lower cholesterol levels. No other vitamin or drug available today can significantly oppose all three of these major cardiac risk mechanisms. An action to reduce the clumping of platelets is an important mechanism of various pharmaceuticals.

However, this is not to suggest that tocotrienols would provide equal benefit as the antithrombotic drugs; comparative data are unavailable. In addition, studies have shown that tocotrienols have exceptional anti-inflammatory properties. Tocotrienols come from several sources, including rice bran oil and wheat germ oil.

VITAMIN TOXICOLOGY

Vitamin excess is especially possible from supplementation of the fat-soluble vitamins and B_6. Excessive intake of vitamin A or D during pregnancy may result in injury to the fetus, and A, D, E, and K taken to great excess anytime may provoke serious adverse effects. Despite such exceptional occurrences, reviewers Fairfield and Fletcher (2002) reached the conclusion that vitamin supplements are a low-cost and low-risk way to avoid illness because an inadequate intake of vitamins has been linked to significant chronic diseases including coronary heart disease, cancer, and osteoporosis.

Vitamins A and D

Only in the latter 1990s was it first recognized that excessive dietary intake of vitamin A can be responsible for reducing bone mineral density and for increasing the risk of hip fractures. As previously indicated, hypercalcemia provoked by an excess of vitamin D can have various adverse effects that can be serious enough at the very rare extreme to be life-threatening because of a negative circulatory impact.

Vitamin K

The synthetic molecule, menadione (vitamin K3), was found in the 1950s to be toxic to newborn infants by means of a tragic incident. When given to pregnant women too late in pregnancy before their time of delivery, an excessive level reached the unborn child, persisted in the neonate, and caused abnormal, toxic oxidative stress. This resulted in hemolytic anemia (RBC breakdown), which caused hyperbilirubinemia (an excess of bilirubin, a metabolite of hemoglobin from high RBC breakdown). This led to a toxic state known as kernicterus, and it caused a number of fatalities in an outbreak at a U.S. hospital nursery. Pregnant women should receive only the safe natural vitamin K_1 or K_2 forms. This is one exceptional case in which the frequent dire warnings of dangers from a synthetic form of a natural substance was fulfilled.

CONCLUSIONS

This viewpoint from one who is described as "a counseling specialist in natural healing" (Saul, 2003) may deserve consideration, though one would be reluctant to agree:

> Most confusion over what constitutes proper health care arises from partisans. Bias against vitamin supplements proceeds from people who stand to lose when cheap, natural health care succeeds. Hospitals, physicians, dieticians, politicians, pharmaceutical companies, and others have a vested interest in disease.

Chapter 22

Marvelous Micronutrients: Essential Minerals

INTRODUCTION

Selected minerals, such as zinc, selenium, iron, and magnesium, are the subject of monographs developed by registered dietitians at the Warren Grant Magnuson Clinical Center. The monographs were produced in conjunction with the NIH Office of Dietary Supplements (ODS). (See www.cc .nih.gov/ccc/supplements/ intro.html.)

If vitamins are seen as the glamorous micronutrients, minerals would be seen as blue collar nutrients (Davis, 1993). Nevertheless, they are equally vital to bodily health and strength despite their lagging in achieving the spotlight of attention awarded to the vitamins, whose name acclaims that they are "vital" to our health.

VITAL MINERAL ELEMENTS

Calcium

This element is one that has many vital roles in both structure and function of the human body. Certainly the most obvious role is the deposition of calcium salts that are fundamental to all bony structures of the skeleton. Well-controlled studies consistently have shown that calcium supplements with or without vitamin D significantly reduce the risk for hip fractures. Calcium must be available in a narrowly controlled range of blood level. An imbalance leading to an excess is called *hypercalcemia,* which has several serious consequences, such as milk-alkali syndrome from a person drinking milk and/or taking antacid medications excessively and compulsively. Problems occur also from a state of deficiency, *hypocalcemia.* At the cellular level it is known that a proper balance must be maintained between the calcium levels outside and within the cells. Moreover, the release of cal-

Consumer's Guide to Dietary Supplements and Alternative Medicines

doi:10.1300/5698_22

cium from a sequestered supply within the cell (where it is bound to a special protein, calmodulin) serves a vital role of signaling and control of ongoing intracellular biochemical activities.

Absorption of the calcium found in external dietary sources is highly dependent upon the action of vitamin D. A deficiency of vitamin D activity will greatly hinder adequate deposition of calcium in normal bone structure for its formation (in childhood) or its maintenance (the remainder of life). Such inadequacy of vitamin D (and thus calcium) results in rickets in children or osteomalacia (bone softening) in adults. Inadequacy vitamin D in turn depends upon a dietary precursor and its activation in vivo that occurs upon exposure of the skin to an adequate amount of sunlight. A sufficient intake of calcium is needed in young adult years of life to reach an optimal state of the bones when one enters the period of age-related decline of gonadal hormone secretion, which favors an inadequate bone replacement (osteoporosis) in elderly persons.

Recent findings (Cho et al., 2004) support a conclusion that the amount of calcium ingested by drinking at least a glass of milk a day can cut the risk of developing polyps that all too frequently may turn cancerous in both men and women (but slightly more for women) by as much as 12 percent. The calcium supplied by two or more glasses a day reduced the rate of colon cancer in test subjects by 15 percent. These were not conclusions from a small-scale research but rather from a meta-analysis combining data from ten nutrient studies that encompassed more than half a million people. Because vitamin D is often added to milk, Cho and colleagues (2004) believe that the vitamin contributed to these cancer-preventative effects either by its ability to help the body to absorb calcium, or perhaps by its own nutritive action.

An illustration of the complexity of nutritional science, and that needful agents may be "good" but may not always beneficial to us, is shown by another finding on dietary calcium intake.

Chromium (Chromium Picolinate Salt)

In the 1980s the idea began that salts of chromium could be a useful complement to conventional therapies for diabetes mellitus, especially type 2. By the year 2000 NCCAM issued an invitation for both basic and clinical research proposals for studies of the role of chromium as adjuvant therapy in type 2 diabetes and/or states of prediabetic impaired glucose tolerance. It was acknowledged that the use of chromium supplements has become a fairly common practice among persons with diabetes, and that accumulating evidence from small, uncontrolled clinical trials suggested that chromium supplementation might indeed alleviate symptoms associated with diabetes and reduce the need for insulin injections for patients with type 2 diabetes.

However, in the 1990s chromium picolinate was hailed as "a medical miracle," and the claims made for it went wild—that it could regulate blood sugar level, increase metabolic rate, increase energy and stamina, enable long-term weight loss, reduce cholesterol and body fat and levels, build muscle, and control appetite, in addition to preventing diabetes! In late 1996 the Federal Trade Commission brought charges against certain distributors of chromium picolinate for false and misleading advertising claims, and required a change in advertising behavior to quell the rampant unverifiable health claims.

Absorption of chromium as the chloride salt is very low (0.4 to 2.5 percent) and that the usual dietary sources are very poorly absorbed by the body. However, chromium picolinate is a more readily absorbed source in the normal digestive process. It is remarkably stable and unaffected by water, buffers, or blood serum proteins. A chromium-containing (small) oligopeptide has been found called "low molecular weight chromium-binding substance," which appears to be the likely mediator of action to enhance the effect of insulin.

Cobalt

The sole need for this element is for the complex cobalamin molecules that we call vitamin B_{12} into which it can be incorporated by bacteria. Its definition as a vitamin recognizes that human beings cannot synthesize the cobalamin molecules. Thus, humans do not actually need cobalt per se.

Copper

Copper enzymes play a role in many biological processes, but in ordinary conditions a person developing a copper deficit is not likely. One exception occurs if a person goes overboard on zinc supplementation. An excess of dietary zinc can so interfere with the intestinal uptake of copper as to produce an actual deficiency in tissues despite an adequate amount of copper in the diet. If a person is thus deprived of even a very small intake of copper they can develop a rare form of anemia. On the other hand, an excessive intake of copper may arise from a faulty water system that includes copper pipe if there is some acidity of the water to solublize some copper. Dissolved copper can cause toxic symptoms such as vomiting. Nonetheless, either extreme rarely occurs in usual situations.

Iodine (As Iodides)

In former times a lack of iodine in the diet of many Americans who lived far removed from the oceans caused a disease known as goiter in which the thyroid gland in the neck becomes quite enlarged. Most people living near coastal areas obtained enough iodine from their occasional meals of marine fish to avoid a deficiency state. Because table salt came to be iodized by the addition of sodium or potassium iodide, people everywhere were no longer hindered from producing the tiny amount of thyroid hormone (known as tri-iodothyronine). Therefore, goiter and even more harmful results of early childhood deficiency were essentially eliminated. However, interior areas of Third World countries on continents such as Africa still have a problem of thyroid-hormone deficit because the people do not receive prophylaxis via iodized salt. It has been said that a most tiny pinch of thyroid hormone (and of needed iodine molecules in it) per year makes the difference between normality and imbecility.

Iron (Ferrous Salts)

The biological necessity of iron is as great and as well-known to the general public as is our need for calcium. Iron-deficiency anemia should be a condition known to almost everyone because it is a problem for childbearing women, especially those with multiple pregnancies at short intervals. This is caused by two factors: the extra nutritional demand for iron as gestation proceeds to fulfill the needs of the developing baby, and absorption of iron from the intestinal contents that is subject to a strict limitation. Often the bar to entry of iron is too high during pregnancy to allow adequate extra uptake, assuming that an adequate amount exists in the diet.

Iron deficiency anemia is a common but not as yet completely understood condition during pregnancy. The exact prevalence of this disorder is not certainly known, but it has been cited as occurring in as many as 50 percent of pregnant women in the United States who did not use iron supplements. A higher risk for this problem with pregnancy has been found to occur in women of the following characteristics: poor socioeconomic status, low iron intake, high number of pregnancies, adolescent pregnancy, and women who regularly use aspirin, which may promote gastrointestinal blood loss. Anemia in pregnancy has been linked to an increased risk for premature onset of labor, and delivery of low birth weight infants who have a less favorable prognosis than those having a normal-range birth weight.

Many pharmaceutical forms of single-ingredient iron tablets exist that trade claims as to which of the iron salts is better absorbed. The only form of pharmaceutical that can claim absolutely no problem of getting iron into the patient's body is the one solution (Imferon) that is given by intramuscular injection. However, based on animal research it has been tainted by fears of a possible injection-site cancer-causing action.

Iron absorption depends on appropriate acidification of the stomach contents by gastric acid secretion. This raises a therapeutic problem when a patient turns up with anemia, tissue iron depletion, and a gastric erosion responsible for the former two.

Case Report 1

An 83-year-old woman presented with fatigue that was found to be the consequence of anemia, with a low hemoglobin level and an MCV (mean corpuscular volume). A GI endoscopic examination showed gastric erosions, but was negative for *Helicobacter pylori,* as a cause for ulcer. The patient was treated with omeprazole and an oral iron formula. After six months of such treatment her hemoglobin had failed to increase to the expected degree. Stool studies and repeat GI endoscopy revealed no sign of overt bleeding. A bone marrow evaluation at the time of her initial hematology examination had been normal except for the lack of iron stores. Malabsorption of iron as a result of the omeprazole was suspected, so the agent was discontinued. Within two months, receiving the same dose and formulation of oral iron, the patient's hemoglobin improved an MCV rose to normal. This confirmed the belief that the omeprazole had seriously reduced the bioavailability of the iron preparation (Sharma et al., 2004).

Iron supplementation in pregnancy is more generally accomplished now in the United States by means of prenatal vitamin-mineral supplements rather than the former usage of sole-ingredient iron products. A dose-related tendency for gastric irritation and discomfort exists whenever iron supplements are employed.

Anemia is a generic term that refers only to a quantitative or qualitative deficiency in the red blood cells. Sometimes people recognize such a deficit through the symptoms of abnormal fatigability, pallor of the skin or mucous membranes, and numerous other ill feelings. However, if a person makes a correct *(partial)* diagnosis of iron-deficiency anemia, the condition still requires the attention of a physician, not a self-chosen course of iron supplementation. The reason? Various causes for an iron deficit exist, and the one applicable to the case needs to be differentiated from others, especially for men in middle to upper age levels.

Men do not experience the loss of blood as women do at menstruation, which can explain most women's anemia. Barring a traumatic injury with blood loss, a man must be examined for blood loss through bleeding in the alimentary canal, which could occur from a peptic ulcer (though gastric pain should point to that possibility) or from a cancer growing silently (without pain) in the GI tract. In either case, treatment is required. If a cancerous growth exists, attention leading to a proper *full* diagnosis is highly urgent. Being alerted by a sign of anemia, a physician may do the necessary test for a GI tract cancer as the possible source and perhaps bring about surgical removal that may be lifesaving.

Another favorite teaching item regarded the iron levels in the body relating to the proposition that "extra" levels increase one's risk for heart disease. This was cause for an early call by Dr. J. L. Sullivan (1981) for men to keep their body iron store at the low to normal range via periodic blood donations because doing so might lower their heart-attack risk. Years later a mechanism for such benefit was recognized via an oxidation hypothesis of heart disease. This focused on the strong capacity for "free" iron to promote the generation of oxidative free radicals. The oxidation of LDL-cholesterol molecules of the blood that is favored by free iron indeed increases the risk for men (and postmenopausal women) of developing coronary artery atherosclerosis and heart disease.

A January 2004 report in the *American Journal of Clinical Nutrition* found that men who ate red meat, which contains the natural form, heme iron, had an increased risk of type 2 diabetes compared to men who consumed foods containing heme iron from sources other than red meat (Jiang et al., 2004). Heme iron is more efficiently absorbed by the body than nonheme iron. About 40 percent of the iron in meat, poultry, and fish is heme iron, whereas the iron in dairy, egg, and plant foods is mostly nonheme. The research was conducted in 1986 on 38,394 men between the ages of 40 and 75 who were free from diabetes, cardiovascular disease, and cancer. After a 12-year period the researchers tracked the men, noting their dietary habits, and found 1,168 new cases of type 2 diabetes. Most men have a problem with excess iron because it is not readily excreted via the usual excretory routes of urine, bile, and sweat. Instead, the primary means for men to lose iron is through the shedding of epithelial cells from the skin and the lining of the gastrointestinal tract, unless they have abnormal blood loss. For premenopausal women, the menstrual blood loss suffices to ensure against accumulation of an excess of iron.

That iron toxicity can occur is not adequately appreciated. This may be an acute overdose problem from accidental overdose (children) or rarely an intentional overdose for suicide by an adult. Before child-resistant packaging, childhood iron poisoning was a serious problem arising from a mother taking coated ferrous sulfate tablets that looked to a child similar to candy.

Thus, we find an example of a mineral element that we cannot live without, yet which in above-optimal levels may in excess actually threaten our life! We are left with good advice that blood donation is a healthful behavior for men, barring any health condition that might disqualify. Moreover, men *should not* supplement themselves as generously as may be appropriate for women, unless it is prescribed by a physician for a rare, serious iron need. The minimal amount incorporated into many multivitamin-mineral formulas (18 mg) is as much as men should supplement their dietary intake, and it would be best to volunteer for regular blood donations as well. The oxidizing free radical concept of degenerative diseases and aging (covered in Chapter 14) carries a basis for the use of antioxidant supplements. Besides taking antioxidants, a complementary approach to avoiding free radical injury would be to keep one's iron levels from being above low to normal and thus tending to cause more radicals to be generated. The presence of iron in elevated or excess levels may be detected by testing the blood level of ferritin, which is not a part of routine blood chemistry screens.

However, it is suggested by Doctor Joseph Mercola (2002) that such a measurement of ferritin is not only desirable but very essential for some persons. Those would be people having an infection with viral hepatitis C (HCV) or having a family history of liver disorders. He suggests that excess iron levels may greatly worsen HCV injury to the liver, and that hepatic iron toxicity may be misdiagnosed as HCV hepatitis.

Magnesium

Magnesium regulates cellular enzymatic and metabolic processes throughout the body through its involvement with more than 350 enzymes. It acts as an essential cofactor for these many magnesium-requiring enzymes. Almost all enzymatic processes utilizing phosphate groups as an energy transfer mechanism employ magnesium for the activation, which enables production of ATP (adenosine triphosphate), the vital energy molecules of all cells. Magnesium is needed for nearly every aspect of body biochemistry, e.g., the synthesis and stabilization of deoxyribonucleic acids (DNA) and proteins.

Electrophysiologic studies have shown slowing of cardiac conduction and increasing of the period of cardiac refractoriness (unresponsive state between beats) after the administration of magnesium. Thus, depletion of body levels of magnesium (known as hypomagnesemia) is manifested in hyperirritability leading to tremors, muscle spasms, and seizures as well as cardiac rhythm abnormalities including atrial fibrillation, ventricular tachycardia, and possibly ventricular fibrillation, which is likely to be fatal. When it is diagnosed, hypomagnesemia can be easily and quickly treated by injecting a solution of magnesium sulfate.

Formerly, the prolonged administration of magnesium-free parenteral fluids to intensive care patients was cause of hypomagnesemia. Persons with diabetes mellitus who have chronically poor blood glucose control may develop a total-body magnesium deficit. Chronic alcohol abuse with reduced intake plus malabsorption also can lead to serious hypomagnesemia; the occurrence rate among people with alcohol dependence is about 25 percent. Excretion of magnesium also is increased in alcoholism to favor a deficit, and the same is true for users of diuretic drugs. Other medications said to be causes of hypomagnesemia are some antibiotics (ticarcillin, amphotericin B, and aminoglycosides), and two anticancer drugs, cisplatin and cyclosporin. One hypothesis of the cause of Alzheimer's disease suggests that an abnormal protein acts to promote the uptake of aluminum over that of magnesium, which causes a neurotoxic element to be substituted for an essential one and results in loss of important nerve cells.

A tissue deficiency of magnesium without a low blood level of magnesium has been found to be a factor in the pathology of migraine. This discovery was made in a curious fashion, by Don R. Swanson (1988) a professor emeritus of information science at the University of Chicago. In the 1980s he decided to take a deep look at medical literature on migraines by a process known as text mining. Starting only with the word *migraine,* he downloaded the abstracts from 2,500 articles in the MedlinePlus database and looked closely at their titles. When certain concepts caught his eye, he designed new searches to determine whether that concept could be found in the texts of other articles related to migraines. In one instance, a reference to a nerve phenomenon called spreading depression caused him to look for articles with that term in their titles. Reading those pieces, he found magnesium being described as preventing spreading depression. More connections with a magnesium deficiency appeared, causing him to search further. He published his research in 1988 saying, "One is led to the conjecture that magnesium deficiency might be a causal factor in migraine." Dr. Swanson's work now is considered significant both to migraine studies and to the aspect of information science known as text mining. A link between migraine headache and magnesium deficiency has been supported by subsequent experiments by medical researchers, but a large-scale study should be conducted to quantify the value of a magnesium supplement for migraine prophylaxis.

Another therapeutic role for magnesium being considered is for the prevention of postoperative atrial tachyarrhythmias (excessively rapid and abnormal pattern of heartbeats), including atrial fibrillation and flutter (Piotrowski and Kalus, 2004). Magnesium has an accepted role in the treatment of ventricular arrhythmias, including torsade de pointes, however, its role for treatment and prevention of atrial tachyarrhythmias is not well defined. Studies on the use of magnesium against atrial arrhythmias have produced conflicting results, probably owing to differences in study design. Judging from the limited data available it appears to possess inherent antiarrhythmic properties. Limited patient populations may benefit from magnesium treatment for atrial tachyarrhythmias. However, more research is needed to define its role in treatment or prevention of those conditions.

The U.S. recommended daily allowance for magnesium in adults ranges between 310 and 420 mg depending on age, sex, and whether a women is pregnant or lactating. A well-rounded diet should provide adequate magnesium. Foods rich in magnesium include dark green leafy vegetables (spinach), whole grains (wheat germ and cereal), nuts (especially almonds and cashews, but also peanuts and others), fruits (bananas, dried apricots, and avocados), and potatoes baked in the skin. The question remains without a final answer as to whether use of a magnesium-containing supplement should be recommended. A large-scale study of the magnesium benefit should be conducted using a supplement.

On the other hand, the likelihood of hypermagnesemia is small because of the gastrointestinal wall acting to limit absorption of magnesium. Less than 40 percent of dietary magnesium is absorbed by the intestine. However, hypermagnesemia may occur if sustained exposure to the mineral exists for a person whose urinary excretion is much below the usual rate. Thus, hypermagnesemia can occur after repeated intake of some vitamin-mineral formulas, certain antacids, or laxatives by persons with unrecognized, untreated renal deficiency. It also could occur in patients who receive excessive therapeutic intravenous infusions of magnesium. Very rarely it may occur in a tumor breakdown syndrome when many cancer cells are killed by therapy with the dying cells may release massive amounts of cellular magnesium. When a rare excess of magnesium occurs, a depression of all excitable cells occurs. Its manifestations include nausea and vomiting, weakness and flaccidity of skeletal muscles, hypoactivity of the cardiovascular system, and depression of the nervous system in general, and respiration in particular. A mutual antagonism in excitable cells exists between magnesium and calcium; thus, a solution of a soluble calcium salt can reverse many symptoms of hypermagnesemia. An exceptional fatal overdose case was described in Chapter 12.

Potassium

The rather small amount of potassium in the human body is very essential for basic physiological functions at the cellular level. In supporting activities of all excitable cells, nerve, and muscle, its concentrations must be regulated within a rather narrow range. Hypokalemia, a state of potassium deficiency, and hyperkalemia, a state of potassium excess, are both inconsistent with normality. An occurrence of hyperkalemia is relatively difficult to encounter. One way would be excessive use of a low-sodium salt substitute consisting of potassium chloride. More likely to occur is hypokalemia because dietary intake must be adequate to avoid a deficit. Some good sources of potassium include the following:

- *Vegetables and fruits in general:* especially potatoes, sweet potatoes, spinach, Swiss chard, broccoli, celery, winter squashes, parsnips, and dried peas and beans.
- *Fruits:* dates, bananas, cantaloupe, mangoes, plantains, dried apricots, raisins, prunes, orange juice, and grapefruit juice.
- *Milk and yogurt:* these have less sodium than cheese, which has much less potassium and usually has added salt.

Selenium

The main useful aspects of this element are discussed at greater depth in Chapter 15 among other chemical components supporting the antioxidant systems of the body. It should be acknowledged immediately that this is a mineral that has a two-faced status, with excessive exposure causing toxicity despite that a deficiency also can cause a rare but serious illness.

Vanadium (Vanadyl Sulfate)

This is another metal salt for which reports from animal experimentation support the idea that it opposes a diabetic metabolic state. Rats made diabetic by experimenters were given vanadyl sulfate (VS), and it was found that their hyperglycemia was eliminated within two days. It is inferred from this that VS has an insulin-like action in pharmacological doses. When tested in persons having type 1 diabetes a consistent effect on blood glucose control did not occur, but the daily insulin requirement fell by 14 percent. Moreover, oral VS supplementation in persons with type 2 diabetes was followed by an increase in insulin sensitivity. This is said to result from a lower level of glycogenolysis and better glycogen storage so that blood glucose is less prone to be excessive. Also reported is a tendency for weight loss, which would be beneficial for the common problem of obesity among type 2 diabetics. Vanasul is a VS product that is being promoted to CAM-oriented physicians for use in a complimentary fashion along with conventional therapy for type 2 diabetes.

Zinc (Zinc Sulfate)

In human chemistry numerous important proteins require interaction with zinc for their proper function(s) to be performed. These include more than 300 zinc-containing enzymes and more than 2,000 transcription factors that determine protein synthesis. Dr. A. S. Prasad (2003), distinguished professor of medicine at Wayne State University School of Medicine, deplored the nature and cause for zinc deficiency disease being recognized for 40 years but ignored by the global health organizations, which allow continuation of a very preventable problem of illness in the Third World that results in growth retardation, elevated susceptibility to infection, and cognitive impairment, which are known to be common in developing countries.

According to Dunea (2001) it has also been recommended for treating numerous afflictions from A to W: "acne, alcoholism, Alzheimer's disease, angina, anorexia, anthrax, body odor, bulimia, cavities, Crohn's disease, depression, diabetes, eye disease . . . viral infections, Wilson's disease, and wound healing." Confirming these multiple supposed benefits of zinc is made difficult by its tending to cause a bad taste, nausea, and mouth irritation, all incompatible with a double-blind, placebo-controlled trial.

Zinc is said to be very useful in maintaining functional health of the immune system, which enables it to support repair of tissue damage and inhibit abnormal clotting that may be a factor in cardiovascular disease. It has been said that eating a diet of bread and water long enough will lead to death, whereas a diet of egg and water will support life for an indefinite period. That eggs, unlike bread, have no vegetable phytate to impair zinc uptake is one reason for this difference. Most multivitamin supplements provide well under 50 mg of zinc, suggesting that it is indeed a micronutrient.

Most multivitamin supplements provide well under 50 mg of zinc. Unless a person goes out of their way to add extra zinc to a multivitamin-mineral supplement, chances are slight of getting anywhere near 100 mg per day. This situation illustrates what has been said earlier, that one should not blindly take dietary supplements without first being properly informed, and that more is better is a myth, and a dangerous one at that (Chapter 11).

Chapter 23

Marvelous Metabolites: Amino Acids, New Biochemicals, and New Health Benefits

> Alpha lipoic acid is more than just another hot supplement you can buy over the counter of your local natural food store; it is indispensable to the proper working of the human body.
>
> Burt Berkson, MD, PhD (1998)

Amino acids (AAs) are assuredly nutrients, as fundamental as possible, but for nearly two decades they have begun to find usage as pharmacologic agents. The first and best example began in the 1970s as L-dihydroxyphenylalanine (L-DOPA) became critical to the therapy of Parkinson's disease by promoting synthesis of dopamine in the brain. Other early applications included L-lysine against symptoms of herpesvirus infection (cold sore, genital lesions) and L-tyrosine for boosting production of the brain catecholamines in psychopharmacology (Davis, 1987, 1991; Braverman, 2003).

COMBINED AMINO ACIDS AS SUPPLEMENTS

Mixed Amino Acids

These combination products (sometimes labeled "protein hydrolysates") are indeed produced by the breakdown of a protein by hydrolysis into its AA components. They are supplied to serve as an overall AA source for restoration after serious starvation, but are mostly of interest as a supplement to promote anabolism for a muscle-building program by athletes or "bodybuilders."

Consumer's Guide to Dietary Supplements and Alternative Medicines

doi:10.1300/5698_23

ESSENTIAL AMINO ACIDS

L-Tryptophan (LTP)

It was formerly made widely available as a single-ingredient product obtained from microbial biosynthesis rather than from AA mixtures produced by protein hydrolysis. It was used to promote higher levels of brain serotonin 5-hydroxytryptamine (5HT) prior to a 1987 toxic disaster in the United States owing to a temporary, now corrected, error of industrial manufacturing. It had been used to oppose insomnia and aid sleep and to reduce symptoms of the premenstrual syndrome. Although the exact nature of the problem was still uncertain, the FDA caused all LTP single-ingredient products to be withdrawn. (See Chapter 30 for a full account of the 1987 event.) Later, LTP was superceded by its 5-HT precursor (5HTP), obtained through a nonmicrobial production process. In 2003 LTP became available again without any fanfare but is not available widely. It may not recover its previous popularity since most former users have changed to 5HTP. Alternatively, foods might be chosen so as to maximize one's intake of LTP. Carbohydrates (starches) in meals help LTP to cross the blood-brain barrier to better gain access into the brain.

Meats are generally regarded as a good source of LTP, organ meats (e.g., liver, heart, and kidney) supposedly being the highest. However, most meats are in the range of 160 to 260 mg/100 g (chicken is about 250), with organ meats ranging between 220 and 330. These levels do not compel meat eating when compared with soybeans, split peas, cheese, and cashews.

L-Lysine

It has been used for treatment of the viral infection that causes herpes of either lip or genital areas. It also is promoted as being crucial to the formation of collagen, a major component of the body's connective tissues.

DL- and D-Phenylalanine

The L-isomer is promoted as an energy-enhancer based vital neurotransmitter in the brain. However, the unnatural D form acts as an enzyme inhibitor that enhances the level of naturally occurring neuropeptides (enkephalins, endorphins) that act similar to morphine in the brain to suppress pain. Products are on the market that contain either the D form or the DL mixture in equal amounts for use in pain relief, as a mild mood elevator, and for an anti-inflammatory action on the basis of animal data. These are especially promoted as an answer to addiction, for opposing the craving of persons with drug dependence, both for stimulants and depressants. The toxicology of DLPA preparations has not been fully investigated. They should not be taken by persons with phenylketonuria (who cannot properly metabolize phenylalanine), by children, by pregnant or lactating women, by people with high blood pressure, or by those taking antipsychotic medications or MAO inhibitors.

L-Isoleucine and L-Leucine

These are known for their structure as branched-chain essential amino acids. They are promoted for stimulating protein synthesis in muscles and as being the major fuel involved in anabolism (tissue-building) actions.

L-Methionine

Being a "methyl donor" it contributes to the internal synthesis of various vital compounds in the human body by transferring a methyl group ($-CH_3$), which is called methylation. That reaction is involved in the basic process of activating the DNA that contains our genetic information. Methionine also functions as a sulfur donor for critical detoxification processes, through its being converted to another sulfur amino acid, cysteine, which in turn is incorporated into glutathione, an essential tripeptide (i.e., composed of three amino acids) that has great importance as an "internal antidote."

Sunflower seeds, commonly fed in winter in the United States to wild birds, are a very good source of methionine, but soy protein is very deficient in it. Thus, some Americans may be feeding the wild birds in their neighborhood a better quality of protein than they are feeding to their family! Diets deficient in methionine may result in a destructive breakdown and metabolism of existing proteins as a means to obtain it. L-Methionine plays a key role in maintaining the availability of folic acid/folate in its active, functioning form. For this reason a methionine deficit can lead to a "functional" folic acid deficiency because the folate is not recycled and reactivated adequately.

A tendency exists for allergic persons to be deficient in methionine. They may respond favorably to additional methionine because it lowers blood histamine levels. A deficient capacity for methylation has been implicated among causes of depression. Methionine is also a precursor to S-adenosylmethionine (SAMe), which is shown to act in humans as an antidepressant and anti-inflammatory material. In Europe other reasons for using L-methionine are recognized including alcoholism, withdrawal symptoms or depression from drug dependence (to barbiturates, opiates or stimulants), allergies and asthma, for lowering copper when it occurs in toxic levels, opposing radiation toxicity, for improved healing from surgery or other wounds, as an adjunct to L-dopa treatment for Parkinson's disease, and in liver disorders.

L-methionine was tested in a double-blind, placebo-controlled study among AIDS patients having myelopathy (spinal nerve injury), but was not significantly beneficial in contrast to a preliminary study. The subjects received L-methionine 6 g/day in two divided doses, which was well tolerated. However, the study found that this dose of methionine was associated with an increase of SAMe (S-adenosylmethionine) levels in CSF (cerebrospinal fluid). The researchers noted that the correlation between degree of nerve conduction time improvement and SAMe level increase in the CSF was close to statistical significance. Direct administration of SAMe seems worthy of testing.

L-Threonine

It is found in eggs, milk, gelatin, and other proteins. Its vendors claim L-threonine to be critical to the synthesis of collagen, tooth enamel, and elastin. It aids the liver and its lipotropic function by also helping to avoid fatty buildup when combined with aspartic acid and methionine. It acts as a precursor of the amino acids glycine, which has an inhibitory role in the central nervous system, and serine, which has fundamental roles in nerve cell structure and function. L-threonine is said to enhance the immune system by aiding in the production of antibodies. It has also been suggested to benefit attention deficit disorder and some types of depression, but minimal evidence for this exists. Treatment of amyotrophic lateral sclerosis (Lou Gehrig's disease) via L-threonine or branched-chain amino acids was tested in six studies. A review of their results concluded that no benefit occurred, instead some indication of an unfavorable influence was found. Thus, no clear indication exists for supplementing the diet by L-threonine.

L-Valine

A third essential branched-chain amino acid (BCAA) similar to the other two is promoted as stimulating protein synthesis (anabolism) for muscle builders. All three branched-chain amino acids are used medically at times by enteral feeding (via a tube) and parenteral feeding (intravenous) for management of hepatic encephalopathy, a brain dysfunction arising from abnormal metabolites in the blood of a person having liver failure. The BCAAs are also occasionally used both enterally and parenterally in management of persons having extensive burns and/or other severe traumas because of their supposed anticatabolic action in these conditions. Several years ago the BCAAs became of some interest to neurological researchers when a pilot study showed that ALS (amyotrophic lateral sclerosis) patients showed symptomatic improvement when given large doses of BCAAs. It was theorized that BCAAs protect against neuronal damage from an excitatory neurotransmitter, glutamate. Based on the pilot study, BCAAs were given orphan drug approval by the FDA for treatment of ALS. Unfortunately, most of the follow-up studies found no benefit, one even suggesting that BCAAs may increase deaths among persons with ALS. The BCAAs may have some action against tardive dyskinesia, an adverse response to the chronic use of antipsychotic drugs.

NONESSENTIAL AMINO ACIDS

L-Taurine

This is a sulfur amino acid, meaning it has a sulfonic acid group rather than the carboxylic acid group of all the other amino acids described herein. It is an essential amino acid for human newborn infants, especially so for the preterm or premature infant. It occurs and is needed throughout the body; however, it is especially concentrated in and often is the most abundant AA in the central nervous system, heart, white blood cells, muscles, and eyes. Taurine can be synthesized from cysteine, but it is unclear whether the resulting amounts are sufficient. In addition, these amounts are higher in men than in women.

Despite it not being a component of proteins, taurine has vital activities in the regulation of ions (potassium, sodium, calcium, and magnesium) with respect to their distribution across the cell membranes of all excitable cells. It also has an inhibitory neurotransmitter action similar to that of gamma-aminobutyric acid (GABA) and glycine. Dr. E. Braverman (2003) calls taurine a "seizure fighter" because it is especially concentrated in the parts of the brain most prone to hyperexcitability in epilepsy. Indeed, its inhibitory influence tends to oppose the excitatory activity of glutamate, which may dispose a brain to epilepsy when an excess of glutamate's action exists. It seems likely that an excess of glutamate in epilepsy may arise from insufficient taurine to activate the enzyme that destroys the activity of glutamate according to research data from an epileptic strain of mice. Limited data support a claimed use of taurine as a protective agent against eye disorders, namely cataract.

L-Tyrosine

As for L-phenylalanine, L-tyrosine is used as an enhancer of brain activity via its supposed ability to promote production of brain dopamine and norepinephrine.

L-Cysteine

This is a sulfur-containing amino acid that similar to methionine bears the vital chemical group sulfhydryl (-SH). Although most cysteine is found in proteins, small amounts of free cysteine are found in body fluids of animals and in plants. L-cysteine can be considered a conditionally essential amino acid under certain circumstances, for example, in preterm infants. L-cysteine is much needed as a precursor for the synthesis of not only proteins, but also glutathione, taurine, and coenzyme A. It also is a source of sulfate groups that are used to increase the water solubility of metabolites of drugs and other molecules, thus improving their urinary excretion. Glutathione has many vital biochemical functions of protective metabolism. Thus, depletion of hepatic glutathione subjects tissues to greater oxidative stress, which can result in loss of cellular integrity and lethal injuries.

N-acetylcysteine (NAC) is a preferred derivative and delivery form for L-cysteine because of its greater stability and possibly higher absorbability. It has been claimed that L-cysteine has anti-inflammatory activity, that it can protect against toxins, and that it might oppose osteoarthritis or rheumatoid arthritis. More research will be needed before NAC can be considered useful for any of these conditions. However, it is in clinical use as a complementary agent in heart surgery to avoid ROS-induced injury. Research to date has mostly been in animal models, with cysteine-supplemented mice and guinea pigs having a more extended life span. Other animals challenged with various toxins but presupplemented with cysteine survived considerably longer than nonsupplemented controls. It has been hypothesized to have an ability to participate in DNA repair.

L-Glutamic Acid (Glutamate)

In the form of monosodium glutamate it is used as a flavor-enhancing agent for foods; thus, human exposure in the United States has been increasingly significant over the past half-century from a major increase in Chinese food preparation practices. Therefore, when an adverse consequence of such exposure for a minority of persons became known it was dubbed in the pharmacological and medical literature as the "Chinese restaurant syndrome." MSG has been well established as a teratogen for lab animals having exposure during pregnancy; thus, it should not be supplemented by pregnant women.

L-Glutamine

This is a conditionally essential amino acid that finds application at times in medicine as a primary energy source for rapidly proliferating mucosal cells of the digestive tract, the enterocytes. This makes glutamine supplementation important for use during cancer chemotherapy for its reduction of gastrointestinal injury that results from administration of many anticancer drugs. This applies especially to severe mucositis that may result from treatment with various cytotoxic antimetabolites. For example, the severity and duration of diarrhea resulting from therapy with etoposide and cytosine arabinoside were lowered significantly for a group of eleven patients given oral doses of 6 g of glutamine three times daily from three days before chemotherapy and continuing for an average of 18 days.

As a dietary supplement, glutamine is not in itself a radical scavenger, but it can be converted in vivo to glutamate, which is necessary for the synthesis of glutathione, the foremost peptide protectant against free radicals. However, it is unclear that persons can ordinarily so lack glutamine as to need supplementation. Moreover, controversy is ongoing as to whether oral glutamine supplementation is helpful or potentially toxic to healthy people. Dr. Russell Blaylock (1997), a board-certified neurosurgeon and author of the book *Excitotoxins: The Taste That Kills* expresses great concern about safety of high intake of glutamine as a supplement. He acknowledges that glutamine per se is not an excitotoxin as is MSG but contends that glutamine is converted within neurons into the excitotoxin glutamate. Indeed, the major source of brain glutamate is from glutamine.

Although serving as a vital excitatory neurotransmitter in the brain, glutamate has a dark side in that its excessive release can be toxic to brain cells, hence the term *excitotoxin.* Two major excitotoxins are the amino acids glutamate and aspartate (whereas some others are metabolites). If they cause particularly susceptible brain cells to become excessively excited the cells will quickly die. Excitotoxins can also cause a loss of brain synapses and connecting fibers. Food-associated sources of these excitotoxins include food additives such as the taste-enhancer MSG (monosodium glutamate) and the synthetic sweetener aspartame as well as hydrolyzed protein and soy protein extract. It is currently arguable whether the use of these is as hazardous as they are accused to be by Blaylock (1997).

Persons having serious liver failure tend to accumulate ammonia in their blood and brain and to develop signs of brain malfunction (encephalopathy). Until recently, it was assumed that the elevated ammonia level caused the liver-disease-associated brain injury and that glutamine was protective. However, newer research indicates that it is instead an excess of glutamine that causes the encephalopathy. Supplementing the glutamine intake would tend to aggravate this problem significantly. Moreover, an accumulation of glutamine has also been found in the brain pathologies of Alzheimer's and Huntington's diseases, and high levels of brain glutamine have also been associated with a more grave prognosis in Lou Gehrig's disease or ALS. Likewise, recent research showed that high brain glutamine levels increase the brain levels of free radicals and impair the ability of brain mitochondria to produce energy, which soon leads to cell death. Thus, it appears that supplementation of glutamine intake is ill-advised (or worse!) with regard to it helping to oppose free-radical-associated disease states. Thus, a simplistic assumption that all essential amino acids are both necessary and safe as a supplement would be grossly and dangerously wrong in the case of glutamine.

The major value for high-dose glutamine would be to aid in repairing gastrointestinal injury on a short-term basis. Dr. Blaylock (1997) recommends that persons having a history of the following conditions need to avoid glutamine supplementation, even for short-term use (http://mercola.com/2004/may/1/glutamine.htm):

- Stroke
- Neurodegenerative disease
- Pregnancy
- Malignancy
- Recent vaccinations
- ADHD
- Hypoglycemia
- Autism
- Multiple sclerosis
- Other neurological disorders

L-Glycine

Besides its being an amino acid component of peptides and proteins, glycine serves in the nervous system as a neurotransmitter, which is especially well established for the spinal cord. Recent reports suggest that it plays a role in pain regulation, and that new analgesic agents may be forthcoming that act via the glycine receptors of the central nervous system. No clear need for supplementation exists.

L-Histidine

Besides the usual role in peptide and protein structure, histidine serves as the precursor for the physiological amine histamine. Allergy sufferers will recognize histamine as at least a partial mediator of their woes, for which reason a great many of us have taken antihistamine drugs, OTC and/or Rx. Many readers will have taken another type of histamine antagonist known as an H2 blocker, which causes the original allergy-aimed histamine antagonists to be called H1 blockers. However, histamine also has some CNS activities as a neurotransmitter at H3 receptors; therefore, we can't suppose that we'd be all better if we could just do without histamine. During the late 1990s one research company was pursuing possible application for an H3 blocker in the treatment of ADHD or other brain disorders. As of yet efforts to develop a therapeutic agent from among antagonists at this brain-located H3 receptor have not borne fruit, but it isn't safe to suppose that such failure will indefinitely prevail. After all, Nobel Prizes in medicine were twice awarded for the researches that produced the H1 and H2 blockers. Can an H3-related Nobel Prize be yet to come?

L-Proline

This is the third most abundant of the AAs in the human body, especially in its structural role in collagen, which comprises 30 percent of the total protein. Therefore it is very essential for healthy skin, connective tissue, bone, and joints. It is much involved in the healing of wounds. Currently, it does not have any particular therapeutic roles and is little noted as a supplement. It does serve as a diagnostic indicator for alcoholism by its blood level being elevated owing to impaired liver function.

D, L-Serine

Phosphatidylserine (PS) is an important phospholipid because it is a structural component of biological membranes of both plants and animals. Chemically, the PS molecule consists of a glycerolphosphate backbone, serine, and two fatty acids, polyunsaturated ones if from soy. Although it was originally obtained from bovine brain, the source of PS was changed to soy lecithin because of concern for contamination by the prion agent responsible for mad cow disease (or bovine spongiform encephalopathy

[BSE]). Thus, as phosphatidylserine, a chemically activated form of the amino acid, serine has come into use for its metabolic value to nerve cells, which is believed to make it a supplement useful against age-related memory impairment. It is a compound that has particular relevance to such cells because of their requirement to form large amounts of phosphatidylcholine for the structural integrity of cell membranes.

For soy PS from one manufacturer, the product's components other than PS have been found to range from 15 percent to 80 percent. This sort of uncertain composition of supposed uniform preparations of "phosphatidylserine" hindered FDA approval of therapeutic claims for current (soy) PS, as all but one study submitted for review used bovine brain PS. Moreover, the clinical studies constituting "scientific evidence" available consisted of mitigation studies, i.e., testing whether PS reduced preexisting dementia or other cognitive dysfunction. It can easily be argued that these were irrelevant to a preventive use of PS to reduce risk of such outcomes. The FDA declined to approve a request for therapeutic claims and responded with approval for only the conditional claims listed in the following excerpt:

> Dementia claim and disclaimer:
>
> Consumption of phosphatidylserine may reduce the risk of dementia in the elderly. Very limited and preliminary scientific research suggests that phosphatidylserine may reduce the risk of dementia in the elderly. FDA concludes that there is little scientific evidence supporting this claim.
>
> Cognitive dysfunction claim and disclaimer:
>
> Consumption of phosphatidylserine may reduce the risk of cognitive dysfunction in the elderly. Very limited and preliminary scientific research suggests that phosphatidylserine may reduce the risk of cognitive dysfunction in the elderly. FDA concludes that there is little scientific evidence supporting this claim. (FDA, 2003)

COENZYME Q10

In the latter 1950s researchers in the United States and in England discovered a new organic molecule in beef heart, other animal organs, and yeast (thus it is available sparingly from food sources) that originally was named ubiquinone. This term came from its having a quinone group in its chemical structure, and from its being ubiquitously distributed, i.e., in the cells of all organs and tissues. This distribution was found to stem from its being required and intimately associated with fundamental cellular functions. The enzymes of intracellular organelles called mitochondria, which are also known as the "powerhouses" of cells, have a fundamental role in energy release from food molecules. It is with those enzymes that CoQ10 acts as a facilitator, a coenzyme. Put very briefly, CoQ10 is necessary for the production of ATP, adenosine triphosphate, which is the foremost "power molecule" necessary for all activities of cells that require energy input for their operation. In addition, research has indicated that CoQ10 has antioxidant and membrane-stabilizing actions, which endue it with further vital physiological roles.

Because CoQ10 can be synthesized internally, it is not classified as a vitamin despite its biochemical actions being very similar to those of several vitamins. However, some authors argue that it deserves vitamin status, and suggest that situations exist in which internal production may not suffice to meet the needed quantities. Although it may never be considered a vitamin, CoQ10 certainly is an essential metabolite. It adds to the nutritional value of certain foods—for example, beef, poultry, and broccoli. Currently, CoQ10 for supplements is produced by the fermentation of beets and sugarcane.

Although no clear deficiency disease has been identified, low levels of CoQ10 seem to be inversely correlated with the symptoms of heart failure. Supplementation of this vital molecule may lend assistance to various other bodily functions by reducing the necessity for its multistep internal synthesis. Thus it is promoted as a component of nutrient formulas for athletes as a legal performance enhancer.

Some evidence shows that either an increased requirement, a decreased endogenous production of CoQ10, or both occurring with advancing age can contribute to a shortfall from optimal levels in older persons. Low levels of CoQ10 could also be a result of poor nourishment, a genetic defect in its biosynthesis, or a depletion of the vitamins, trace elements, or other factors necessary for its biosynthesis. This is commonly suggested as a reason for its use by elderly persons to ensure adequacy of CoQ10 supplies. Dietary supplementation with CoQ10 is commonly practiced by physicians in Europe and in Japan. A great many published studies are available from those areas. As long ago as 1974, the Japanese government approved CoQ10 for therapy of chronic heart failure, and about 250 preparations that contain CoQ10 are on the market there for treatment of cardiovascular diseases.

A review article in 2001 concentrated on clinical studies that evaluated CoQ10 usage in patients diagnosed with heart failure, angina pectoris, or hypertension. Most clinical trials of CoQ10 have focused on these three cardiovascular diseases, all of which are common in the United States. The reviewers evaluated available data concerning the safety, efficacy, and dosing of CoQ10 for management of heart failure, angina, and hypertension. Some

U.S. cardiologists do prescribe CoQ10 for their heart disease patients. It is said to be used to reduce vascular damage during bypass surgery. For the many other proposed applications much less information is available on which to base an evaluation of efficacy or recommendations for dosing schedules. It is an FDA-approved orphan drug for certain rare genetic mitochondrial disorders.

CoQ10 and Statins

The primary biosynthesis of CoQ10 depends on a reductase reaction of 3-hydroxy-3-methylglutaryl coenzyme A (HMG-CoA), a reaction that is also involved in cholesterol synthesis. The statins are a widely used class of therapeutic agents used for lowering (excess) blood cholesterol levels by their inhibiting its biosynthesis. The inhibition of this biosynthesis depends on opposition to the same cofactor, HMG-CoA, that is essential for the biosynthesis of CoQ10. Thus, concern exists that use of the statins is causing patients to develop a deficiency of CoQ10. Indeed, one manufacturer of a statin is said to have considered adding CoQ10 to their product, but they unfortunately decided against that course. Perhaps this was a result of concern that doing so would expose their product to liability for an unwanted side effect, but other more technical factors may have been responsible.

ALPHA-LIPOIC ACID (THIOCTIC ACID)

Alpha-lipoic acid (alpha-LA) is a natural metabolite and coenzyme as well as a minor food constituent.

Alpha-LA is proposed to be a unique nutrient also for its having also an insulin-like effect by which it promotes glucose transport into cells. A concentration-dependent increase in glucose uptake was observed in humans cells treated with alpha-LA in vitro. Based on U.S. research showing that it facilitates the metabolism of glucose, alpha-LA is medically approved in Germany for treating type 2 diabetes (non-insulin-dependent diabetes mellitus), and for opposing its potential complications. Obviously, it should be expected to act similarly and to be equally useful on both sides of the Atlantic Ocean.

In Europe, alpha-LA has also been used for decades (usually under the name thioctic acid) to protect the liver against toxicants and to antidote (detoxify) certain poisons, such as mushroom toxin, or excessive iron, copper, or heavy metals such as cadmium, lead, and mercury (see also Chapter 20). This is possible because the alpha-LA molecule contains sulfur (thiol groups) that can bind and facilitate the excretion of such metals while minimizing their toxicity. alpha-LA also has been considered useful in Europe for treating elevated liver enzymes from various other liver injuries besides metals, such as from radiation poisoning and alcoholic hepatitis. It has also been used to reduce the painful symptoms of diabetic neuropathy.

Evidence suggests that alpha-LA, alone or combined with vitamin E is an effective therapy for radiation exposure by lowering oxidative damage and helping to maintain normal organ functions. Such therapy was applied and was said to be effective for treating children living in areas affected by the Chernobyl nuclear accident in the former Soviet Union. However, these were uncontrolled observations that do not satisfy evidence-based medicine criteria.

The potential therapeutic uses of alpha-LA for its direct radical scavenging, for recycling of other antioxidants, for accelerating the synthesis of glutathione, and for its opposition to inflammation-related factors have not been given much attention. Such mechanisms support a sometimes dramatic experimental effect of alpha-LA against the injurious effects of oxidative stress conditions. A significant potential application would be to prevent ischemia-reperfusion injury, e.g., cellular injury that occurs in the brain or heart when a blood-flow interruption (ischemia) is followed by restored blood flow (reperfusion). This problem may occur with stroke, cardiac arrest, subarachnoid hemorrhage, or head trauma.

One must wonder if alpha-LA might also be able to reduce the rate of POCD (postoperative cognitive dysfunction), a potentially devastating brain disorder, especially impairing the memory, that occurs after surgical anesthesia. It is a problem of progressively higher frequency as the age of the patient increases. The absence of adverse effects of alpha-LA would seem to avoid questions of safety and ethics in performing a placebo-controlled trial.

THE SAMe STORY

SAMe and the Nervous System

S-Adenosylmethionine (SAMe) was described in Chapter 12 as a metabolite that was developed in Europe, where it has proved very useful as an antidote for agents that are injurious to the liver, to oppose joint symptoms of osteoarthritis, and to overcome depression. To reiterate, it plays a pivotal biochemical role in methylation reactions that are essential for many biological events. Thus, it is widely distributed throughout the body tissues in every living cell, with particularly high levels in the brain and liver. The endogenous synthesis of SAMe depends upon both folic acid and vitamin B_{12}.

Deficits of B_{12} seem to be especially associated with reduced levels of SAMe in the brain, which may be an explanation for the occurrence of neuropsychiatric disorders associated with inadequate tissue levels of B_{12} (Lindenbaum et al., 1988). The persons who develop pernicious anemia sometimes initially show neurological signs and symptoms of brain disorders or behavioral alterations that may even include psychosis. Many elderly persons show motor or behavioral deviations that appear to be improved by injections of B_{12}. It seems as if SAMe might be another mode of dealing with these problems more directly, as they likely arise primarily from SAMe not being synthesized efficiently by such persons. It may be critical to determine whether adequate bioavailability of SAMe exists in elderly persons. Poor intestinal absorption could hinder the efficacy of oral products and require a more bioavailable approach (e.g., sublingual), or an injectable form, as is true for B_{12}.

Because SAMe is rather free of adverse effects or supplement-drug interactions, it is highly desirable for clinical studies to be conducted in the United States to confirm those in the literature from European investigators. Unfortunately, it does not appear presently among those dietary supplements for which federal grants are supporting needed studies. Prominent among uses of SAMe in Europe is depression. Thus, it might be an effective complement to pharmaceutical antidepressants that could permit a lowering of their doses so as to avoid their unwanted effects, e.g., hindrance to sexual function in both men and women. Indeed, a high degree of synergism occurs with concurrently used pharmaceutical antidepressants of different classes.

Chapter 24

Bioflavonoid Benefits: Chemoprevention of Cancer

> What are bioflavonoids? They make oranges orange, blueberries blue, and cherries red.
>
> Anonymous

A prominent theory as to the origin of malignant neoplasms (literally, new growths, or cancers) is that they arise from damage to genetic material, the DNA of the genes borne on the chromosomes. Strong evidence for this concept long has been that certain rare congenital deviations in chromosome structure are clearly associated with and responsible for persons developing several varieties of cancers. In more recent times it has become known that certain genes have the capacity to promote cancerous transformation of cells and the uncontrolled growth known as malignancy, whereas other genes act to oppose this. Although some genetic deviations causing cancer are known to exist from the point of conception, most cancers are a consequence of cellular events that occur after birth. Among the factors that can act to this end are physical stimuli, such as ionizing radiation that damages the genetic material (DNA), chemicals called carcinogens that also alter the DNA, and some oncogenic (cancer-causing) viruses.

One mechanism whereby radiation and chemicals are believed to disturb the normal structure of DNA is by the generation of several chemical agents known as ROS, which stands for *reactive oxygen species* (see Table 14.1). These ROS are also called free radicals, and molecules that can act to neutralize them are referred to as free radical scavengers. However, because the ROS cause injury through oxidative (oxidizing) actions, most of the agents that oppose and neutralize them are commonly know as antioxidants.

Consumer's Guide to Dietary Supplements and Alternative Medicines

doi:10.1300/5698_24

Naturally occurring antioxidants from food sources are many and varied. Among the vitamin component of foods we benefit from the antioxidant actions of vitamins A, C, and E. The array of antioxidants available from the diet is summarized in Exhibit 14.1. The relationship of this general group to opposing disease is broad and varied, including nervous system degenerative disorders, cardiovascular disease, and neoplastic diseases—cancer.

As Exhibit 14.1 indicates, the actions of the antioxidants are not confined entirely to an opposition to the ROS. Some have other mechanisms of action that may complement the former, as for example quercetin and genistein inhibiting the enzyme known as topoisomerase. This is a mode of action for a certain few compounds among all of the classical pharmaceuticals known as cytotoxic antineoplastic drugs.

The role of environmental exposure to carcinogenic chemicals in one's risk for developing cancer has been a topic of great concern for several decades. One response to the perceived problem of unavoidable exposures, as from metropolitan air pollution, has been to search for protective agents among dietary supplements. Thus, for many years considerable interest has existed in the possibility of reducing cancer rates through increasing the intake level of cancer-preventing chemicals. Whatever the source and origin, natural or synthetic agents able to decrease the effects of exposure to cancer-promoting chemicals are known as chemopreventive agents. The major chemical group thought to have such a capacity are the naturally occurring polyphenolic compounds, which share strong antioxidant and anti-inflammatory activities. Each of these actions seem to exert chemopreventive activity against cancer-promoting conditions.

Population-based (derived from a whole citizenry of a state or nation) epidemiologic research can test for an effect of certain dietary items by a comparison of rates for a type of cancer in groups of people who do or do not eat them. Finding that certain human groups have lower rates of cancer than the general rate throughout the world can point to certain dietary components as being protective. Thus, epidemiologic evidence may be suggestive of but cannot confirm an anticancer benefit. When laboratory animal studies testing food components for an ability to reduce or prevent experimental cancers support the epidemiologic data, grounds exist for claiming benefit from increasing their ingestion or for adding such components to the diet via supplements. *Prospective* clinical trials to seek confirmation of long-term benefit would be quite difficult and expensive because of their long-term nature—ten years at least. Consequently, human research to validate supposed cancer chemoprotective actions is lacking, and likely will continue to be so.

A major example of this sort of situation is the cruciferous vegetables, which include broccoli, cabbage (as in coleslaw and sauerkraut), cauliflower, brussels sprouts, and kale (which encompasses mustard greens and chard). This group of vegetables turned out not only to be a rich source of vitamins and minerals but also to contain a multitude of various phytochemicals having anticancer properties. The means for their benefits are believed to include antioxidant properties known to oppose carcinogens, enzyme actions that detoxify carcinogens, and inhibition of tumor cell growth.

Among the individual cruciferous vegetables, broccoli and cabbage appear to provide the best defenses against cancer. That bladder cancer hits about 39,000 men and 15,000 women annually in the United States makes it is important to know that we can change our diet to improve our odds in favor of *not* being one of these statistics, but this fact is not being as highly publicized as it warrants.

CHEMOPREVENTIVE CANDIDATES

The search for cancer chemopreventive agents is ongoing among pharmaceutical industry researchers. It is not clear to what extent natural substances may enter their consideration. It is possible that a synthetic or semisynthetic analogue of certain dietary supplement components might be part of industrial investigations. However, a journal that is much more pharmaceutical-industry-oriented than CAM-oriented recently showed candidates for use as cancer chemopreventive agents (Table 24.1).

It is clear from Table 24.1 that only a few pharmaceuticals believed to oppose cancer onset are now available in contrast to the large number of currently available nutrients and botanicals containing phytochemicals viewed to act as cancer chemopreventives. Much of the basis for this characterization is their preventive action in rodent tests against model carcinogens. For example, in regard to polyphenols very many additional foods and herbal products (especially highly colored ones) could be named as sources besides green tea and grape. Similar statements could be made for the other phytochemical classes listed without sources because they are such widespread components. Proponents of the supplement scene would likely say that nutrients and botanical supplements offer Now what the pharmaceutical industry can only hope for some day—efficacy that essentially lacks toxic drawbacks. The currently available pharmaceuticals, the NSAID class of anti-inflammatories, do not score well for low toxicity, as seen by the Fall 2004 withdrawal of Vioxx. We will take a closer look at some botanicals, bearing in mind that clinical data required to validate them is far from satisfactory yet.

TABLE 24.1. Current candidates for possible cancer chemopreventive use.

Nutrients	Phytochemicals (sources)	Pharmaceuticals
Calcium	Carotenoids (vegetables)	Anti-inflammatory agents:
Fiber	Curcumin (turmeric)	NSAIDs (aspirin, ibuprofen, etc.) and COX-2 inhibitors
Folate	Diallyl sulfide (garlic)	Chromatin modifiers[a]
Selenium	Genistein (soy)	Nuclear receptor ligands[a]
Vitamin D	Polyphenols (Green tea, grape seed)	
Vitamin E	Indole-3-carbinol	
	Isoflavones (soy products, etc.)	
	Isothiocyanates	
	L-perillyl alcohol	
	Saponins	
	Terpines	

Source: Modified from Lewis (2003).

Note: Also significant would be MSM (Chapter 23) and ascorbic acid (Chapter 14).

[a]Not yet available.

BIOFLAVONOIDS

Flavonoids or bioflavonoids are natural products widely distributed in the vegetable kingdom and currently consumed in large amounts (up to several hundred milligrams per day) in the average Western diet. They are sometimes called vitamin P, indicating that they cannot be produced in the animal body, but they are not associated clearly with a deficiency disease, which disqualifies them for the title of vitamin. The main source of bioflavonoids is the citrus fruits—lemons, grapefruits, oranges, and to a lesser extent, limes. Other fruit sources are apricots, cherries, grapes (especially grape seeds), black currants, plums, blueberries, blackberries, pears, and papayas. They are generally found in the edible pulp of the fruit more than in the strained juices. Good vegetable sources of bioflavonoids are onions, red cabbage, green pepper, broccoli, parsley, tomatoes, peas, and even pine bark extract. They can also be found in teas (especially green tea), cocoa, red wine, and beer. The flavonoids are also called polyphenols for their sharing a major chemical feature of multiple phenolic hydroxyl groups. They have a variety of significant physiological or biochemical roles important to the plants, so it is not surprising that they tend to have bioactivity also in mammalian tissues or organs.

Botanicals containing flavonoids have been used since ancient times by healers and laypeople alike to treat a great variety of human illnesses. Recent research supports the idea that diets rich in fruits and vegetables oppose the onset of much age-related illness, i.e., to lower the risk of cancer and cardiovascular disease. A wide variety of flavonoids exert similar protective actions against the oxidation of low-density lipoprotein both in vitro and in vivo in some human and animal experiments. This is thought to oppose the development of atherosclerosis and cardiovascular disease. Flavonoids also have been demonstrated to modulate the activity of various enzymes and to modify the behavior of many mammalian cell systems.

Much laboratory research suggests that members of this large and diverse group may possess significant antihepatotoxic, antiallergic, anti-inflammatory, antitumor, and even antiosteoporotic activities. In some cases both animal experimental data and Phase I human data are available, but few if any have yet to be validated via the controlled testing of modern Phase II and III clinical trials. However, one such agent, flavopiridol, in 2000 was undergoing Phase II single-agent human trials and Phase I combination trials (with paclitaxel and cisplatin) for cancer chemotherapy. Flavopiridol seems promising, especially in a combination with paclitaxel, for which preclinical studies showed a synergistic antitumor effect. Flavonoids have also been considered to be potential anti-HIV agents.

Research in the field of flavonoids has been stimulated by discoveries suggesting that a flavonoid component of red wine might explain the "French paradox." This phrase denotes the low cardiovascular mortality rate observed in the French populations despite their high intake of saturated fats. This advantage has been attributed to consumption of a particular flavonoid, resveratrol, obtained by drinking red wine.

Certain flavonoids are potent inhibitors of the production of prostaglandins, which are a group of powerful proinflammatory signaling molecules. Researchers have found that this effect arises from the flavonoids' inhibiting several key biosynthetic enzymes (i.e., lipoxygenase, phospholipase and cyclooxygenase) essential to the production of prostaglandins. The flavonoids also tend to inhibit phosphodiesterases, enzymes necessary for the biosynthesis of other proinflammatory proteins (cytokines) that mediate cell activation and adhesion of circulating leukocytes at sites of cellular injury.

The high levels of antioxidants present in certain fruits, vegetables, grains, and beverages may have an important role in protecting the gastrointestinal (GI) tract itself from oxidative injuries and in opposing the development of stomach, colon, and rectal cancer. Because the flavonoids (also, carotenoids) do not seem to be as well absorbed from the gut as are the dietary antioxidant vitamins C and E, their levels and activity can be much higher within the lower intestinal tract than can ever be achieved in the blood or body tissues. This points to their antioxidant action in the intestinal tract as generally being more significant than in other organs.

SPECIFIC FLAVONOIDS

Green Tea Extract

Each year several million tons of tea are produced from dried leaves and leaf buds of the oriental shrub *Camellia sinensis.* Black tea, which accounts for about 78 percent of production, is prepared by first drying and then fermenting the leaves. It is the type of tea most widely drunk in Europe and North America. Green tea, which is not fermented, is made by steaming or panfrying tea leaves and then drying them; this destroys enzymes so that fermentation cannot occur. About 20 percent of the world tea crop is devoted to production of green tea, which is mostly consumed in China and Japan, where it has been used both as a stimulant beverage and medicinally as a digestive remedy for about 5,000 years. Scientific research into the effects of green tea has focused largely on its potential to prevent cancer. This focus arose from many epidemiologic studies in Far East populations that showed a low rate of cancers. They suggested that the regular drinking of tea (particularly green tea) might decrease the risk of cancer, especially of the upper digestive tract.

Borrelli and colleagues (2004) performed a systematic review of green tea and gastrointestinal cancer risk. Twenty-one epidemiological investigations met their criteria for inclusion. Those studies seemed to suggest a protective effect of green tea existed against development of benign adenomatous polyps and chronic atrophic gastritis. By contrast, no clear epidemiological evidence supported the hypothesis that green tea has a role in prevention of stomach and intestinal cancers. No prospective randomized human trial has been reported.

However, several rodent studies have confirmed a suspected anticarcinogenic effect. For example, extracts of green tea applied to mouse skin have been found to inhibit the development of skin cancer in response to known skin carcinogens. Green tea extract given orally or by injection has been shown to inhibit the growth of transplanted tumors and to lower the development rate of tumors in animals exposed to cancer-producing agents. A few studies have reported that green tea or green tea extract reduces the potential of cancer cells to metastasize (spread via blood or lymph) in some animal systems. Other data suggest that green tea serves to oppose the cumulative genetic damage necessary for a cell to become transformed from normal to aggressive metastatic cancerous activity.

As with most botanicals, the chemical composition of green tea varies with geographic origin of the leaf, the time of its harvest, and the subsequent processing. Constituents of black tea differ from those of green tea because the actions of fermentation and oxidation on black tea lowers the content of catechins (flavonols) and flavonoids and lowers the concentration of total polyphenols, which research suggests are responsible for the chemopreventive effect of green tea.

The antioxidant actions of flavonoids in tea, which include prevention of oxidative effects on LDL, are among several potential mechanisms that could be responsible for cardiovascular protective effects. Other possible mechanisms include an opposition to the inflammatory process in atherosclerosis, reduction of thrombosis, promoting normal endothelial functions, and blocking production of cellular adhesion molecules. Collective antioxidant effects of multiple components in a flavonoid-rich diet may more effectively reduce the risk for cardiovascular disease than could any one antioxidant alone.

With respect to anticancer activity, a catechin in green tea that has generated the most scientific interest is the potent antioxidant component, epigallocatechin gallate (EGCG). The mechanism of action of EGCG and other similar substances is uncertain, but they may function in several ways. They surely act as antioxidants, and also may act by inhibiting enzymes involved in cell replication and DNA synthesis. They may hinder cell-to-cell adhesion or may inhibit some intracellular communication pathway required for cell division.

Turmeric and Curcumin

Turmeric *(Curcuma domestica; Curcuma longa)* is a member of the ginger family that is thought to be indigenous to the Indian subcontinent but which is grown and harvested commercially also in China and many regions of tropical southeastern Asia. It has active constituents that are yellowish-orange volatile oils known as curcuminoids. It is best known for its culinary use, being a major component of curry powder that is widely consumed in southeast Asia. Moreover, indigenous systems of medicine, including the ayurvedic and traditional Chinese medicine systems, used turmeric extensively for centuries in the treatment of inflammatory conditions and other diseases. Turmeric has been used in India mainly for arthritic and muscular disorders. In China it has been used as a topical analgesic and for a wide variety of other conditions, ranging from flatulence and colic to ringworm and to even hepatitis and chest pain. In the United States turmeric is an approved food additive that is commercially available at low cost. It has been used as a coloring agent in pharmaceuticals, yellow mustards, and cosmetics.

In Europe a major turmeric constituent known as curcumin has been applied for relief of dyspepsia, loss of appetite, feelings of excessive fullness after meals, and liver and gallbladder complaints. Curcumin also is used for systemic treatment of rheumatoid arthritis and the eye disease chronic anterior uveitis. Topically it has been used against conjunctivitis, skin cancer, smallpox, and chicken pox.

More significantly, curcumin recently has been the subject of considerable interest as it has shown immunosuppressive, antineoplastic, antioxidant, anti-platelet-aggregation, and antiviral activities both in vitro and in whole animal research. It is being investigated as a potential adjuvant therapy for several types of cancer, because of both its expressing immunosuppressive activity and its action as a cancer chemoprotectant for the colon and perhaps other organs. Curcumin also has antibacterial and antiparasitic activities, and it preferentially inhibits platelet aggregation induced by platelet-activating factors and arachidonic acid.

Curcumin has shown several activities that may mediate an anticancer action. One is causing apoptosis ("programmed cell suicide") in various human cancer cell lines and animal tumor cells. Another action is known as antiangiogenesis, inhibiting formation of blood vessels to supply the needs of a tumor. A third action is its inhibition of the cyclooxygenase (COX) enzyme. This has been associated with a reduced risk for colon cancer, as well as having useful anti-inflammatory effects. Feeding curcumin to rodents has resulted in a chemopreventive action against cancer formation in the forestomach, colon, duodenum, and skin. Curcumin also has a weak estrogenic effect characteristic of phytoestrogens. This has opposed the carcinogenic action of DDT (dichlorpiphenyltrichloroethane) and has synergized with phytoestrogens in opposing induction of breast cancer by DDT-like compounds.

Unfortunately, neither turmeric nor curcumin has been extensively studied by human trials. For treating arthritis, fresh turmeric root dosages of 8 to 60 grams three times daily, or 400 to 600 mg of curcumin three times daily, have been recommended. For dyspepsia, a dose of 1.5 to 3 grams of turmeric root is recommended. Root preparations should be standardized to contain not less than 3 percent curcumin and not less than 3 percent volatile oils. Recently marketed is an anti-arthritic combination of turmeric, for its COX-inhibitory action, jointly with *nine* other herbal components. This complex mixture confounds any possibility of identifying the basis for the possible benefits of the product. Other applications mentioned previously as being under clinical investigation should not be considered appropriate reasons for self-medication.

Curcumin exposure has apparently occurred safely in its use as a culinary spice for centuries. It is estimated that adults in India ingest 80 to 200 mg of curcumin daily without adverse effects. Thus, the only reported adverse effects of curcumin or turmeric are rare cases of allergic contact dermatitis among persons working in a spices shop. Some Indian women apply turmeric to their skin to minimize unwanted hair growth, but few experience dermatitis as a consequence. The German Commission E Monographs cited no known interactions of curcumin with medicines. Because of a possible additive antiplatelet activity, caution should be exercised with respect to a joint use of curcumin with anticoagulants, or with other medications or dietary supplements known to impair coagulation. Turmeric should be avoided by patients with bleeding disorders or bile duct obstruction, and should be used only with the approval/supervision of a physician in patients having gallstones. The American Herbal Products Association classifies turmeric as a menstrual stimulant, and some sources recommend the avoidance of curcumin in pregnancy and during breast-feeding.

A very encouraging amount of basic research with curcumin and related materials is ongoing. Although the quantity and quality of the currently available clinical studies are both insufficient, turmeric appears to be safe for self-medication. Well-designed clinical trials are needed and warranted to clarify the possible contribution of turmeric/curcumin in the prevention or treatment of several varieties of cancer as well as in treatment of rheumatoid arthritis and several ocular conditions.

RESVERATROL (RED WINE EXTRACT)

Although resveratrol is found in other plants, such as eucalyptus, spruce, and lily, and in foods such as mulberries and peanuts, its most abundant natural sources are grapes of the *Vitis vinifera, Vitis labrusca,* and muscadine types, all of which are used to make wines. It occurs in the vines, roots, seeds, and stalks, but its highest levels are in the grape skins. Grapes grown in cooler climates have higher concentrations, and the unfermented grape juice has much less resveratrol than does red wine, which has more resveratrol than white wine because of the longer length of time that the grape skins are present during the fermentation process.

The main claim to fame for this compound associated with grape skins and red wine has been its reputed benefit to the cardiovascular system, as supposed (but unproven) basis for "the French paradox." The high intake of wines by the French people became a focus of inquiry, and experimental data were found suggestive of a heart-protective component in wine. Most protective was red wine, and from this was identified the flavonoid constituent resveratrol as a likely mediator of that protective effect. Although this may not be a fully established fact, it has been sufficient grounds for developing supplement products based on their supposed content of resveratrol, i.e., "red wine extract." To this time most research on the antioxidant and anti-platelet properties of resveratrol has been done in vitro. Thus, additional studies in animals and humans are needed to confirm whether resveratrol supplementation is truly beneficial. A recent study found that even red wine that was dealcoholized was capable of decreasing atherosclerosis, as were red and white wines. Researchers concluded that moderate consumption of nonalcoholic red wine, which provides the usual amount of resveratrol-related polyphenolic compounds, can oppose atherosclerosis.

Another area of suggested health benefit is cancer chemoprevention. Data indicate that resveratrol may trigger the process of apoptosis in tumor cells, as for curcumin. A Singapore research group is reported by to have found it active against human leukemic and breast cancer cells in vitro by its induction of apoptosis (Pervais, 2001). Moreover, the same action was seen in vivo against skin tumors in mice. Not only are these actions well confirmed, but also their mechanistic details have been elucidated.

Recently, resveratrol was described by James A. Crowell and colleagues (2004) as having antimycotic, antiviral, and beneficial cardiovascular and cancer preventive activities, and being under development for several clinical indications as a pharmaceutical agent. They pursued a broad basic toxicologic evaluation, which found most adverse events to have occurred in the group of rats administered the highest level of 3,000 mg per kilogram body weight per day, whereas a 300 mg level of resveratrol per kilogram body weight per day caused no observed adverse effects. Clinical signs of toxicity included reductions in final body weights, hemoglobin, hematocrit, red cell counts, and food consumption; elevation of six clinical chemistries; and increased white cell counts and in kidney weights. Clinically significant renal lesions were observed, including an increased incidence and severity of nephropathy. This shows that, similar to a drug, resveratrol can show high-dose toxicities.

Cancer-Related Effects of Resveratrol

Resveratrol has been studied to see whether it alters the initiation, promotion, and progression of cancerous growths. Baht and Pezzuto (2002) colleagues reported that resveratrol was indeed effective during each of these phases of the cancer-onset process. Resveratrol appears to decrease tumor initiation by three mechanisms—both antioxidant and antimutagenic activities and increasing the levels of a drug-metabolizing enzyme capable of detoxifying carcinogens. It opposes tumor promotion activity by its anti-inflammatory effects and an ability to inhibit cyclooxygenase-1 (COX-1). COX-1 increases the levels of proinflammatory substances, which may also stimulate tumor cell growth. Studies on the progression of cancer have found that resveratrol caused favorable changes in human leukemia cells and inhibited an enzyme needed for DNA synthesis in proliferating cancer cells. Moreover, resveratrol inhibited the development of preneoplastic lesions in mouse mammary glands in culture and inhibited tumor formation in mice when treated with a carcinogen.

In September 2004 investigators at Fred Hutchinson Cancer Research Center in Seattle reported that drinking one glass of red wine daily may reduce a man's risk for prostate cancer by 50 percent. Moreover, the protective effect appears strongest against the most aggressive forms of prostate cancer. Schoonen et al. (2005) found that men who consumed four or more glasses of red wine per week reduced their risk of prostate cancer by one-half. They found no significant effects, either positive or negative, associated with consumption of beer or liquor, and no consistent risk reduction was found with consumption of white wine. This supports the inference that red wine must contain a compound that is lacking in other types of alcoholic beverages. They believe this compound to be resveratrol. These researchers postulate five possible mechanisms:

1. As an antioxidant, it helps scavenge and remove cancer-causing free radicals.
2. As a potent anti-inflammatory agent, it blocks some enzymes that act to promote tumor development.
3. It reduces cell proliferation, reducing the number of cell divisions that could lead to cancer or to the continued growth of cancer cells.
4. It increases apoptosis (programmed cell death), thus helping to rid the body of cancerous cells.
5. It may act as an estrogen, reducing the level of circulating male hormones such as testosterone that promote growth of prostate cancer cells.

Despite these varied signs of anticancer activity, no toxic effects have been observed. An especially appealing characteristic of resveratrol's anticancer potential is this minimal toxicity, especially to blood-forming cells, in contrast to a great majority of anticancer drugs. (The same advantage applies for turmeric and green tea.) More studies on both cellular and animal models are required for the findings truly to be applicable to humans.

The similarity in structure between resveratrol and a well-known synthetic estrogen (diethylstilbestrol) has prompted research concerning its activity as a phytoestrogen. However, it is unclear whether such properties might oppose or enhance the growth of estrogen-dependent human breast cancer cells. As weaker agents than the normal internal estrogens, they might reduce activation of breast cancer cells by a woman's own secretions. However, in the postmenopausal woman this action might be lost, and an unwanted effect to increase the risk for breast cancer would seem possible.

In spite of any possible health benefits, using red wine for these purposes poses health risks (as for other alcoholic beverages) if its use should progress to chronic abuse and dependence, which adds many health risks of overindulgence such as brain and liver damage or even cirrhosis as causes for illnesses or death.

PROSTATE CANCER

Prostate cancer is the second most common cause of cancer death in men. More than one-third of recently diagnosed prostate cancer patients utilize some form of CAM therapy, but the quality of their sources of information has been questioned. Vitamin E appears to be particularly effective in opposing prostate cancer when used along with other dietary supplements such as selenium and vitamin D. Other possible prostate cancer preventives include whole flaxseed, milk thistle, curcumin (turmeric), and red wine or its component resveratrol, discussed previously. To the contrary, those supplements promoted for raising testosterone levels may be harmful (surely some physicians dispute this) because higher androgenic hormone levels have been blamed for an increased prostate cancer cell growth. The widely used saw palmetto products have been shown to benefit prostate health, but without their increasing testosterone levels. Data for saw palmetto have been published that indicate it shows good promise for inhibiting prostate cancer in addition to its value for reducing the symptoms of benign prostatic hyperplasia.

Lycopene

Lycopene is a carotenoid phytochemical that gives tomatoes their red color. It is the prevalent carotenoid in the Western diet and the most abundant carotenoid in human serum. Lycopene ranks highest among major natural carotenoids in its capacity for neutralizing singlet oxygen, i.e., it acts as a powerful antioxidant and scavenger of ROS. In addition to its antioxidant activity, its other biological activities include enhancing of cell-to-cell communications and growth control. Research indicates that lycopene is most effective when accompanied by other nutrients to be found in the fresh, raw vegetable. It has been especially associated with beneficial effects for men on the prostate gland. In vitro and in vivo studies on the growth of tumor cells suggest that it can exert protective effects against specific cancers, including those of the prostate.

A review was conducted on 72 epidemiological studies that investigated a possible link between cancer risk and consumption of tomato products. Of these, 57 found tomato intake to be associated with a trend for reduced risk, with 35 of the studies showing a statistically significant association. A major prospective study (Gann et al. 1999) examined the relationship of plasma levels of several antioxidants to prostate cancer risk using plasma samples obtained in the Physician's Health Study. The study found that lycopene was the only antioxidant associated with a significantly lower occurrence of prostate cancer.

These findings support other study results that identified lycopene as the carotenoid with the most definite opposing relationship to the development of prostate cancer. Although research results appear promising, the findings are not yet conclusive. Most have consisted of epidemiological studies focused on an association of lower prostate cancer risk with consumption of lycopene-rich foods. Determining an optimal level of lycopene intake to be a cancer chemopreventive and testing for possible adverse effects of its chronic use as a supplement remain to be accomplished. Enough evidence presently exists to warrant use of lycopene in prospective clinical trials to examine its efficacy as a chemopreventive agent for prostate cancer.

A recent report of importance concerning cardiovascular risks and lycopene intake was the ongoing Women's Health Study conducted by researchers at the Brigham and Women's Hospital and Harvard Medical School. This study followed more than 28,000 middle-aged and elderly women for nearly five years with collection of blood samples to permit measurement of plasma lycopene levels. At the beginning of the trial none of the women had any form of heart disease, but when the test period was completed, 483 women were diagnosed with cardiovascular disease. The subjects were divided into quartiles for plasma lycopene levels, ranging from those with the lowest lycopene level to those with the highest. Women in the upper three quartiles had a 50 percent reduction in the risk of cardiovascular disease compared to women in the lowest quartile. The researchers note that even though the study clearly showed that higher lycopene levels were associated with lowering of the risk of cardiovascular disease in women, additional trials are needed to test women at a younger age level, and also men, in order to determine the generality of the results.

Tomatoes are the best natural source of lycopene, but the benefits from tomatoes may depend on how they are prepared. Surprising research data from Cornell University indicated that the body absorbs lycopene more efficiently and benefits from a higher antioxidant activity when tomatoes are cooked as opposed to eating them raw. Studies suggest that eating cooked tomatoes along with a source of fat—such as cheese or meat—may also improve lycopene absorption.

Soy Isoflavones

Evidence suggests that the dietary consumption of isoflavones found in legumes (e.g., soy) is related to lower rates of benign prostatic hyperplasia and prostate cancer among Asian men. Four to five times more men die of prostate cancer in the United States than in Japan. One interpretation is that this reflects a greater intake of red meats in the U.S. diet, but another explanation offered is that the higher intake of soy isoflavones by the Japanese has a beneficial effect, lowering prostate cancer rates. This was supported by the results of epidemiological studies testing the idea that soy products and constituents (primarily isoflavones) are partly responsible for lower rates of occurrence and mortality from prostate cancer.

Isoflavones have been shown to influence not only hormonal status but also protein synthesis, intracellular enzymes, growth factor action, cell proliferation, and angiogenesis (forming of new capillaries). Genistein is a major isoflavone of soy that has received much attention owing to its having antiproliferative, estrogenic, and antiestrogenic effects. More recently genistein has been found to promote apoptosis (cell suicide) by lung cancer cells. The isoflavones, specifically genistein, have shown enough evidence to warrant clinical trials to test its efficacy as a chemopreventive agents for prostate cancer. However, animal evidence shows detrimental effects on rodent offspring from exposure to genistein during gestation. In rats, exposure to genistein during pregnancy and lactation exerts long-lasting modifying actions on the function of the endocrine and immune systems in adulthood (Klein et al., 2002). Whether such exposure to phytoestrogen in early development alters the occurrence of infectious or autoimmune diseases as well as cancers in later life requires investigation. An unpublished study found that early postnatal exposure of mice to genistein caused obesity, their adult weights being nearly three times greater than normal (personal communication, J. Heindel, March 25, 2005).

Pycnogenol

This agent is an extract of pine bark harvested from a coastal forest in southwest France. As it contains a variety of polyphenols, it acts as a natural antioxidant that has been shown to exert anti-inflammatory actions that may provide wide-ranging benefits, but especially to the cardiovascular system. M. Putter and colleagues (1999) at the Arizona Prevention Resource Center compared the effects of Pycnogenol to those of aspirin in a group of 38 cigarette smokers because smoking increases the risk for dangerous aggregation of blood platelets. Thus, the researchers were able to assess how platelet aggregation might be affected. Subjects were given either 500 mg of aspirin or 125 mg of Pycnogenol before they smoked in order to increase the clumping of blood platelets. Within two hours blood was drawn from all subjects to evaluate platelet aggregation. Both Pycnogenol and aspirin lowered platelet aggregation significantly, but aspirin also had an undesirable response of increased bleeding time whereas Pycnogenol did not.

NONFLAVONOID CHEMOPREVENTIVE AGENTS

Conjugated Linoleic Acids

Conjugated linoleic acids (CLAs) describes a group of compounds that are variants of the substance linoleic acid, which is one of the essential fatty acids. Variants of linoleic acid differ in the type and arrangement of their unsaturated chemical bonds. The specific structure of chemical bonds in the CLA is crucial to the compounds' ability to oppose the risk for cancer, i.e., to act as anticarcinogens or cancer chemopreventives. Indeed, at high intake levels, the base compound, linoleic acid, is said instead to act oppositely to *increase* the rate of cancer growth in laboratory animals.

Researchers have become excited about CLA because they are anticarcinogenic at much lower levels than many other naturally occurring anticarcinogens—agents found in plant sources. It is effective in animals at levels as low as 0.05 percent of the total diet. Dairy products are the main dietary source of CLA for people, other than from certain meats. However, according to the October1996 Cornell Nutrition Conference, the usual human intake of CLA from dairy products provides merely one-third of the amount of CLA that provides protection against cancer in experimental animal models. Lamb, beef, and veal—in descending order of levels—contain higher levels in terms of milligrams of CLA per gram of fat than do other meats, e.g., pork, chicken, turkey, and seafoods.

CLA found in dairy products depends upon microbes in the cow's rumen secreting enzymes that causes a breakdown of the cow's dietary linoleic acid from plant food to form CLA. The many variables affecting this process cause the concentration of CLA in milk fat to vary greatly. One survey of different herds found more than a sevenfold variation of CLA levels. Cow's milk in summer contained twice the CLA as was found in the winter, which indicates a higher level when feeding on grass in pastures. Neither processing nor storage has much effect on the CLA levels of dairy products. However, producing reduced-fat dairy products obviously would cause a lowering of CLA. In contrast, processing and cooking of meat tends to increase its levels of CLA. One study showed a nearly fivefold increase in CLA content of ground beef after grilling.

One approach to increasing the bioavailability of CLA is to boost the proportion of CLA in milk fat without increasing the proportion of fat in milk products. A method is under research for seeding the cow's stomachs with improved or engineered bacteria that produce more CLA; another is to elevate their intake of unsaturated fatty acids.

CLA may have other physiological effects that can benefit human health. Research has shown that CLA can oppose the development of atherosclerosis in arteries of rabbits. However, both the short- and long-term human health consequences from the eating of an increased level of CLA are unknown.

Chapter 25

The Pharmacology of Ascorbate

THE FEARED, UNAPPRECIATED TOMATO

The tomato plant was one of the New World's unknown bounties waiting to be collected and added to the European settlers' indigenous food sources. The explorers of South America took it from Peru to Spain, from whence it spread to Italy and beyond so that tomatoes were a staple of the continental diet by 1560. However, it had not been known by the early British colonists, and it was not native to North America. Thus, among those who settled on the Atlantic coast, it was a species not adopted as a food, in contrast to the acceptance of New World species such as corn and the potato. When the tomato plant first came to be grown in the United States in the early 1800s its fruit was regarded as poisonous, apparently because it was thought to be a member of the family *Solanaceae* to which belonged species known to be poisonous, e.g., deadly nightshade, *Atropa belladonna.* It is said that acceptance had to await a day when Robert Gibbon Johnson ate a tomato on the steps of the Salem, New Jersey, courthouse to demonstrate an absence of poisonous effects. This negative reputation was difficult to overcome by virtue of it being "common knowledge" that one takes a great risk by eating the tomato fruit. (The history of the tomato as a medicinal, substituting for calomel in treating "bilious" states, is recounted more fully by Smith [1991].)

Two physicians, J. S. and J. M. Goodwin, in 1984 drew upon this history to suggest a worthy new phraseology, "the tomato effect," which is defined for medicine as occurring "when an efficacious treatment for a certain disease is ignored or rejected because it does not make sense in the light of accepted theories of disease mechanisms and drug action." This can be seen as the opposite of the placebo effect, which may have been responsible for an enthusiastic and widespread acceptance of therapies later shown to be useless or even harmful.

The tomato effect represents a mind-set that favors the rejection of a new and seemingly implausible therapy, or at the very least an unconventional one. Goodwin and Goodwin (1984) gave historical accounts of the tomato

Consumer's Guide to Dietary Supplements and Alternative Medicines

doi:10.1300/5698_25

effect occurring for colchicine, gold compounds, and aspirin, all later accepted as well validated, valuable therapies. They also suggested that modern medicine is particularly vulnerable to the tomato effect. Pharmaceutical companies "have increasingly turned to theoretical over practical arguments" to support their new wonder drugs. Thus, ascorbate qualifies for being called a "tomato" because of its being an underappreciated and much maligned chemical when it is used in pharmacological rather than physiological doses, because in actuality much evidence supports it as having great usefulness, relatively untroubled by safety problems.

It may have been unfortunate that the term *orthomolecular* was devised to describe such nonvitamin uses for chemicals familiar as vitamins or other nutrients. The term carries more than a hint of nonconformity or downright quirkiness that may have been too off-putting for comfort to the generally conservative, or even staid, medical profession. An unfounded or at best a grossly exaggerated idea exists that ascorbate may exert injurious effects upon the kidneys if used in megadoses for its pharmacologic benefits. Various physicians who now and in earlier times have dared to put it into action have seen no such renal effects of the sort darkly warned against by sources disapproving of or outright opposing usage of ascorbate for nonnutritional effects. Levy (2002) presents an extremely broad array of literature on ascorbic acid that supports the medical value of ascorbate, but he avows that his intense literature searches revealed no published record for occurrence of the renal damage "commonly known to occur," only the raising of that hypothetical possibility, mainly for persons having a rare excretory problem. Clearly the mention of ascorbate being a useful chemotherapeutic agent for infectious or neoplastic diseases has also represented a new idea that consequently has been thoroughly rejected, as would have been predicted by Dr. Peter Medawar's principle.

BASICS ON ASCORBIC ACID

Vitamin C is a simple compound having the chemical name of ascorbic acid, or ascorbate when in a salt form. It is chemically related to the simple sugar glucose. It is not widely available in foods, except for the citrus fruits as well as peppers and broccoli. When dissolved in physiological fluids, ascorbic acid occurs in the ionized ascorbate form. Some supplement products utilize salts of ascorbic acid, e.g., sodium, potassium, magnesium, or calcium ascorbates, because they avoid potential gastric hyperacidity from using the acid form. Most animals do not need to obtain ascorbic acid in their food—only human beings, nonhuman primates, guinea pigs, and one bird species cannot synthesize the molecule. Other species are able to produce ascorbate in their own cells. Having a vital metabolic role, ascorbic acid became known as a vitamin, but some authors think that this classification actually understates its importance in maintaining health and life.

This view is well expounded by Levy (2002), who describes how the human species lacks only one final enzyme in a metabolic sequence that would otherwise allow us to produce the needed ascorbic acid. If that enzyme were not lacking, it would not be a vitamin but would still be a metabolite having critical functions for the maintenance of health. He expounds on the idea that human resistance to the stressful circumstances of infectious diseases or encounters with poisons would be highly improved if we were able to produce more ascorbic acid "on demand" in the amounts needed. Levy also embraces the view of Nobel laureate Albert Szent-Gyorgi that life itself is vitally supported by the electron-transfer activities of ascorbic acid.

Equally interesting is the possibility raised by Levy that for some individuals ascorbic acid may not be a vitamin. If indeed the gene for the missing enzyme is active, i.e., is "turned on," for a small minority of people, then they would be producing their needed ascorbic acid rather than requiring it in the diet. One must agree with Dr. Levy that the missing research to test this possibility is a vast oversight and is neglect on the part of the biomedical research community. This is true because the hypothesis that some persons do indeed produce ascorbate was published as long ago as 1981. The identification of individuals whose ascorbate-producing enzyme activity has been turned on would open vistas of research that would facilitate testing of the reputed anti-infective and antitoxin role of vitamin C. Positive findings would have revolutionary implications for medical practice. Perhaps that is one reason the research has not been and is not being done—revolution is seldom welcomed by followers of the prevailing power structure or scientific paradigm. A likely population in which to test for ascorbate producers might be exceptionally healthy, extremely elderly individuals. It could turn out to be a key aspect of survival to exceptional age.

Because ascorbic acid is prone to chemical alteration and is water-soluble, the body is not able to store very much from an excess intake beyond what is immediately needed and used. If it is taken in at a rate beyond what can be used, the excess is excreted, mainly via the kidneys. However, what might be considered an excess for normal conditions may not be excess when the body is undergoing adverse circumstances. Many conditions of illness, injury, or other stresses can acutely increase the need for a continuing high intake; otherwise, a state of depletion can readily occur. An example of stress-related ascorbate depletion is the adrenal cortex. Many mid-twentieth century animal studies on stress responses employed as an index of stress a rapid fall in the amount of ascorbic acid that could be measured in the adrenal cortex of rodents.

One highly important role of ascorbic acid in our basic physiology is for maintaining collagen, which is a protein that plays a fundamental structural role in the formation of connective tissue and in the repair processes following tissue injury. When this compound is not sufficiently available, adverse changes are found in skin, ligaments, and bones. In scurvy, the classical vitamin C deficiency disease, the amount of "cement substance" is insufficient, preventing the cells of the capillary vessels from holding together fully and causing leakage of blood. This may be noted as small petechial hemorrhages in the skin, and possibly overt bleeding from the gums plus hidden bleeding into the joints, which likely leads to inflammation and tenderness. If not treated effectively, the scorbutic condition may progress to death, as it did among the crew of sailing ships in days past.

Ascorbic acid is also well-known for its activity as an antioxidant, which serves to protect critical molecules from damage. Ascorbate has other varied roles in the biochemistry of the body. The inactive form of folic acid must undergo conversion to the active form (folinic acid), a process that depends upon ascorbate. Moreover, it serves to protect thiamine, riboflavin, folate, pantothenic acid, vitamin A, and vitamin E from oxidative and inactivating reactions caused by oxidizing free radicals. Thus, ascorbate is highly valuable for its antioxidant properties, which oppose the actions of free radicals to cause the injuries of oxidative stress.

For this reason, vitamin C should be used after a myocardial infarction (heart attack) or stroke to oppose the action of free radicals formed under the condition of reperfusion stress after tissue hypoxia (inadequate oxygenation) and the damage they may cause. Other uses might include treating victims of electrical shock and lightning strikes. Such varied conditions as leukemia, asthma, and pancreatitis also may benefit from ascorbate treatment using levels of ascorbate intake that are considerably higher than the RDA for its vitamin role. Because uses described in the following sections appear to go beyond the normal, accepted nutrient roles of vitamin C, the chemical name *ascorbate* will be emphasized over its vitamin name.

ASCORBATE AND THE CARDIOVASCULAR SYSTEM

Ascorbate Against Heart Failure Risk

Oxidative modification of low-density lipoprotein cholesterol (LDL) is thought to contribute directly to the formation of dangerous atherosclerotic plaques in the walls of larger arteries. The antioxidant vitamins and other antioxidants have been theorized to oppose and possibly reverse the process. Ascorbic acid therapy may help heart failure patients by improving the health of their blood vessels. Congestive heart failure (CHF) occurs when the pumping action of the heart is so inefficient that it cannot meet the body's needs, which leads to symptoms such as fatigue and shortness of breath. CHF is most commonly a consequence of an underlying heart condition such as coronary artery disease and possibly a current or past heart attack that has injured the heart muscle and significantly reduced its efficiency.

German and French researchers (Rossig et al., 2001) reported that ascorbate appeared to stop cells in the blood vessel wall from dying. They suggested that this protection could explain previous study findings that vitamin C improve blood vessel flow rates in people having CHF. Research suggests that the damaging forms of oxygen called reactive oxygen species (ROS) accumulate in the blood as the state of heart failure progresses. Their injurious action known as oxidative stress may contribute to dysfunction in the lining of the blood vessel wall, the endothelium, by killing endothelial cells. Ascorbate helps to eliminate cell-damaging ROS from the body.

Rossig and colleagues (2001) gave 34 patients either ascorbic acid treatment or an inactive placebo. Treated patients first received an intravenous dose of ascorbic acid, followed by three days of oral supplementation. All were taking the standard heart drugs used for CHF. Previously, the researchers found by in vitro experiments that cultured endothelial cells exposed to ascorbate did not respond as usual to certain proinflammatory proteins. Those proteins cause such cells to die by the process called apoptosis or programmed cell suicide. Similarly, when they examined blood samples from these patients they found that the patients receiving ascorbate had far less evidence of apoptosis among their endothelial cells than they had before ascorbate treatment. Patients receiving a placebo showed no such benefit.

Another possible mechanism for ascorbate protecting patients with coronary heart disease (CHD)—impaired blood flow via the coronary arteries to the heart muscle—is through its counteracting the adverse effects of a high-fat meal. The serum triglyceride level rises after a high-fat meal, and high triglyceride levels play a critical role in the process of atherogenesis (forming of fatty plaques in the arterial wall). A 2002 study (Ling et al., 2002) was designed to evaluate the effect of a single 2,000 mg oral dose of vitamin C on impaired endothelium-dependent vasodilation after a high-fat meal in patients with CHD. It included 74 patients with coronary heart disease and 50 people without CHD but who had risk factors. The two groups were split into subgroups—those who took 2,000 mg of vitamin C and those who did not—with all groups eating the high-fat meal (800 cal, 50 g fat). Serum levels of triglyceride, low-density lipoprotein cholesterol, high-density lipoprotein cholesterol, and total cholesterol were measured in the fasting state and at two, four, five, and seven hours after the high-fat meal.

At two to five hours after the meal in all groups the serum triglyceride levels rose significantly. Vasodilation was assessed in the brachial artery of the arm by means of an ultrasound method at baseline while fasting, and at 4 hours after the meal. The capacity for patients with CHD to show vasodilatation when fasting was impaired in comparison to persons without disease. Arterial dilatation was significantly hindered after the meal in people not taking vitamin C (both with and without CHD), but was not hindered in patients or control subjects who received ascorbate; they showed no significant change after the meal. It appears that the oxidative stress mechanism operates during the interval following a high-fat meal so as to cause failure of the vasodilator function via injury to or malfunction of the blood vessel endothelium (the lining cells that secrete a vasodilator, nitric oxide [NO]). As an inhibitor of such oxidative stress, ascorbate may serve to block whatever pathological process is responsible. These data support the idea that vitamin C can provide a significant protection against an adverse reduction in blood vessel dilatory function that predispose a person to heart attack or stroke. Vitamin C intake shows promise of being a valuable benefit to CHD patients.

Ascorbate Against High Blood Pressure

Researchers at Emory University School of Medicine in Atlanta, Georgia, examined data from the Third National Health and Nutrition Examination Survey (NHANES) to assess the relationship between serum levels of antioxidants and blood pressure in 15,142 individuals. The study sample was considered to represent adequately the U.S. adult population. After adjusting for a variety of factors, increasing levels of serum vitamin C were associated with significant reductions in diastolic but not systolic blood pressure. Increasing levels of serum beta-carotene were associated with a significant reduction in systolic blood pressure. In contrast, serum levels of vitamin E were associated only with significant elevations of diastolic blood pressure. The factors that were controlled for in the analysis included age, sex, race, education, high-density lipoprotein levels, history of myocardial infarction, angina, diabetes, body mass index, smoking status, physical activity level, antihypertensive drug use, and their serum levels of other antioxidants. This research has overcome the faults of prior studies, including too small-samples, specialized subgroups that were not broadly representative of the general population, and failure to compare the effects of different antioxidants on blood pressure. Moreover, those studies produced conflicting results.

In spite of the findings just described, the United States Preventive Services Task Force (USPSTF) (2003) stated that they found insufficient evidence to recommend for or against using vitamins A, C, and E for the prevention of cardiovascular disease, saying that "definitive evidence of the role of vitamin supplementation on altering cardiovascular outcomes is lacking." Currently ongoing clinical trials should provide a basis for more clear recommendations, but they will require many years of follow-up to be valid.

Ascorbate Against Stroke

Research was conducted at the University of Kuopio in Finland in view of evidence for vitamin C reducing atherosclerosis. The aim was to test for a correlation between vitamin C intake and the risk of stroke, especially associated with high blood pressure. The research team followed 2,419 randomly selected men ranging in age from 42 to 60 years at the outset of the study with no prior history of stroke. Over a period of ten years blood samples were taken and blood pressure and body weight were measured. At the end of the study 120 men had experienced a stroke. After adjusting for various factors such as alcohol intake and history of smoking, the data supported two important conclusions: (1) subjects who showed the lowest level of ascorbate in their blood were almost 2.5 times more likely to experience a stroke than subjects having the highest amounts of ascorbate and (2) subjects who had high blood pressure, who were overweight, and who had low levels of ascorbate were three times more likely to suffer a stroke than were overweight subjects having high blood pressure but whose blood showed the highest levels of ascorbate.

Beyond these very favorable results remains the question of what mechanism operated to produce them. The Finnish investigators believe that the antioxidant action of vitamin C had helped prevent a buildup of plaque in the arteries, and thus allowed the maintenance of normal strength of the arterial walls. A major point of interest concerns the intake of vitamin C by the subjects. Subjects with high ascorbate levels and those with low levels differed remarkably little in their eating habits. The researchers estimated that the difference between the two groups was equal to the equivalent of only about 1.5 glasses of orange juice per day. This suggests that one need not take extraordinary steps to reap the benefit of extra ascorbate. Drinking one glass of orange juice for breakfast each day, and then another at lunchtime or dinner should suffice to help a person to be equal to the group that showed reduced risk of stroke—certainly a worthy aim. If a person maintains a reasonable body weight, controls blood pressure, does not smoke, and keeps alcohol consumption at a low to moderate level, their cardiovascular system health will be much better for the efforts. Of course, if a person cannot enjoy orange juice, supplemental ascorbate (despite it's being synthetic) will likely have similar effects. Natural sources of ascorbate from citrus fruits do provide other active nutrients, the citrus bioflavonoids, that may contribute by enhancing the ascorbate activities.

ASCORBATE IN TREATMENT OF CANCER

Around 1970 the Nobel laureate chemist Linus Pauling and a physician colleague were audacious enough to use ascorbic acid as a therapy against cancer. In 1976 this was reported in a prestigious journal, *Proceedings of the National Academy of Sciences USA* (Cameron and Pauling, 1976). The physician, Ewan Cameron, carried out such tests in Scotland on patients whose cancer was too far advanced for any hope of survival for more than a short time to exist. They were given intravenous doses of 10 grams (10,000 milligrams) per day of sodium ascorbate. The initial small-scale trial was later followed by a more substantial study, Cameron and Campbell (1991), after undergoing long delays followed by ultimate rejection by four medical journals. The critics quibbled over matters of design of the study while not providing objections that could fully explain away the clear results—that cancer patients regarded as beyond help had a significantly greater survival time after they received ascorbate therapy than did patients who received no ascorbate.

In the study 294 patients were assigned to receive ascorbate whose median survival time was 343 days, and 1,532 patients without ascorbate whose median survival time was only 180 days. The statistical probability of such a difference between the groups occurring by chance alone was calculated to be one in 10,000. In one series 13 of 100 terminally ill patients reached a five-year survival criterion of "cure." Moreover, the need for doses of morphine or heroin (legal drug in the United Kingdom) was greatly reduced, indicating significant pain reduction produced by ascorbate dosing.

Ascorbic acid and its salts have been shown in several different laboratories to exert preferential toxicity toward neoplastic cells in vitro and in vivo, beginning as early as 1980 (Bram et al., 1980). Given in high enough doses to maintain plasma concentrations above levels that have been shown to be toxic to tumor cells in vitro, sodium ascorbate has the capacity to kill tumor cells selectively in a manner rivaling that of conventional cancer chemotherapeutic agents. Most studies of ascorbate and cancer failing to show benefits did not employ sufficiently high doses of ascorbate to maintain the known tumor-killing plasma levels of ascorbate.

Dr. Hugh Riordan and colleagues (2000) presented data that demonstrate the ability to sustain plasma levels of ascorbate in human subjects above the concentrations shown to be toxic to tumor cells in vitro. This supports the feasibility of using ascorbate as a safe but cytotoxic cancer chemotherapeutic agent. Ascorbate has shown in vitro anticancer efficacy, alone or in combination tests with alpha-lipoic acid, vitamin K_3, phenyl ascorbate, or doxorubicin (an anticancer agent). The two-day treatment assays with a 10 mM concentration of ascorbate increased the percent of cancer cells dying in apoptosis.

Alpha-lipoic acid greatly enhanced the ascorbate cytotoxicity, reducing its median effective dose at two days against hollow-fiber tumors from 34 mM to 4 mM. Lipoic acid, unlike ascorbate, was equally effective against both proliferating (reproducing) cells and cells not in the proliferative state. Ascorbate levels in human blood plasma were measured during and after intravenous ascorbate infusions. Infusions of 60 grams produced peak plasma concentrations above 20 mM, which means that they achieved the level that killed cancer cells in vitro along with lipoic acid. Thus, tumoricidal plasma levels clearly are achievable in vivo. The ascorbate efficacy was enhanced in an additive fashion by phenyl ascorbate or vitamin K_3. The effect of ascorbate on doxorubicin efficacy depended on concentration; low doses opposed the doxorubicin cytotoxicity, and high doses increased the kill rate.

ASCORBATE AND PANCREATITIS

The levels of ascorbic acid in fasting plasma samples from 30 healthy volunteers were compared with those found in admission samples from 29 consecutive patients having acute pancreatitis and 27 patients with other acute abdominal crises. The results showed that the stress of an acute abdominal crisis is accompanied by a decrease in the plasma level of ascorbate. In acute pancreatitis, early and profound oxidative stress complicates the illness by denaturing the available vitamin C. A cause may exist for a judicious administration of ascorbate injections to patients with acute pancreatitis in order to boost plasma antioxidant defenses. An evaluation of the use of ascorbate added to usual therapies versus those therapies alone would be desirable to determine if the outcomes would be improved. Some NCCAM studies of this sort are now going forward on other CAM agents.

QUESTIONS ABOUT ASCORBATE'S SAFETY

Both short- and long-term administration of ascorbate have been questioned with respect to their safety by those opposed to such practices, without their actually citing instances of significant adverse responses. On the other hand, at clinics such as that of Hugh Riordan, MD in Wichita, Kansas, patients are reported to have received with impunity daily doses intravenously of 50,000 mg for up to eight weeks (Casciari et al., 2001). Dr. Levy (2002) quotes Kalokerinos and colleagues (1982a) as stating that in Australia some 100 physicians have administered as much as 300,000 mg of ascorbate per day to their patients, and that "in most cases the results have been spectacular, the only side effect is 'chronic good health.'"

AIDS patients of Dr. Cathcart (1984) have taken extremely large daily oral doses (25,000 to 125,00 mg) after escalation guided by increasing "bowel tolerance." This means that they increase their dosage at a rate to minimize bowel intolerance shown by gas and diarrhea. Not only Cathcart but also other physicians have noted that the more sick the patient the more ascorbate they can tolerate without such adverse symptoms. The main bogeyman regarding megadose ascorbic acid is the idea that kidney stones will result from the high renal output of one of the four ascorbate metabolites, oxalic acid/oxalate. Kidney stones usually consist of primarily calcium oxalate. Levy (2002) states, "Cathcart's extensive clinical experience directly contradicts the widespread but mistaken belief that large doses of vitamin C will result in kidney stone formation." By 1993 Cathcart's patient count had exceeded 20,000 according to Levy (2002). It would seem obvious that a patient known to have an elevated urinary oxalate level might be at greater risk for kidney stone development with sustained ascorbate in large doses. However, Levy's (2002) review found "a strong suggestion in some studies that regular supplementation with vitamin C actually decreases the chances of kidney stone development." His review provides a thorough listing of abnormal conditions that are possible factors favoring a kidney stone problem. Many are avoidable by voluntary actions, but some are disease states. Others reaching a similar conclusion are Prasad and Prasad (2001) who stated that "there are no published data to support the conclusion that high doses of vitamin C produce kidney stones in healthy people" (i.e., those without rare predisposing conditions, as per Levy [2002]).

Cathcart (1985) stated that he had seen no aggravation of gouty arthritis, only benefit, with megadose C. This indicates that renal excretion of urate, which is inadequate in gout patients, was not further hindered by the high urinary output of ascorbate and its metabolites. Persons should not attempt self-directed oral megadosing with ascorbic acid rather than one (or a mixture) of the ascorbate salts—sodium, calcium, magnesium; should avoid dehydration by maintaining high water intake; and should be mindful of Cathcart's (1985) bowel tolerance principle. He reports occasional patients out of thousands showing heartburn, small sores in the mouth, or a light rash.

Riordan and colleagues (2000) has mentioned a possibility for an adverse response to excessive amounts of breakdown products from cancer cells being killed extensively and rapidly. In the summary of his safety review in his book, Dr. Levy (2002) states, "It can certainly be concluded that vitamin C is an exceptionally safe supplement, which has already been given in very large doses for extended periods of time with no significant problems occurring" (p. 376).

CONCLUSIONS

The material in this chapter presents examples from the extensive literature supporting the idea that pharmacological dosing with ascorbate has much to offer as an essentially nontoxic therapeutic practice. The first major problem is that few allopathic or osteopathic physicians currently in practice have learned about the possibility of a major therapeutic value existing from high oral doses or injection with ascorbate. Neither in medical school, their internship or residency, or subsequent postgraduate education (the latter frequently subsidized by the pharmaceutical industry) were they likely to be exposed to unorthodox, nay, *revolutionary* ideas of this ilk. Or if they were, it was delivered with a dismissive, "well of course those ideas have been proved false, and besides the treatment risks serious toxicity." The problem is that such derisive allegations aren't supported by hard facts. In this situation, concepts that seem revolutionary cause discomfort if they are allowed serious consideration. It is much more comfortable to regard the available facts as being nonexistent.

What is the second and perhaps the main obstacle to ascorbate? Simply put, the problem is that it cannot become a "blockbuster" or "cash cow" for a pharmaceutical manufacturer; it cannot be patented and it is too cheaply produced to make an acceptable profit (or to boost values of a company's stock) by the standards of the contemporary pharmaceutical industry. The economic factor likely also applies to contemporary medical oncology practitioners' usage of expensive cytotoxic and/or hormonal drugs. Indeed, a widespread use of ascorbate against cancer would reduce the manufacturers' income and profits from currently used chemotherapy or anti-infective drugs and might attack oncologists' incomes as well. For such reasons the costs of developmental research to test, define, and confirm its efficacy for these important applications are quite unlikely to be made available from the private sector. Hope exists only for federal funding to these ends via NCCAM, who supports similar tests on even less promising supplements.

Making the Attempt

However, it costs relatively little to purchase an ascorbate product ready to be put in solution and used for intravenous administration, or even for a sterile solution to be prepared "from scratch" in a well-equipped hospital pharmacy. This means that "big pharmaceutical business" need not be involved. Any medical oncologist who says of a patient that they aren't a candidate for conventional chemotherapy—too much for them to tolerate (too toxic) with no prospect for significant benefit—could try ascorbate as others have, with the potential for a positive nontoxic outcome. If no positive outcome were to result, great expense and suffering from the therapy would not have occurred. However, this option will not be offered and won't likely happen other than by persistent outspoken insistence of the patient or their family members.

Advice on how to "work the system" to obtain intravenous ascorbate therapy for one's loved one is provided by Andrew Saul, PhD, in his 2003 book, *Doctor Yourself* (pp. 194-197). (See www.doctoryourself.com/strategies.html.)

Chapter 26

Marvelous Aloe Vera

I don't see the logic of rejecting data just because they seem incredible.

Sir Fred Hoyle
English astronomer

BACKGROUND

The medicinal use of aloe vera (mainly from *Aloe barbadensisis,* but also other *Aloe* species) may be as old or older than any of the other medicinal plants discussed in this book; it has been known for thousands of years as having therapeutic value. In the early twentieth century several medical researchers examined it in the context of modern medical practice and found it still to be valuable. In contrast to most botanicals, aloe vera has seen its major use by external application. Except for the mid-twentieth century discoveries of synthetic antimicrobial agents and the antibiotics, aloe vera would likely have become a more widely used anti-infective therapy for superficial injuries and infections. In more recent decades its usefulness when taken internally has been much explored.

Whereas in ancient times it was quite an ordinary practice to use the aloe vera gel directly from the fresh succulent plant, this is a folk medicine approach with which few if any modern clinicians could be comfortable. Atherton [1998] is an exception.) Still, the impressive medical evaluations that were published in the 1930s and 1940s were indeed based on using the fresh plant materials especially against severe burns to body surfaces. At that time a good alternative to using the fresh gel did not yet exist. Some of those cases were not ordinary burns but rather extraordinary ones produced by overexposure to radioactivity.

So-called radiation burns are actually skin surface ulcers resulting from

Consumer's Guide to Dietary Supplements and Alternative Medicines

doi:10.1300/5698_26

excessive radiation exposure. In that era such lesions generally were from an X-ray source, whereas many other potential sources now exist, including radiation release from nuclear reactor accidents, as happened a few years ago in Japan and earlier at Chernobyl in the Ukraine. Radiation burns commonly progress to ulcerated skin lesions that are very long-lasting. Such injuries often fail to heal indefinitely because radiation suppresses the normal essential healing processes—especially the regrowth of capillaries and small arteries in the area of injury needing repair. Repeated findings by various research teams showed that healing of such lesions could be substantially speeded by their being treated constantly with wraps wetted with aloe vera gel. These gave a significant boost to its credentials as a healing remedy for various types of skin lesions that even reduces or eliminates scarring.

It would be quite inappropriate to do a placebo-controlled clinical trial of this therapy in humans, but it could be evaluated as an add-on to another standard therapy to determine whether it could produce a significant synergistic improvement. Apparently it has not been so tested. However, experimental validation of prior clinical observations was provided by studies on swine, rabbits, and guinea pigs in experimental designs that were considered appropriate in that era (but would not be today), using untreated control groups. Aloe treatment (fresh whole leaf) was found to hasten both the degenerative and regenerative-reparative phases of the response of animals to radiation at a standard level.

Healing of the resulting ulcers was achieved in two months, whereas the untreated lesions were incompletely healed even after four months. Similar benefits were seen for surgical wounds in mice or experimental freezing of the skin (frostbite) in rabbits. More recently, evidence has been obtained to indicate that aloe reduces the local inflammatory mediators, including thromboxane A_2 and histamine. Thus, aloe vera preparations are offered for opposing burns, inflammation, itching, swelling, and pain, or for promoting the healing of all sorts of superficial wounds. Aloe exerts a valuable anti-infective action as well. Decubitus ulcers (bedsores) exemplify another difficult-healing condition for which aloe vera greatly aids healing and recovery. It has not been claimed that aloe vera can *prevent* radiation burns; thus, it is not surprising that a Cochrane review on aloe vera concluded that it was not found to be an effective preventative for radiation-induced injuries (Vogler and Ernst, 1999). They did allow that it might be effective for genital herpes and psoriasis, but found the question of whether aloe vera promotes wound healing was not clearly answered.

The pharmacological profile of aloe vera as determined by animal experimentation, and in part confirmed by human medical observations, has included the following:

- Local anesthetic
- Wound debridement (proteolytic enzyme removal of dead cells and debris)
- Healing facilitation by stimulating cell division
- Anti-infective (bacteria, viruses, fungi/yeasts; also internally)
- Immunologic stimulation (especially when taken internally)
- Anti-inflammatory
- Antiarthritic

This listing is derived from the informative 1984 and 2003 books by Coats and Ahola. A well-nigh ecstatic endorsement and exposition on aloe vera in his medical practice and personal use by a British physician, Peter Atherton, is available at www.positivehealth.com/permit/articles/aloe%20vera/atherton.htm. He describes two main targets of aloe's action—epithelial surfaces both externally (skin) and internally (mucous membrane surfaces of alimentary canal, respiratory tract, and the genitourinary tract), and the immune system components.

However, it became quite a problem that the fresh plant gel was not readily able to be preserved while still retaining its full activity. Although many products are on the market labeled as containing aloe vera, measures of their activity in comparison to the fresh plant gel indicate that many are unable to retain the original therapeutic activity. This causes great difficulty in providing a convincing research picture, when negative outcome data from impotent products are mingled with the positive data from fresh plant gel or from one of the few products that achieve a high degree of stabilization of the gel's intrinsic therapeutic activity. Bill C. Coats of Texas (and Coats Aloe International) has devoted his professional career to aloe vera basic research and clinical applications, as well as international marketing, and has received U.S. patents on processes for achieving high-quality stabilized products (see http://www.coatsaloe.com/coatsmain.htm and Coats and Ahola, 1984, 2003). Robert H. Davis, PhD, (n.d.) has conducted various biomedical researches on aloe vera that are accessible on a Web page titled "Whole Leaf Aloe Vera—Polysaccharides and Wound Healing" Davis's article describes the biologically significant components, especially those providing its wound healing and immunomodulatory activities (http://www.wholeleaf.com/aloeverainfo/aloeverapolysaccharide.htlm).

Regardless of the possible variations in efficacy of aloe vera components, for some years aloe vera has been increasingly used in cosmetic products, for its antiaging and wrinkle-reducing action, or in anti-inflammatory skin products, e.g., for sunburn or accidental burns. Topical formulations also are available to meet the needs of athletes for a cream or lotion that opposes inflammation and soreness and penetrates to promote quick recovery from traumatic injuries to skin, muscles, tendons, or joints. Clinical evaluations of these uses may not be adequate for scientific evidence, but many NFL athletes report being greatly benefited by use of those products at the impetus of their athletic trainers (see Coats and Ahola, 2003).

THE NATURE AND CONTENTS OF ALOE VERA

Considering the broad range of beneficial biological activities attributed to aloe vera, its is no surprise that the plant contains a complex mixture of bioactive agents. Many nonspecific components probably do not contribute greatly, if at all, to the healing benefits, such as vitamins A, B-complex (including folate, but only a trace of B_{12}), C, and E; eight physiologic minerals, as the chlorides; and seven essential with 11 nonessential. More specific to the aloe plant are the anthroquinones, which include the once-valued cathartic agent aloin (acting as its metabolite, emodin, produced in the intestine). This portion now is separated and removed in the processing for preparations useful in many other respects. Several active enzymes are included that give aloe vera activity as a digestive aid internally as well as aiding shin surface debridement.

Very therapeutically important are the mucopolysaccharides and glycoproteins that have a mucilaginous character. This enables them to protect, soothe, and moisturize skin, especially when burned or scraped, but also when uninjured (thus, used in cosmetics). This fraction also exerts a pro-wound-healing action, perhaps in part through a growth factor known as gibberellin. This agent activates the fibroblast cells essential to tissue repair in wound healing. Internally, the mucopolysaccharide component of aloe vera also can soothe injured mucosal surfaces in various disturbances of gastrointestinal balance. When taken internally some polysaccharide components also are absorbed and modulate the ongoing immune system activities systemically in a favorable fashion.

ORAL ALOE VERA GEL

Evidence exists that when taken internally, when it qualifies as a botanical dietary supplement, aloe vera gel exerts a significant anti-inflammatory action on the mucosal surfaces of the gastrointestinal tract (GIT). For this purpose the preparation is free of the laxative component of the whole plant gel. Furthermore, it has been found to exert antimicrobial actions in vitro that can be expected to be helpful in vivo for treating mild to moderate infectious problems of the GIT. An FDA-approved indication for improvement of digestion by aloe vera exists as well.

Based on the FDA certification, the Medicaid Vendor Drug Program of the State of Texas in 1991 gave an exclusive approval and listing of the Coats stabilized aloe vera gel drink for GIT therapy as well as the several topical formulations. Many physicians in Texas have prescribed such aloe vera products for their patients, including the internal form, and an international scope exists for its use in the Third World. The oral product has been widely used for various GIT maladies or dysfunctions—especially for infectious intestinal problems in children, but also in adults for inflammatory states.

The spectrum of inhibitory efficacy against microorganisms demonstrated in vitro has been extensive enough to include *Helicobacter pylori,* the prime causal factor of peptic ulcer disease. Dr. Peter Atherton has endorsed aloe vera for gastritis, colitis, diverticulitis, the diarrhea and/or constipation of irritable bowel syndrome, and for leaky gut syndrome from his practice experience despite a lack of scientific research data. One early report regarding use of aloe vera in treating peptic ulcer was found (Blitz et al., 1963).

A Cochrane review found ten studies suggesting that oral aloe vera might be a useful adjunct for lowering blood glucose in diabetic patients as well as for reducing blood lipid levels in patients with hyperlipidemia (Vogler and Ernst, 1999).

PROTECTIVE ALOE VERA POLYSACCHARIDES

Simple sugars, monosaccharides, and complex carbohydrates—polysaccharides—are all components of aloe vera. Some of these are of a mucilaginous nature that enables them to exert soothing and protective effects on skin, which has made aloe extract a popular components of cosmetic skin products. It is the larger polysaccharide fraction of aloe vera whole leaf juice that is responsible for immunostimulating effects, whereas others that are somewhat smaller exert an anti-inflammatory action. Together, these are able to provide symptomatic improvement for illnesses that have an autoimmune basis, such as rheumatoid arthritis, a debilitating condition of painful, stiff, swollen joints caused by a misdirected attack by one's own defense mechanisms.

Even if taken internally the polysaccharide molecules can be active systemically by being taken into cells of the intestine by an active process of engulfing them called pinocytosis or "cell drinking." This enables certain cells acting as part of the immune system to deliver intact large molecules for a "viewing" by the immune system—checking whether or not they are dangerous. This facilitates the large polysaccharide molecules acting to trigger positive changes in immune system activities that can modulate ongoing reactions that may be responsible for actions that are detrimental to the organism.

As one example, medical researchers in 1994 at the University of Texas in Galveston and Houston, Texas, reported tests of an aloe vera gel extract for an ability to modify the response of mice to four daily UV skin exposures (Strickland et al., 1994). Ordinarily, such exposures would suppress delayed-type hypersensitivity responses (which represent cell-mediated immune system activity) to a provocative microbial or chemical stimulus applied to the skin after the four exposures. However, treatment of the exposed skin with aloe gel after each exposure to UV radiation was found to block any suppression, maintaining the normal immune reaction. Moreover, aloe-treated animals did not lose the quantity and quality of immune cells in the skin that was shown by the unprotected control mice.

LIFELONG ORAL ALOE VERA INGESTION

A rather unusual *lifelong* feeding study was published in 2002 from the San Antonio University of Texas Health Sciences Center by Dr. J. T. Herlihy and colleagues (Ikeno et al., 2002), who tested for a benefit of dietary aloe vera on age-related disease. They used male specific pathogen-free rats that were assigned to one of four experimental groups: Group A (the controls) fed a semisynthetic diet without aloe vera; Group B, fed a diet that contained 1 percent freeze-dried aloe vera plant filet; Group C, fed a diet containing 1 percent freeze-dried, charcoal-processed aloe vera filet; and Group D, fed the control diet and given whole leaf charcoal-processed aloe vera (0.02 percent) in the drinking water.

Ikeno et al. (2002) showed that lifelong aloe vera ingestion resulted in "neither harmful effects nor deleterious changes. In addition, Aloe vera ingestion appeared to be associated with some beneficial effects on age-related diseases" (p. 712). Group B rats exhibited "significantly less occurrence of multiple causes of death, and a slightly lower incidence of fatal chronic nephropathy compared with Group A rats" (p. 712). Rats from both Groups B and C rats showed the same trend by slightly lower rates of atrial blood clots in the heart than did the Group A controls. The study findings suggest that aloe does not cause any obvious harmful adverse effects, and could also be beneficial for the prevention of some age-related pathology. Very few dietary supplements have been put to such a safety test.

Chapter 27

Eye Health

Mad dogs and Englishmen go out in the midday sun.

Noel Coward
English playwright, actor, and director

Our world is defined by what we see, beginning in infancy, and continuing to our end of life. One of the most disastrous disabilities is loss of vision—physical blindness. The seriousness of that disability was emphasized centuries ago by scriptural use of analogy between physical lack sight and spiritual blindness—lack of spiritual insight. Loss of the ability to walk can be more readily and effectively compensated, as can loss of hearing, especially if it occurs after childhood. Granted that people make remarkable adaptations to a loss or lack of vision, it is still a disability much to be avoided.

PHOTOTOXICITY

The vast majority of all organisms on the earth depend directly or indirectly on the energy provided by sunlight for life (certain deep-sea or subterranean microbes being the exception). Thus, sunlight is a necessity of our living, one of many necessities that are helpful under correct circumstances but that can be harmful when encountered to excess or inappropriately. Ironically, one of the greatest hazards to eye health is over-exposure to sunlight, without which we wouldn't see much at all! The retina of the eye can be severely and irreversibly burned by even brief direct exposure to the sun's rays, a hazard for people seeking to view an eclipse of the sun without special lenses to greatly filter and weaken the exposure. However, reflected rather than direct sunlight is the important source of exposure to the eye. An extreme level of reflection overexposure from snow or ice is responsible for causing temporary "snow-blindness." Inuit people long ago realized that re-

Consumer's Guide to Dietary Supplements and Alternative Medicines

doi:10.1300/5698_27

flection must be reduced so they invented bone goggles that allow only a narrow slit of light to pass. High reflection at a light-colored sandy beach can also cause the corneal injury known as photokeratitis—damage of the outer corneal layers that causes severe pain and reversibly impaired vision.

Although outdoor work causes many persons to receive occupational sun exposure and to be at risk for long-term adverse effects, it is a current paradox that for most Western nations the greatest sunlight overexposure arises from recreational activities. Foremost in the irony is that fair-skinned peoples of industrialized nations tend to practice sunbathing or use of tanning salons for merely cosmetic purposes. Although education against this as a risk factor for skin cancer is prevalent, equal attention needs to be paid to eye protection against injury from sunlight. A local ophthalmology clinic provides patient information stating a common view that UV light from the sun has been implicated (but not proven) to be a cause of degeneration of the retina. Other diseases such as high blood pressure, diabetes, and kidney disease may also affect the macula.

Ultraviolet (UV) radiation, the light rays at longer wavelengths than those that we perceive in the visible spectrum of sunlight, are its most hazardous component. Their mechanism of injury to the eye is believed to be promoting excess oxidative reactions in the visual cells of the retina. The injury arising from UV exposure is known as phototoxicity, a consequence of light-promoted photooxidative chemical reactions. Although UV type B (UVB) has been mainly implicated as the source of dangers (the sun-blockers for skin protection act mainly against UVB), concern that the UV type A (UVA) rays are also injurious to eye structures is growing. Use of UV-attenuating sunglasses (with side shields) whenever outdoors in sunlight, as well as wide-brimmed hats, would decrease eye exposure and risk for injury. They should be worn for optimal protection of the eyes from UV injury to the eyes regardless of one's iris color or skin type. Merely tinting eyeglasses do no good. If they do not carry a label saying they are 99 percent or 100 percent UV effective, they are not worth buying. On the other hand, if truly protective, they are worth wearing throughout the year in most of the temperate zone as well as in the tropics.

Age-Related, Sunlight-Related Eye Disease: Cataract

During aging abnormal chemical complexes that accumulate in the lens of the human eye cause cataract, in which the lens of the eye loses full transparency and vision is reduced. It is accepted that the risk for cataract rises in proportion to a person's habitual outdoor time and thus their sunlight exposure. The mode of injury by sunlight to the lens and retina is believed to be the generation of ROS (reactive oxygen species). Thus, a deficiency of exogenous (dietary) or endogenous (internally produced) protective chemicals is likely to increase the risk of injury. A 1998 report showed that light near the extreme of the UVA, where sunlight had been thought to be harmless, is even more prone to produce oxidizing free radicals than rays in the UVB range. Such radicals are blamed not only for premature skin aging but also for damage to cellular DNA and the suppression of the immune system caused by UV exposure.

Cataract prevalence also rises with age. With the contemporary aging trend in the U.S. population, the rate of visual impairment or even blindness stemming from cataract increases. People who live in the southern United States have a four times higher rate of cataracts than people residing in more northern areas. A growing worldwide challenge is to avoid or delay cataracts and to treat those that occur. Cataracts in the outer portions of the lens are associated with general outdoor exposure, whereas amount of UV radiation exposure correlates better with changes within the nucleus of the lens. Genetic factors are believed to make a contribution to cataract formation as well as environmental ones. However, reducing one's eye-exposure to UV rays from sunlight and reducing one's smoking are two steps that may lower the risk for cataract. Fortunately, cataract is an eye disease for which a surgical correction has become routinely available in the United States. Unfortunately, the same is not true of macular degeneration.

RISKS FOR AGE-RELATED MACULAR DEGENERATION

Age-related macular degeneration (AMD) is a disease of aging that robs the sufferer of normal vision in later life because of a progressively reduced retinal function. This condition has been growing more common in the United States in recent decades. According to one reviewer, the typical person vulnerable to AMD is a smoker who eats a high-fat diet and shows a history of high sunlight exposure, all of which are known or suspected to elevate one's risk. The combustion of tobacco smoking generates significant quantities of one ROS, nitric oxide, and perhaps others. Metabolism of the hundreds of foreign chemicals (xenobiotics) of tobacco smoke undoubtedly tends to generate more ROS.

Indulgence in alcoholic beverages appears to be another risk factor for AMD. Adults who drank at least four "standard drinks" per day were found to be seven times more likely to develop AMD than were nonindulging persons in a control group (Klein et al., 2002). The normal metabolism of alcohol comprises a source of one important ROS, superoxide. Worse yet, persons who are drinkers may also be heavy smokers, in such instances the combination puts them at an additional risk for oxidative injury to the retina (to say nothing of the brain, liver, and other organs). Those two lifestyle factors define individuals whose need for nutritional supplements are the highest among the general population, because of an additional tendency for ingesting a poor diet.

Two pharmaceuticals have recently been reported to lower one's risk for AMD—aspirin and members of the group of lipid-lowering agents known as statins. Wang and Del Priore (2004) presented observations comparing the rate for developing the more severe "wet" form of macular degeneration among users versus nonusers of these medications. The scientists found that the patients already taking statins were only one-half as likely as those without statins to develop wet AMD, which is caused by a growth of new blood vessels underneath the retina. (However, van Leeuwen et al. [2003] refuted two earlier preliminary reports of statins lowering risk for macular problems.) Persons already taking aspirin were about 40 percent less likely to develop this new blood vessel growth. For individuals not required to take a statin by their metabolic and cardiovascular status the use of aspirin would be the least risky approach. To persons wishing to avoid even aspirin for its adverse gastric effect, a natural COX-2 inhibitor (e.g., curcumin) might be desirable, considering that researchers suppose an anti-inflammatory action is responsible for the statin/aspirin ocular benefits.

Not surprisingly, eye structures also are at risk of toxicity from the use of certain drugs. High doses in the therapeutic range for prednisone, other corticosteroids, and allopurinol are a well-known risk for elevating intraocular pressure, i.e., precipitating glaucoma. Injury to the macula, almost always irreversible, is associated with use of the antimalarial agents chloroquine and hydroxychloroquine (also used for rheumatoid arthritis). The breast cancer agent tamoxifen (Nolvadex D, Soltamox, Tamofen) in high doses is said to favor maculopathy (macular disease). Findings of a French analysis of drug histories of AMD patients suggested that severe neovascular AMD is associated with long-term thiazide diuretic treatment. Damage to the optic nerve is attributed to use of the antiarrhythmic drug, amiodarone (Cordarone), and to the antitubercular agent also sometimes used for HIV-infected persons, ethambutol (Myambutol), which is known for causing sudden decrement of (color) visual acuity. Less threatening, soon reversible changes in color vision are caused by Viagra. Botanicals are not exempt from adverse effects on the eye.

Recently, the American Macular Degeneration Foundation stated that it believed millions of unsuspecting Americans may go blind from macular degeneration and that no cure is available for this little-understood disease.

Their Web page (http://www.macular.org/) also declares that "zeaxanthin is important to healthy eyes—especially for people with macular degeneration."

What is zeaxanthin, and why is this substance given such a positive endorsement? We will consider next the answers to these questions and related topics.

DIETARY ROLE IN EYE HEALTH AND DISEASE

The importance of the vegetable components known as carotenoids to health of the eyes is inferred partly from their properties as antioxidants combined with knowledge that retinal cells are at high risk for potentially quite injurious photooxidation reactions. Generation of oxidizing free radicals (ROS) by the UV rays is believed to play a central role in the production of age-related eye disease. This includes not only cataract but also AMD—the most important causes of impaired vision in older adults. Nonetheless, some medical writers still say that the causative role of UV rays in such problems is "suspected but unproven."

Carotenoids and the Eye

In the center of the retina, the layer containing the visual receptor cells, is an area known as the macula lutea, or commonly just macula. The term lutea comes from a Latin root meaning yellow or yellowish. In human anatomy we find it also describing the corpus luteum, a yellow structure that forms upon the surface of the ovary where an egg has been released, and that contains cells synthesizing progesterone during the month-long ovarian cycle before it dies away. The use of *lutea* for the central macula spot on the retina comes from the yellow color of the macula.

What makes the macula yellow? Carotenoids, a variety of vegetable pigments that were named for the carrot, which we know as being very orange-colored. Lutein and zeaxanthin are the two carotenoids distinctive from other major dietary carotenoids in that they are present in high concentration throughout the human retina. Others found there include lycopene, alpha-carotene, beta-carotene, and beta-cryptoxanthin. In fact, their concentration in the macula is nearly three times higher than levels in blood plasma. This is not without a purpose; it appears that carotenoids do indeed performs an essential function to the retina. Pigments of the retina absorb blue light waves and thus oppose their penetration, which may both increase the sharpness of our vision and give protection to the retina against oxidative injury.

Although antioxidants, including the carotenoids, have been hypothesized to lower the risk of age-related cataracts by preventing oxidation of proteins or lipids within the lens, prospective epidemiologic data to confirm this are limited. The ophthalmology research group at Harvard tested prospectively the hypothesized association between carotenoid and vitamin A intakes and cataract extraction in men (Brown et al., 1999). Male U.S. health-related professionals (36,644) who were 45 to 75 years old in 1986 were the study population. Others were later included as they reached 45 years of age. A detailed dietary questionnaire was used to assess their intake of carotenoids and other nutrients.

During eight years of follow-up, 840 instances of age-related cataract extraction were documented. The data showed a moderately lower risk for needed cataract surgery among men with higher intakes of lutein and zeaxanthin, but not of other carotenoids (lycopene, alpha-carotene, beta-carotene, and beta-cryptoxanthin) or vitamin A. This was after other potential risk factors, including age and smoking, were controlled. Among the specific foods high in carotenoids eaten, broccoli and spinach were the ones most consistently associated with a lower risk of cataract. The data from such research hinges greatly upon the reliability of the dietary questionnaire, which surely is less than measures of the blood levels of target compounds would be.

For a similar study in women, after age, smoking, and other potential cataract risk factors were controlled for, the women with the highest intake of lutein and zeaxanthin had a 22 percent lower risk of cataract extraction compared with those in the lowest 20 percent by intake. Other carotenoids (alpha-carotene, beta-carotene, beta-cryptoxanthin, and lycopene), vitamin A, and retinol were not significantly associated with cataract risk. An increased rate of eating spinach and kale, foods rich in lutein, was associated with a moderate decrease in risk of cataract. These studies support a conclusion that daily meals of vegetables and fruits high in carotenoids may enable cataract avoidance. The findings support a recommendation that persons to lower their cataract risk should consume daily vegetables and fruits with a high carotenoid content.

Other eye structures—the iris, ciliary body, and the choroid layer—also show high levels of carotenoids. Moreover, a deficiency of lutein and zeaxanthin now is suspected of contributing to the process of macular degeneration, which is the leading cause of vision loss among adults aged 65 years and older in both Europe and the United States. Foods from which lutein and zeaxanthin may be obtained include egg yolks, orange juice, corn, honeydew melons, orange pepper, kale, spinach, collards, turnip greens, and broccoli.

Lutein and zeaxanthin are not essential in the same fashion as are the vitamins for support of health, normal growth, and survival, or for avoiding a deficiency disease that might lead to illness and ultimately death. However, they may soon qualify for being classed as conditionally essential nutrients, which might be interpreted as being "quasi-vitamins." For this classification to apply a criterion would need to exist that upon deficient intake of the factor some chemical, structural, or functional abnormality must appear that will be clearly corrected by dietary supplementation with the factor in question.

Isothiocyanates for Eye Health

This is another group of food chemicals that has proven to be of special significance to eye health. In particular the compound sulforaphane has become a "hot" new agent for this purpose. It has been identified as a constituent of broccoli sprouts.

Sulforaphane provides a new indirect approach to protecting against oxidative injury as an alternative or adjunct to the use of direct-acting antioxidants for neutralizing free radicals. It acts to stimulate selectively some gene expression, i.e., to activate the gene-directed synthesis of certain valuable proteins. Those are products of phase 2 genes, which consist of detoxifying enzymes that perform phase 2 detoxification reactions on certain foreign molecules, but very important, also against the ROS molecules that are the cause of oxidative injury, e.g., to the RPEs (retinal pigment epithelial cells) as shown recently by Gao and Talalay (2004). They suggest that this should prove to be a capable protective action against retinal degenerative states, e.g., AMD, that can be obtained by dietary (or dietary supplement) means. Other works from Johns Hopkins and elsewhere have confirmed that sulforaphane exerts the same inducing action on human cells in vitro toward enzyme production as in animals. Research from Stanford University that used broccoli sprouts also found a protective action in respect to experimental prostate cancer in animals, and other data showed an ability to oppose risk factors for heart disease. This indeed is a dietary approach showing great promise for disease prophylaxis.

Fats in Our Foods

A multicenter eye-disease research project was conducted among five ophthalmology centers to determine the risk level for AMD relative to the level of dietary fat intake. Higher vegetable fat consumption was associated with an elevated risk for AMD; the odds-ratio for AMD was more than twice as high (2.22) for persons in the highest 20 percent versus those in the lowest 20 percent of fat intake. Higher intake of specific types of fat to include vegetable fats, monounsaturated and polyunsaturated, and linoleic acid (omega-6) instead of total fat intake may provoke a greater risk for advanced AMD. Diets high in omega-3 fatty acids or fish were associated with a lower risk for AMD when the intake of linoleic acid was low.

Body Weight Weighs in As Risk Factor

The same research group evaluated whether anthropomorphic (bodily measures), behavioral, and medical factors were associated with progression to advanced stages of AMD associated with loss of vision. The 261 participants at outset were 60 years or older, with some sign of nonadvanced AMD in at least one eye. The average follow-up time was 4.6 years. A higher body mass index (BMI) correlated with a higher risk for progression to the advanced forms of AMD. The relative risk was 2.35 for a BMI of at least 30, and 2.32 for a BMI from 25 to 29, relative to the lowest category (BMI less than 25). Both overall and abdominal obesity correlated with a higher risk for progression to advanced AMD, and greater levels of physical activity tended to decrease the risk. These data point to a likely importance of weight control in preventive measures against AMD.

Obesity increases significantly the risk of developing cataract overall, and especially of posterior subcapsular (PSC) cataract in particular. This was demonstrated in a study of 87,682 women and 45,549 men aged 45 years and older at the outset, who did not initially have diagnosed cataract. The cause of PSC cataract may be mediated at least in part by prediabetic factors—glucose intolerance and insulin resistance—in the absence of overt clinical diabetes.

NONDIETARY LIFESTYLE RISK FACTORS FOR AMD OR CATARACT

Cigarette smoking has been found to be an independent, avoidable risk factor for AMD in women in the United States via an 11-state prospective study with a 12-year follow-up. Risk for AMD increased very significantly with an increasing number of pack-years smoked. Among women who smoked for 65 or more pack-years, the risk was 2.4 times the risk of never-smokers. Compared with current smokers, little reduction in risk was seen even after cessation of smoking for 15 or more years. Thus, it is critical to avoid, rather than hoping to reverse, this risk of smoking.

Similarly, the smoking of cigarettes was examined by the authors for an association between time since quitting smoking and incidence of cataract extraction. The study participants were women and men enrolled in the Nurses' Health Study and the Health Professionals Follow-Up Study, respectively. In comparison to current smokers, the former smokers (who had quit smoking 25 or more years before) had a 20 percent lower probability of cataract surgery (after adjustment for age, average number of cigarettes smoked per day, and other potential risk factors). However, the risk among past smokers did not decrease to as low a level as that seen among those classed as never-smokers. Again, never smoking beats cessation of smoking for health's sake.

Alcohol consumption has been implicated in the pathogenesis of cataract in some but not all studies, and no prospective analysis of the relationship between alcohol consumption and cataract had been conducted in women. Therefore, the Harvard ophthalmology group (Chasan-Taber et al., 2000) performed a prospective study in female registered nurses that began in 1980 with more than 50,000 included, and others were added as they became 45 years of age for a total of 77,466 women. Information on alcohol consumption and occurrence of cataract extraction was gathered over 12 years. When compared to nondrinkers, female nurses consuming alcoholic beverages were not at increased risk of cataract, even up to intake levels of 25 grams or more per day (two or more drinks) after controlling for risk factors such as cigarette smoking, body mass index, and diabetes. This does not refute prior evidences of an adverse effect, which were mainly based on men, who very probably had higher average levels of exposure to alcohol.

CLINICAL APPLICATIONS

Many nutritional writers have pronounced that supplemental intake of antioxidants will be a protection against phototoxic retinal injury. However, this hypothesis has not yet been fully validated by the available research. Limitations are suggested by the study described in the next section. Nevertheless, caution should dictate an increase in one's level of intake of dietary antioxidants with advancing age. This calls first and foremost for eating foods that best supply the carotenoids, but it also should elicit serious consideration of using supplements that provides sulforaphane and vitamins A, C, D, and E, plus selenium, and antioxidants such as alpha-lipoic acid.

Age-Related Eye Disease Study

This project, results of which were published in the October 2001 issue of *Archives of Ophthalmology,* was designed (1) to learn more about the natural history and risk factors of AMD and cataract and (2) to evaluate the effects of high doses of antioxidants and zinc on the progression of AMD and cataract (AREDS, 2001). Briefly, the results from the AREDS (Age-Relate Eye Disease Study) showed that high levels of antioxidants and zinc significantly reduced the participants' risk of advanced AMD and its associated loss of vision, compared to patients receiving a placebo. The same nutrient factors did not significantly modify the development or the rate of progression of cataract.

A high-level intake of antioxidants and zinc lowered the probability of developing AMD in an advanced form by about 25 percent. These nutrients also reduced the risk for loss of vision from advanced AMD by about 19 percent; however, they had no significant effect on the development or progression of cataract. The specific daily amounts of antioxidants and minerals used for the research were as follows:

500 milligrams of vitamin C
400 international units of vitamin E
15 milligrams of beta-carotene
80 milligrams of zinc (as zinc oxide)
2 milligrams of copper (as cupric oxide), added to avoid a copper deficiency arising from the zinc supplementation, which tends be competitive with copper uptake

This formulation was prepared and supplied by Bausch and Lomb, which marketed it for general use under the name Ocuvite. Equivalent products are available from other manufacturers, and the components could, of course, be taken other than through such a combination product.

People who are at special risk for developing advanced AMD (as with a clear family history) should consider taking from an early age a formula similar to that used in the AREDS study. Only an eye care professional can diagnose whether you have AMD, and if you are at risk for developing the advanced form of disease. That doctor should conduct a dilated-eye examination for visualization of the interior of the patient's eyes. This allows for careful searching to detect signs of AMD. If the reader already is taking a multiple vitamin-mineral supplement daily, review it with your doctor or pharmacist for adequacy in comparison to the AREDS formula's recommended ingredients.

Concerning possible unwanted effects of such multivitamin-mineral usage, AREDS participants reported few side effects from the regimen. About 7.5 percent of the participants assigned to the zinc treatments had urinary tract problems that required hospitalization, compared with 5 percent of those not taking zinc in their assigned treatment. The zinc group also reported anemia at a slightly higher rate than the controls level, but this was not a significant difference. However, it is important to be certain that any person using a zinc supplement also receives supplemental copper because of the competition between the two minerals for absorption, because copper deficit is one cause for anemia. Slight coloration of the skin is a well-known and harmless side effect of large doses of carotenoids. It was noted slightly more often among the participants taking antioxidants that included beta-carotene. It is compared to tanning, and usually regarded as supplying a healthier look. This study supports a conclusion that the nutrients are not a cure for AMD, nor will they restore vision already lost from that disease. However, they may play a critical role in persons at high risk for AMD in avoiding the development of advanced AMD.

CONCERN ABOUT ADVERSE EFFECTS OF SOME NATURAL PRODUCTS

An Oregon Health and Science University researcher, Frederick W. Fraunfelder, MD, presented a review in the *American Journal of Ophthalmology* in October 2004 on cases of ocular adverse effects associated with dietary supplements (Fraunfelder, 2004). He found reported side effects ranging from simple dry eye to retinal hemorrhages and transient visual loss. Most of these effects were with high doses or topical application. Although none of the reported cases caused permanent damage, he speculated that many could have if the patient had not discontinued use of the product.

Ginkgo biloba was associated with two cases of hemorrhaging into the anterior chamber of the eye, plus other reports of retinal hemorrhages in patients taking it. This is concordant with the known inhibition by ginkgo of platelet aggregation, which favors bleeding, both externally and internally, especially in combination with aspirin or other drugs that inhibit clotting processes. Reports of eye irritation and conjunctivitis have been associated with *Echinacea,* especially its topical use. Chamomile tea is used by some persons topically in and around the eyes to treat styes and runny, irritated eyes. Fraunfelder found reported cases of severe conjunctivitis with such topical use.

American Indians are said to have used licorice to treat inflammatory eye diseases. Fraunfelder found cases of transient vision loss after licorice ingestion, similar to what occurs in an ocular migraine attack without headache. The side effects appeared to be associated with large doses. Canthaxanthine is a carotenoid used in cosmetics, as a food coloring, and to produce an artificial suntan when taken orally. Deposits of it occur in the retina that appear to be absorbed later but may require years to disappear. Visual changes from canthaxanthine are related to retinal function abnormalities that have been detected with visual field testing and a electroretinography test. Members of the genus *Datura* are well known for containing atropine or similar alkaloids having anticholinergic activities that dilate the pupil, causing mydriasis. An accompanying paralysis of the control of the lens prevents focusing and causes blurry vision for a few days; some persons having a glaucoma state or tendency may have elevated intraocular pressure.

It is said that niacin can cause some of the most severe ocular reactions of all the products reviewed, including decreased vision, cystoid macular edema, dry eyes, discoloration of the eyelids, eyelid edema, and loss of eyebrows or eyelashes. These appear to be a function of high dosage, and would require discontinuation of niacin therapy. Fraunfelder found reports linking high toxic doses of vitamin A to intracranial hypertension, which could lead to an ocular hemorrhage as well as to stroke. In the majority of cases this condition resolves if vitamin A is discontinued. "Ocular side effects from supplement products are often undiagnosed and unreported. Physicians must remain vigilant in recognizing adverse ocular side effects and inquiring whether a patient is using alternative therapies," said Fraunfelder (2004).

CONCLUSION

"Mad dogs and Englishmen" should seek protection in sunscreens, UV-blocking lenses, and a good intake of zinc, carotenoids, and antioxidants, and so should you!

Chapter 28

Functional Fruits

BACKGROUND

It has become commonplace to see or hear media health stories reminding us that the U.S. population is becoming older, and that with this aging will come major increases in the age-associated diseases—not only cancer and cardiovascular disease but also the most dreaded and devastating of these, the brain pathologies of Alzheimer's disease (AD) and Parkinson's disease (PD). It is estimated that within the next 50 years about 30 percent of the population will be 65 years or older. Of those aged between 75 and 84 years, six million will develop some degree of nervous system degenerative disease symptoms, and of those older than 85 years, more than 12 million will develop some form of dementia.

Factors commonly believed to make a significant contribution to the development of these degenerative disorders, as well as to normal age-related declines in memory and motor functions of the brain, are (1) an increased susceptibility to damaging and persisting effects of oxidative stress (caused by ROS), and (2) increased susceptibility to effects of inflammatory conditions. Unless methods are found to prevent age-related decrements in nervous system activity, health care costs will continue to rise at an exceptional rate. Thus, it is very important to explore every possible means to oppose or reverse age-related neuronal damage as well as the subsequent behavioral manifestations. Fortunately, the recent growth of biochemical knowledge of cells has opened avenues of research focused on identifying new therapies that could potentially disrupt the sequence of events involved in these highly detrimental processes. In this regard, many researchers are considering a greater role that certain dietary components may play in alleviating degenerative disorders and are now beginning to pay particular attention to the intake of phytochemicals found in fruits and vegetables (more so than in nuts).

Epidemiologic data demonstrate an association between high intake of fruits and vegetables and a lower risk for chronic disease. For example,

Consumer's Guide to Dietary Supplements and Alternative Medicines

doi:10.1300/5698_28

Verlangieri and colleagues (1985) found that the consumption of fruits and vegetables, particularly those rich in vitamin C (based on content and consumption), may have offered a protective effect against deaths from cardiovascular disease. Several plausible biological reasons explain why consumption of fruits and vegetables might slow or prevent the onset of such chronic disease. Fruits and vegetables are rich sources of various nutrients, not only vitamins, but also trace minerals, dietary fiber, and many classes of biologically active compounds, particularly those having antioxidant and anti-inflammatory actions (flavonoids = polyphenols, and anthocyanins that impart color to fruits). Such phytochemicals can exert multiple actions that are complementary and overlapping, such as modulation of detoxification enzymes, of cholesterol synthesis, or of hormone metabolism, stimulation of the immune system, reduction of platelet aggregation and of blood pressure, plus antioxidant, antibacterial, and antiviral actions.

Although these effects have been examined primarily in whole animal and in vitro cell-culture models, some experimental dietary studies in humans have also shown a capacity for fruits, vegetables, and their phytochemical constituents to improve these potential disease opposing mechanisms. Animal studies have been published from the United States and as far away as Finland and India reporting favorable metabolic effects of fruits found in those regions. The human studies have relied on intermediate and substitute end points serving as an index of disease risk. Various designs for clinical investigations have been used that have included some questionable designs and statistical analyses. Length of treatments have ranged from a single dose to years. Dietary control has varied in stringency from the mere addition of supplements to the habitual diet to provision of all food for the (short) experimental period. Rigorous design and conduct of dietary studies in humans are highly important for validating epidemiologic or animal-based research by means of human data.

MORE DETAILS

Cranberries: Old Wives' Tale Worthy of Believing?

Cranberries *(Vaccinium macrocarpon),* particularly in the form of cranberry juice, have been used widely for many decades for the prevention and/or treatment of urinary tract infections. Patel and Daniels (2000) suggested that science should investigate further the benefits of the humble cranberry. In the same year were two reports of attempted meta-analyses on this very topic.

Jepson and colleagues (2000b) reported an assessment of the utility of cranberries for the *treatment* of urinary tract infections. No clinical trials were found which fulfilled all of their usual inclusion criteria. To be specific, no randomized trial was found that assessed the efficacy of cranberry juice for the treatment of urinary tract infections. Thus, as of 2000 no scientific-quality evidence existed to support the proposition that cranberry is effective for treating urinary tract infections.

In addition, Jepson and colleagues (2000a) report of an analysis of all randomized controlled trials of cranberry juice/products used for the *prevention* of urinary tract infections in susceptible populations of men, women, and children. Four trials met the inclusion criteria, three compared the effectiveness of cranberry juice versus placebo juice or water, and one compared the effectiveness of capsules of cranberry concentrate/extract versus placebo capsules. Their conclusion was that:

> the small number of poor quality trials gives no reliable evidence of the effectiveness of cranberry juice and other cranberry products. The large number of dropouts/withdrawals from the trials indicates that cranberry juice may not be acceptable over long periods of time. Other cranberry products such as cranberry capsules may be more acceptable. On the basis of the available evidence, cranberry juice cannot be recommended for the prevention of urinary tract infections in susceptible populations.

However, subsequent to the Cochrane analyses being published, a more favorable report came from Finland in 2001 on a study that was conducted at the Laboratory of Clinical Microbiology and Oulu University Hospital, Oulu, Finland. It was conducted to determine whether recurrences of bacterial urinary tract infection caused by *Escherichia coli* could be prevented by the intake of a cranberry and lingonberry juice mixture or by taking of a *Lactobacillus* drink designed to favorably alter the intestinal bacterial population (Kontiokari et al., 2001). Besides two groups for the two test drinks was a third no-treatment control group. Assignments to the groups were made randomly. However, it was not possible to accommodate blinding to treatments, so the design is called "open."

The treatments were to be drunk five days a week for one year. A statistically significant 20 percent reduction in absolute risk was found for urinary infections in the cranberry group compared with the no-treatment group. At six months, eight (16 percent) women in the cranberry group, 19 (39 percent) in the lactobacillus group, and 18 (36 percent) in the control group had experienced at least one recurrence of infection. Generally speaking, up to 60 percent of women will have a urinary tract infection and a third of those will have several recurrences. Kontiokari and colleagues (2001) concluded that a 50 mL (2 oz.) serving of cranberry and lingonberry juice concentrate daily reduced the recurrence of symptomatic urinary tract infection by about half compared with the control group, whereas the *Lactobacillus* GG drink had no effect on recurrence. Self-treatment with cranberry juice may help lower health care costs significantly by its reducing the need for Rx antimicrobials against recurrent urinary tract infections.

A very plausible basis exists for clinical antibacterial effects of cranberry. It has been shown to oppose the adherence of bacteria, especially the dominant species causing urinary infections, *Escherichia coli,* to the epithelial cells of the urinary tract. Without adherence the bacteria are relatively hindered in setting up an infection. Two possible components responsible for this are fructose and a polymeric compound of unknown structure. Whereas many fruit juices contain fructose, only cranberry and blueberry are able to provide both components, which is believed to explain the benefits observed for cranberry. A person who cannot tolerate cranberry should perhaps give blueberry a try.

Prunes: A Significant Functional Food

This fruit (consisting of dried plums) would qualify for the health foods section of your supermarket. However, you are most likely to find it in the section of canned fruits and vegetables, because it's no Johnny-come-lately as a self-help remedy for its action against constipation. Prunes have a highly palatable sweet flavor, which facilitates their use as a mild laxative and causes them to be considered the epitome of a functional food, in twenty-first-century parlance. Dried prunes contain about 6.1 grams of dietary fiber per 100 g, but prune juice is devoid of fiber owing to its being filtered before bottling. The laxative action of both whole prunes and prune juice may be explainable by their high content of fiber and sugars, fructose, and sorbitol (14.7 and 6.1 g/100 g, respectively). Prunes serve as a good source of energy because of simple sugars, but they do not provoke a rapid rise in blood sugar concentration. Prunes also contain large amounts of phenolic compounds (184 mg/100 g), which may aid in the laxative action and in the delay of glucose absorption. Research is needed to confirm the levels of carotenoids and other phytochemicals from prunes.

Moreover, the high potassium content of prunes (745 mg/100 g) could be beneficial for cardiovascular health as our current diets tend to favor a deficiency of potassium. Dried prunes are an important source of the trace element boron, which is suggested to play a role in prevention of osteoporosis. A serving of prunes (100 g) fulfills the recommended daily requirement for boron (2 to 3 mg). In vitro data show that phenolic compounds in prunes inhibit the oxidation of human LDL; these might serve as agents to oppose chronic diseases such as heart disease and cancer. In short, the user of prunes in whatever manner may surely experience short-term benefits and long-term ones also. However, as with some other fruit juices, the high potassium content may rarely become a problem if one's intake is overdone (principle of Chapter 11).

Cancer Chemoprevention by Black Raspberries and Cherries

Cancers of the oral cavity represent 2.5 percent of all cancers that occur in the United States, but treatments for them are relatively ineffective. Researchers at the Ohio State University Division of Environmental Health Sciences conclude that new strategies for prevention need to be developed and tested in appropriate animal models. In a 2002 report they showed that the hamster cheek pouch could be used to evaluate the ability of black raspberries to inhibit oral cavity tumors induced by exposure to the model carcinogen, DMBA (Casto et al., 2002). After 12 to 13 weeks of DMBA treatment the animals were sacrificed and the number and volume of tumors were determined. The researchers found a significant reduction in the number of tumors between the black-raspberry-treated animals and control groups, which supports their prior studies also showing chemopreventive activity of raspberries. This exemplifies the numerous animal researches now ongoing that have encouraged the view that cancer chemoprevention can be achieved by proper selections of the human diet.

That cherries are an excellent source of cancer chemopreventive activity is supported by a considerable amount of laboratory data. Cherries are rich in a flavonoid, quercitrin, that has been found by researchers to be a highly potent chemopreventive agent. When one eats cherries the quercitrin is said to be available to oppose any cancerous cells that may be present. (Note that NIH screening for anticancer activity was negative for quercitrin, which is a different matter than chemoprevention.) Cherries also contain ellagic acid, a natural plant phenolic known for acting against carcinogenic or mutagenic agents. Some researchers believe that intake of ellagic acid may be one of the most effective ways to prevent cancer. Another compound found in cherries, perillyl alcohol (POH), is also powerful in opposing the occurrence of various types of cancer in animal tests.

A final bioactive component of cherries is an antioxidant, melatonin, which is also found in the human brain as a neurohormonal agent that aids in maintaining the body's natural sleep patterns. Extensive evidence has demonstrated that melatonin plays a significant role in regulating the 24-

hour (circadian) rhythms of our bodies. Because melatonin occurs and acts in quite low levels normally, a minor increase achieved by taking it in food or as a supplement can possibly produce a significant increase.

Moreover, tart cherries are touted as having an ability to relieve some sources of pain by virtue of their content of anthocyanin and bioflavonoid components that inhibit COX-1 and COX-2 enzymes as do the nonsteroidal anti-inflammatory drugs. Joint pains and migraine headaches should be benefited by such an action. Brownwood Acres supplies tart cherry juice concentrate in a pint or one-quart size; the recommended one ounce (or about 2 tablespoons) per day may be diluted in either water or milk. Brownwood Acres also supplies blueberry and pomegranate concentrates that are stocked by at least one major retail grocery chain. (For more on the anti-aging role of blueberry, see Chapter 14.)

Promising Pineapple

Bromelain refers to an extract from pineapples that contains multiple positive activities that have been demonstrated both in vitro and in vivo to be anti-inflammatory (including anti-edema), anticlotting or antithrombotic (via a reversible inhibition of platelet aggregation), and fibrinolytic (clot dissolving). The active component(s) responsible are determined only in part, but have been associated, among other factors, with several closely related proteases (proteolytic enzymes). Owing to its efficacy after oral intake, to its safety, and to a lack of undesired side effects, bromelain has earned considerable acceptance and usage among patients as a phytotherapeutic agent.

Based on the activities cited, bromelain has been applied against several diseases, such as pyelonephritis, surgical traumas, thrombophlebitis, angina pectoris, bronchitis, and sinusitis. It also has been suggested to enhance the absorption of drugs, particularly of antibiotics. These activities appear in part to be related to the enzymatic component. A recent review states that results of preclinical pharmacological studies support bromelain being an orally active agent for complementary tumor therapy. Bromelain appears to act as an immunomodulator to raise the immunocytotoxicity of monocytes, whose functioning tends to be impaired by cancer when tested against cancer cells taken from patients. Moreover, it was seen to elevate production and secretion of several desirable cytokines and to exert anti-metastatic (anti-invasive) activity, which would be a very desirable clinical action. Arguments that bromelain cannot be effective after oral administration because of its protein nature definitely have been refuted by multiple experimental findings.

Get into Grapefruit!

Compared to other citrus fruits, grapefruit is rich in water-soluble fiber, which has been shown to enhance digestion while helping to slow the absorption of carbohydrates that would otherwise contribute to blood sugar spiking. An added bonus to grapefruit's ability to lower insulin levels is that it tends to avoid the higher insulin levels that promote hunger pangs, so that the appetite is reduced.

Bandolier, a Web site on evidence-based medicine (www.jr2.ox.ac.uk/bandolier/), stated (as of July 2004) that they could find no evidence for such properties for grapefruit. A 1999 German paper (van Woedtke, 1999) presented an analysis of six commercial grapefruit seed extracts, finding that five had antimicrobial properties, activity against a strain of *Candida.* However, all the extracts showing antimicrobial activity contained the chemical benzethonium, and, in some was found triclosan and methyl paraben; all of these are synthetic antimicrobial agents. The only extract without antimicrobial activity contained no such chemicals. Seemingly, the only antimicrobial activity was imparted by the synthetic chemicals used to preserve grapefruit. However, the marketing of grapefruit in the United States may not require adding such chemicals. van Woedtke (1999) concluded that organic grapefruit would have no effect. As noted in Chapter 11, a strong probability exists of a synergistic interaction between grapefruit and many Rx drugs, which may simply require (or permit) the use of a lower drug dosage.

CONCLUSIONS

Children and adults would do well to cultivate a taste for fruits, and even to cultivate the plants that bear them, according to the possibilities open for wherever one resides. Fresh fruits can be delicious as well as highly nutritious. Even if one needs to use a little sugar to cut the tartness, as for grapefruit, this likely would be less than the amount of sugar and calories added for processed forms (e.g., canned in syrup or baked in a pie). When antioxidant nutrients can be so tasty, it seems that we should reduce our need for supplements by eating more fruit. The best approach is to have the best of both worlds—eat freely also of fruits and nuts as a substitute for less-nutritious, sugar-laden snack foods.

PART V: Most Certain Supplement Marvels

To most of us nothing is so invisible as an unpleasant truth. Though it is held before our eyes, pushed under our noses, rammed down our throats—we know it not. In times of change, learners inherit the Earth, while the learned find themselves beautifully equipped to deal with a world that no longer exists.

Eric Hoffer (1902-1983),
The Passionate State of Mind

Chapter 29

Botanical Mistaken Identity

Europe experienced a tragic "Chinese herbal nephropathy" epidemic; have we learned the lessons from it in North America?

BACKGROUND

During the early 1990s a Chinese botanical remedy became widely used in Belgium as part of a slimming regimen dispensed by weight reduction clinics, which included also appetite suppressants from conventional medicine, e.g., dexfenfluramine or fenfluramine and phentermine (fen-phen). Among the estimated ten thousand Belgian women who participated in such practices, some began to be diagnosed with valvular heart disease and kidney pathologies that were attributed to the reducing regimen. The heart problems were ultimately attributed to the dexfenfluramine or fenfluramine exposure. However, the renal pathology was widely recognized by 1998 as arising from the herbal component because of many persuasive scientific findings. Despite the data, some proponents of the herbals continued to argue without scientific basis that another cause of the toxicity exists.

During 1992 and 1993 several dozen patients with renal failure were admitted to Belgian hospitals. Ultimately, more than 100 cases were tallied. Their kidneys were undergoing a progressive degeneration (technically, an interstitial fibrosis with tubular atrophy). These changes were notable for the marked extent of the fibrotic process and for the rapidity of its progression. Although the main suspected source for the pathology initially was the synthetic antiappetite drugs, some circumstance rather supported the view that a herbal component had contributed. Subsequent investigation revealed that two botanical ingredients, *Stephania tetrandra* and *Magnolia officinalis,* were claimed to be included, but instead a plant known to be dangerous, *Aristolochia fangchi,* had been substituted for the *Stephania.* It is likely that this was from name confusion because the latter correct plant is known in Chinese as *fang-ji.* The genus *Aristolochia* contains 28 additional spe-

Consumer's Guide to Dietary Supplements and Alternative Medicines

doi:10.1300/5698_29

cies, but hereafter we will use this name to indicate either *fangchi* or the whole genus. It was subsequently indicated by the FDA that all members of the genus are known, or must be assumed, to contain the toxic factor, aristolochic acid, and thus all are assumed to share the toxic properties of *Aristolochia fangchi.*

Powders labeled *Stephania tetrandra,* but likely consisting instead of *Aristolochia fangchi,* as shown by the presence of aristolochic acid, also were sold in France between 1989 and May 1994 (Stengel, 1998). In May 1994, cases of end-stage renal failure were recognized in Toulouse, France, and were associated with the same Chinese herbal incriminated in the cases reported from Belgium. Ultimately, the same problem of renal toxicity surfaced also in Spain, Britain, Japan, and Taiwan.

Despite that the importation of *Aristolochia* had been banned by Germany in 1981, and a warning also had been issued in 1982 by the World Health Organization, the plant was not banned from Belgium until 1992. Nevertheless, after such developments overseas, *Aristolochia*-containing products were not prohibited in the United States by the FDA until late May of 2000, and continued to be available for sale at least during the summer of 2000. At that time the FDA sent a belated announcement of its being concerned about botanical products, including dietary supplements, containing aristolochic acid to health care practitioners and to six organizations representing the botanical or dietary supplement industry (FDA, 2001b). This warned manufacturers that appropriate steps should be taken to ensure against the presence of aristolochic acid in their products, which would make them subject to seizure by the FDA.

It may not have been coincidental that the notice of the FDA's being "concerned" was issued shortly before the appearance of a highly relevant publication in the June 8, 2000, issue of the *New England Journal of Medicine* (Nortier et al., 2000). It came from Brussels, Belgium, and was authored by eleven specialists in nephrology, pathology, or molecular biology research. Since the end in 1992 of *Aristolochia* marketing in Belgium they had seen 43 cases of end-stage renal failure among women who had used a product containing the Chinese herb. The research group had reported in 1996 that kidneys removed from five patients showed evidence of a chemical interaction between molecules of aristolochic acid and those from cells in the kidneys. Moreover, other physicians had reported instances of urinary tract cancer in several such patients in 1994 (Nortier et al., 2000).

Therefore, the Brussels clinicians had counseled the 43 female patients of their suspicion that cancer might be developing in their retained but nonfunctional kidneys. They suggested that it consequently would be desirable for such kidneys to be surgically removed. After 39 patients underwent the suggested removal, the organs were subjected to histopathologic and biochemical studies. The result was that 18 (46 percent) of the 39 patients were found to have developed urinary tract carcinomas. In 19 others (48 percent) the examination revealed a precancerous state known as dysplasia. Only two of the 39 (5 percent) showed no abnormal findings in their kidneys.

Thus, the injury by *Aristolochia* to the European dieters had included not only the destruction of their kidney function, but also the induction of cancerous or precancerous pathology. Analysis of prescription data indicated that the persons who had taken greater cumulative amounts of the herbal had a greater likelihood of being among those showing cancerous changes. In each of these 39 women's tissues, aristolochic acid was detected in a form bound chemically to the DNA of the kidney cells as adducts. This seems to be a smoking-gun level of evidence for a causal role of the chemical in the kidneys becoming cancerous.

An editorial in the same issue of the journal as the paper from Belgium was written by Dr. David Kessler, formerly the director of the FDA and currently dean of medicine at Yale University (Kessler, 2000). Dr. Kessler warned that similar occurrences in the United States are possible; he found he was able to buy capsules labeled *Aristolochia* in spring of 2000. The "food supplement" classification of herbals had allowed this known (to European medical scientists) hazard to human health to be imported without restriction.

An FDA letter in April 2001 updated a previous letter relating to use of *Aristolochia,* repeating that "at a minimum, we believe that it is absolutely necessary that manufacturers who produce products that contain ingredients that may be contaminated with aristolochic acid test their products to confirm the absence of aristolochic acids" (FDA, 2001b). Even so, the ban might represent closing the proverbial barn door too late.

In July and November 2000, several products were withdrawn from the U.S. market by their producers in response to the FDA communication. They were Nature's Wonderland Virginia Snake Root, powder and capsules; Meridian Circulation tablets and liquid; and Quell Fire tablets.

A further reason for wondering whether the FDA is listening adequately to scientists in other parts of the world stems from its failure to act upon receiving a report that was distributed worldwide in summer 1999. Professor Alasdair Breckenridge, Chair of the United Kingdom's Committee on Safety of Medicines, sent a statement titled "Renal Failure Associated with Aristolochia in Some Chinese Medicines." The letter reported two patients in the United Kingdom developing end-stage renal failure associated with Chinese herbal remedies that contained *Aristolochia,* and more than 70 cases reported in Belgium in 1993 that were associated with a slimming product containing *Aristolochia.* Despite its long usage in Chinese traditional medicine the plants in this genus contain aristolochic acids, which are known to be carcinogenic and associated with kidney toxicity (Breckenridge, 1999).

Furthermore, Australian authorities reported that imported Chinese herbal medicines in Australia were also found in 1999 to contain *Aristolochia,* although labeled to be of the genus *Clematis.* This mixup seems likely to reflect the existence of another *Aristolochia* species named *Aristolochia clematis.* Australia's Therapeutic Goods Administration, which is comparable to the FDA, takes the position on *Aristolochia* that it has no safe application in therapeutic products, and is of such danger to health that it is prohibited for sale, supply or use in Australia.

Yet despite these and many other contrary evidences, millions of Americans continue to hold the opinion that they are completely safe in their use of botanical products because such remedies are composed of "harmless" natural herbal ingredients rather than "dangerous synthetics."

In October 2003 a letter to the editor in *New England Journal of Medicine* cited a high number of Internet Web sites offering botanicals identified as containing the banned component, aristolochic acid (Gold and Stone, 2003).

One can only hope that the FDA will respond with the alacrity and anger at this state of affairs as it warrants. Gold and Stone (2003) contend rightly that the FDA's efforts to protect the U.S. botanical-using public are thoroughly undermined by the availability of such products via the Internet. It is very difficult or impossible to determine whether orders for such sources would be filled from a U.S. location or from another country. The authors present a clearly logical argument, but their proposal that the FDA should have the power to control what appears on the Internet will arouse much opposition by freedom-of-speech advocates. The proposal appears unlikely to gain the support needed for its enactment, even for U.S.-based Web sites, and no prospect that Web sites based outside the United States may be prevented from carrying such material exists. Prevention of the importation of botanicals is another problematic matter. One must infer that the products are already being illegally imported and subject to FDA seizure as adulterated materials.

MORE CASES

Confusion arising from duplication of common names for medicinal plants and herbs is not rare. *Snakeroot* is an English name commonly applied to more than one plant. This clearly can be a source of toxic misadventures. We are unaware that any other so striking as the case of *Aristolochia fangchi* has been recognized in North America, although some may exist among botanical poisoning epidemics in the Third World. Two further example will elaborate on this hazard.

Mandrake toxicity—with severe nausea and vomiting—has resulted from using the wrong plant species because of name duplication. The "real" mandrake, *Mandragora officinarum,* is a European plant (also called love apple) not found naturally in North America. Here another unrelated toxic species, *Podophyllum peltatum,* has been called the mandrake, although it is widely known by the name mayapple.

A Near Miss in 2001

Another possibility for such a toxic mixup was recognized, and apparently avoided. In late April 2001, the U.S. Food and Drug Administration sent out a warning for people to avoid a poisonous plant mistakenly labeled as a harmless herb that could be "tasty in a soup." A Canadian nursery distributed the herb to nurseries in Washington and Idaho as well as to British Columbia. Anyone who might have eaten the plant was advised to consult a physician promptly. The actual plant distributed mistakenly was autumn monkshood *(Aconitum carmichaelii),* which remains quite poisonous even after being cooked. It has caused human deaths. Poisoning from the alkaloid aconitine contained in this plant causes an irregular heartbeat, or paralysis of the heart muscle, which could lead to death.

Other symptoms might include tingling sensations in the limbs, burning or tingling of the mouth or tongue, muscle weakness, and gastric distress. The plants have tall, violet-blue flowers, and they were packaged in blue plastic pots for distribution starting in early March 2001. About 1,500 plants were thought to have been sold, but no known cases of illnesses existed at the time of the notice. Another miracle! This incident illustrates the principal better known regarding mushrooms—that an amateur botanist cannot be certain of a safe selection when confusion between similar-appearing toxic and nontoxic species is possible.

Chapter 30

The L-Tryptophan Disaster

Will the disaster be repeated?

A HISTORY

L-tryptophan (LTP) is an essential amino acid that occurs naturally in peptides and proteins. Relative to many amino acids, it is somewhat less commonly supplied. It has much additional importance as a precursor of small molecules, especially serotonin (5-hydroxytryptamine, 5HT), which has many different roles in the human brain and body. It has long been available as a component of powdered mixtures that contain many amino acids produced by the breakdown (hydrolysis) of common proteins. Such products are sold in health food stores and elsewhere as a nutritional aid to favor muscle growth and are aimed at athletes and bodybuilders. However, because of the difficulty and expense of isolating LTP from such a mixture, products that formerly supplied LTP as a single amino acid in an oral dosage form relied upon an unusual source of LTP, produced biosynthetically by bacteria ("manufactured LTP"), not by chemical synthesis.

In the 1980s, it became popular to take LTP tablets for relief of various common symptoms such as insomnia or PMS (premenstrual syndrome). In summer and fall of 1989 products that supposedly contained only the amino acid LTP were implicated in causing a serious illness known as EMS (eosinophilia myalgia syndrome) in hundreds of people who took the supplement products. At least 37 persons in the United States died, and more than 1,500 were permanently disabled by their developing a serious, often chronic illness that followed using this supplement. The three initial cases all were middle-aged women. Although the severity of symptoms differed, people affected had in common the features of muscle pain (myalgia), weakness, oral ulcers, abdominal pain, shortness of breath, and skin rash. The doses of LTP that they had used were similar, but the duration of use before onset of illness varied from a few weeks to two years.

Consumer's Guide to Dietary Supplements and Alternative Medicines

doi:10.1300/5698_30

Analysis of the subsequent hundreds of cases showed that the onset of the illness was marked by skin symptoms in 57 percent of cases, myalgia in 34 percent of cases, and neuropathy (nerve injury) and dysfunction in 34 percent. A swelling of the arms and legs commonly occurred. Sufferers with EMS were found to show an excess of circulating eosinophils (e.g., eosinophilia), which are a type of white blood cell produced by the immune system to defend against parasites but which also may be increased in some allergies. It is believed that in people with EMS, the excessive numbers of eosinophils begin to attack the body's own tissues as if they were foreign. EMS was frequently characterized by severe joint and muscle pains, swelling, and excess fatigability and shortness of breath, among other continuing symptoms. Generally it was found that 60 percent of EMS sufferers had a slow disappearance of the illness over years. An unfortunate 20 percent, especially older patients, progressed to death in about 18 months. The remaining 20 percent had indefinitely continuing symptoms that were sometimes severe, including muscle weakness or myalgia, skin changes, and even cognitive deficits from apparent brain injury.

The CDC Health Hazard Evaluation Board in March 1990 issued the following statement:

> The risk of contracting EMS due to the consumption of any dietary L-tryptophan product far outweighs any perceived benefit that may be derived from continuing marketing of this product in any dosage form. (Lecos, 1990)

This led the FDA in March 1990 to ban the general importation and marketing of manufactured LTP and supplements containing it. However, an exception exists for material intended for use in an exempt category, as an additive for foods, in the use of which no case of EMS has appeared. In addition, shipments may be considered for release at the request of a licensed physician.

The EMS epidemic was traced to batches of LTP that were produced by one Japanese chemical company, because in 95 percent of all cases of the illnesses the patient had consumed a product using this company's manufactured LTP. After much chemical sleuthing, EMS was tentatively attributed to a low-level contaminant in the incriminated LTP. The contaminant was dubbed "peak X," as its structure was quite difficult to determine. Manufacturing changes seemed to have allowed this toxic agent to appear in batches produced subsequent to an alteration of methods. Peak X evidently served as a trigger for an immune system reaction that treats normal body cells as if they were foreign ones. However, many people who consumed LTP from the incriminated source did not develop EMS, and some cases of EMS (and a related disease, eosinophilic fascitis) occurred before and after the 1989 epidemic. Animal studies in an inbred strain of laboratory rat showed that treatment with LTP and Peak X resulted in some, but not all, of the pathologic effects seen with EMS. In addition, some pathologic changes were seen in rats treated with LTP that was free of peak X. Thus, the situation remains rather confused and uncertain.

THE SEQUEL: 5-HYDROXY-L-TRYPTOPHAN

A few years later, however, supplements consisting of a close relative to LTP, 5HTP or 5-hydroxy-L-tryptophan, were marketed and heavily promoted for a wide range of problems despite that a few scattered cases of what appeared to be EMS were reported for people taking 5HTP in the 1980s. In 1994, a group led by Esther Sternberg of the National Institute of Mental Health (Sternberg, 1996) identified peak X also as being a contaminant in a particular batch of 5HTP that had been associated in 1991 with the development of EMS in one Canadian user. Although a few other cases of EMS have been reported in people who have taken 5HTP, the Canadian case was the first in which the suspected contaminant has been identified. Although it is widely believed that impurities in the LTP were the cause for EMS, some researchers have suggested a role for "pure" tryptophan itself, or for certain susceptibility factors of the persons so affected as being very crucial. Thus, it is not entirely certain that EMS was simply a result of exposure to a single source of L-tryptophan, and that other sources are safe. Similarly, for 5HTP the situation is complex and unclear in that it is produced entirely differently, from fermentation of an African bean.

Further detection of a contaminant similar or the same as Peak X was reported in September 1998 by Mayo Clinic researchers (Williamson et al., 1998). They demonstrated low levels of peak X, which they believe consists of a group of nearly identical molecules, from off-the-shelf bottles of 5HTP that had been bought at health and nutrition stores in New York City and Rochester, Minnesota. Six brands of 5HTP were analyzed by mass spectrometry, which can yield detailed information from extremely small amounts of the compounds. All six brands contained peak X in quantities that ranged from 2.9 percent to 14.1 percent of the level that were associated with the disease in the Canadian woman. Although those amounts may seem small, the authors stated that a real possibility existed that a person could ingest a sufficient quantity of the contaminated 5HTP to obtain a potentially harmful amount of peak X. "It's ludicrous to think that something is safe just because it is 'naturally derived,' some of the most toxic substances known to humans are naturally derived" (Williamson et al., 1998).

In August of 1998 the FDA, based on the Mayo research, confirmed the presence of impurities in some 5HTP products then being marketed. Contaminated samples included both those produced by biosynthetic means and those described as being produced naturally from seed extracts. Since that report some 5HTP packages began to declare their product to be free of peak X. People who are taking 5HTP, or who are thinking about taking it, should know that there *may be* potential health risks associated with it, and that it would be more likely as doses increase. Other analyses have declared 5-HTP to be free of significant contamination as by peak X (Das et al., 2004). Physicians and other health care practitioners have been called upon to report any adverse events associated with 5HTP, but apparently no subsequent wave of illnesses was identified. Uncertainty again!

Both L-tryptophan and 5HTP act as precursors of serotonin, which as a brain neurotransmitter is involved in mood, sleep, appetite, and other functions. Marketers of 5HTP supplements have described it as a "safe" and "natural" alternative to LTP, claiming that it improves headaches, insomnia, obesity, depression, anxiety, and other conditions. These benefits are poorly documented by scientifically valid clinical trials. Concern exists especially because one book currently on the market recommends a dose of 300 to 900 milligrams of 5HTP daily. At that dosage level, exposure to peak X could possibly equal the level of the Canadian case if the product were to contain similar quantities of peak X to those found in the Mayo study. However, subsequent research has failed to agree that such a problem exists for currently marketed 5HTP products.

Another Potential Hazard from 5-HTP?

However, another, quite different hazard of L-TP exists that is also a liability of 5HTP usage, which is the production of a toxic response known as serotonin syndrome because it arises from an excess of 5HT in the brain. This adverse reaction was reported a number of times in the 1980s for persons who took LTP in conjunction with antidepressant drugs of the class known as MAOIs or monoamine oxidase inhibitors. These pioneer antidepressants are now seldom prescribed, but they still find utility for a select few psychiatric patients. The enzyme inhibition allows an accumulation and an enhanced action of serotonin not only in the brain but also in the intestine and circulatory system. By its action as a precursor to promote greater synthesis of serotonin, LTP would amplify an MAOI effect. Within suitable limits this might aid the attaining of a therapeutic response. However, an accumulation of serotonin to excess is what occurs in the serotonin syndrome, which carries a significant mortality risk and can be difficult for an emergency physician to diagnose.

Clearly it is a more risky situation when a person self-treats with a nutritional supplement and may not tell the physician who is prescribing antidepressant medicines. Because of its chemistry being a step closer to serotonin, an even greater risk would seem to be that serotonin syndrome could occur from use of 5HTP with an MAOI. Moreover, a possibility for an adverse interaction between 5HTP and an herbal supplement that has MAOI activity could exist, such as occurs for extracts of *Ginkgo biloba* leaves. Concurrent self-medication with both 5HTP and a gingko product seems to be a likely scenario that is ill-advised.

Incidentally, the supplement SAMe (S-adenosylmethionine) has been indicated as another biochemical besides LTP and 5HTP that can be a cause for the serotonin syndrome. Although a considerable number of cases of serotonin syndrome have been reported, few have been recognized and reported as involving supplements—not what one could call an epidemic, but something to be conscious of nonetheless.

The Other Side of the Coin

A nutrient formula can be subject to errors leading to adulteration, but it can also be dangerous if lacking what it should supply. A tragic example of that played out in news bulletins from Israel in fall 2003 (AHK Israel Newsletter, 2004). An illness identified as severe thiamine deficiency in 17 babies left three dead and caused neurological and other problems in the others. The German manufacturer of infant formula admitted that a kosher, soy-based product it sold in Israel was missing the vitamin ingredient required to sustain infant life. Tests showed that the product contained between 29 and 37 micrograms of vitamin B_1 per 100 grams, less than one-tenth of the product's declared level of 385 micrograms per 100 grams of prepared food.

The manufacturer (Humana Milchunion Everswinkel) fired four executive employees because of mistakes in the production of the infant food formula sold in Israel. Losing their jobs were the head of product development and the directors of the quality control unit and chemical laboratory. The first mistake occurred during product development on a new soy-based formula. The team responsible for development misinterpreted some analytical data with the result that vitamin B_1 was not added as it should have been.

This meant that the milk-alternative product contained only 10 percent as much thiamine as was stated on the label. A second error occurred in the quality control section when outside analytical data on the new product came back without a measure of the vitamin content. However, the scientific staff of Humana Milchunion accepted the product analysis as being complete. The third mistake occurred when it was noticed by chance that the data on vitamins were indeed missing. A query communicated to the analytical laboratory confirmed that no tests were done on vitamins at all. The appropriate intervention did not follow, so the defective formula was exported. Although some infants must be fed an infant formula, the view that "the breast is best" seems to be highly supported by this incident.

Chapter 31

Miracles Promised, Not Delivered: False Hopes, Failed Hopes

> The law of things is that they who tamper with veracity, from whatever motive, are tampering with the vital force of human progress.
>
> John Morley
> British statesman and writer

> A few observation and much reasoning lead to error; many observations and a little reasoning to truth.
>
> Alexis Carrel
> Nobel laureate in Physiology or Medicine

Using self-chosen remedies for some aspects of health care truly may have a rational and justifiable basis. Examples of this include many conditions that have long been the subject of autotherapy in the United States, e.g., symptomatic management of common colds and upper-respiratory tract allergies, "simple" nonvascular headaches, short-term digestive tract upsets, musculoskeletal pain, and mild to moderate skin irritations and injuries. However, other, more severe health problems exist for which modern medicine has answers, and for which neglecting to utilize those options becomes foolhardy and irrational. When purveyors of dietary supplements or other alternative therapies advocate unproven materials as "reasonable alternatives" for certain ailments, a rational view requires one to look the other way. Use of such as complementary to conventional therapy may bear less risk, so long as the unconventional does not act at cross-purposes to the conventional medication. Unfortunately, available data at present are generally inadequate to exclude the risk of an adverse interaction.

What are some conditions for which an alternative therapy might be hazardous from its depriving a person of a likely effective conventional

Consumer's Guide to Dietary Supplements and Alternative Medicines

doi:10.1300/5698_31

therapy? Prime examples would include severe infections, diabetes, asthma, hypertension, epilepsy, and Parkinson's disease. Surely for millions of people around the world the costs of modern medicines to treat such conditions make the medicines unavailable. Those people may by necessity resort to and depend upon traditional remedies of uncertain efficacy compared to modern medicines. But for citizens of a Western society to be encouraged or even solicited to choose an unproven remedy over scientifically proven pharmacotherapies is inappropriate. To notice that solicitation happening is distressing to behold.

Extreme claims for some alternative remedies have been responsible for evoking an attitude of total disbelief toward all alternative remedies in the minds of many medical practitioners and researchers involved in medical science. Numerous authors have called the exuberant claims for some supplements by the contemporary promoters the equal of those by nineteenth-century snake oil vendors. Loss of much credibility is a natural result of many highly questionable claims that clearly are aimed at the most gullible individuals whose desire for high promises is greater than their capacity for discernment. Some outrageous verbatim examples include the following:

- Sexual Function and Potency 100 percent Restored!
- Prostate Problems Eliminated!
- The First Formula That Regenerates the Beta Cells of the Pancreas and Insulin Output for Diabetics
- The Natural Age Eraser—Rejuvenates Every Cell in Your Body!
- Remedy That Cures Heart Disease and Stroke
- Say Goodbye to Allergies! Reprogram Your Body's Immune System!
- Astonishing Cancer-fighting Discovery
- Lose Weight Permanently Without Even Trying
- Do-it-yourself Thyroid Cure
- Alternatives You Can Use Now to Prevent Alzheimer's
- Flu Gone like Magic
- Solved—the Secret Mystery of Aging!
- Renews the Cells That Line Your Arteries and Maintain Flexibility
- Lose Inches of Fat in 48 Hours or Less

Some would conclude that the authors of such claims must rely on their readers being totally ignorant of science for their acceptance. Indeed, many scientists are quite concerned about the widespread scientific illiteracy of the U.S. population. However, some observers would blame the scientists themselves for cultivating gullibility and a "gee whiz, what will they discover next?" attitude by virtue of their frequently premature and overblown press releases concerning research findings from biomedical laboratories. These communications serve more to satisfy the scientist's ego than to communicate true, useful information to the nonscientist public.

SOME MIRACLE CURES EXAMINED

A book having the bold title *Miracle Cures* by Jean Carper (1997) is worthy of consideration to illustrate the rhetorical excesses that exist in the literature advocating natural remedies. The section following this paragraph identifies the agents described in this source and summarizes their supposedly "miraculous" benefits. Even at the best possible outcomes their benefits would mostly warrant only "marvelous" rather than "miraculous." The subtitle of the book includes a phrase, "the healing power of herbs," which clearly raises undue hopes. Healing implies a benefit lasting after the remedy is no longer taken. The one agent of all these that is actually represented so to act is bee pollen, which is said to cause a person's lifelong allergic reactions to cease and disappear, according to a testimonial. It is not made clear and obvious that claimed benefits are only for temporary relief of symptoms while the remedy is being used. Despite this temporary benefit, many authors advocating supplements deride the Rx pharmaceuticals for their inadequacy in not giving a lasting cure, contrasted to supposedly curative natural therapies. One of the most impossible to justify claims is seen in calling fish oils containing the omega-3 fatty acids a *universal* miracle cure.

Documenting Support for These Claims of "Cures"

To give due credit, Ms. Jean Carper (1997) provided extensive medical literature citations backing the avowed benefits she describes in this book. However, this is a proper time to proclaim the principle that all literature references are not created equal. Some of her citations do indeed on their face appear likely to provide valid evidence in support of the claim for health value of the material discussed; however, a good many others are not from recognizable, familiar journal sources, which indicates a probability that no more than an abstract was available for evaluation by the writer. A title and an abstract seldom provide sufficient grounds for accepting the point of the article as having been rightly tested and confirmed.

PubMed is a service of the U.S. National Library of Medicine (NLM) available to the public via the Internet that includes more than 14 million citations to biomedical articles dating back commonly to 1966, and in a lesser degree to the 1950s.

As was discussed in Chapters 2 and 3, it is important what sort of test design was utilized in a medical investigation. Outside of medical journal publications from western Europe and North America, clinical studies that employ randomization with placebo controls and double-blind conditions have been a rarity until quite recently. This history has left a negative bias in the minds of many scientists in medical and biomedical research that may no longer be fully warranted. To be realistic, those journal articles not published in journals known and respected for having a careful (if not zealous) prepublication review will be little recognized. Their contents will not carry as much weight as do journals with reputation for meeting those measures.

Sad to say, altogether too many instances of papers appearing even in highly respected journals have involved fabrication of data and other fraudulent behaviors that passed reviews and were published. Such incidents serve to further reinforce the skepticism toward material published in "lesser" journals, and even more so to the presentation of unformalized observations in channels that are assumed not to exert stringent criteria for acceptance. It is recognized widely among medical/biomedical scientists that a manuscript rejected by several high-ranking journals may ultimately see publication in a lesser or even little-known and obscure outlet. Rarely is a particular work shown after passage of time to have merited publication in a "higher" journal by which it was rejected. However, these few exceptions do not prove that many or most items seen in a "lesser" journal all are meritorious. Exceptions do not prove *that* rule!

SELF-CHOSEN THERAPIES FOR DIABETES

How should one regard the promotion of self-chosen therapies for diabetes? Perhaps as "preying on the gullibility of the public"? Certainly an accusation of irresponsible advertising would seem to be warranted. Does misleading advertising have a potential for harm to those who "fall for it"? That would depend upon the condition involved. For example, a person who relies on alternative remedies for treating insulin-dependent (type 1) diabetes mellitus (IDDM), much less his or her believing that the remedy would totally remove its cause, is likely to be endangering their health and possibly shortening their life. This assumes that they would otherwise be able to obtain the needed insulin therapy. In some recorded instances such claims have misled diabetic persons into discontinuing insulin therapy for the promised benefits of an oral remedy that avoids noxious injections.

Insulin treatment for diabetes can block its adverse metabolic impact. Admittedly, optimal treatment is onerous, often requiring multiple daily checks of the glucose level of one's blood as well as several daily insulin injections. Both of these are a literal cause for pain. Many recent advances have been made toward insulin preparations that improve the control of blood glucose, and even some advances have been made toward alternative administration besides injection. The possibility now exists for noninvasive analysis of blood glucose, but the expense of such an instrument will prevent many patients from taking advantage of it to avoid pricking their finger for blood samples. It is certainly understandable that a diabetic or a parent of a diabetic child would hope for a once-and-for-all solution as is promised by some supplement claims. To offer such a hope without thorough and unquestionable verification is a highly unethical and dangerous behavior that could warrant being called predatory. It certainly seems to take advantage of persons who may have heard forecasts that gene therapy or stem cell therapy may *one day* indeed accomplish such a curative action. However, that day surely has not yet arrived.

The Chinese herbal potions for oral treatment of diabetes, which have found their way into the United States (Chapter 28), are a threat to any who might put their trust in them. Such products' inadequacy as a substitute for insulin is compounded when their true composition may include an orally active hypoglycemic agent pirated from a drug company, as has been observed at times. Those hypoglycemic agents can be effective only for the adult-onset, type 2 diabetes (non-insulin-dependent diabetes mellitus, or NIDDM).[1]

However, a list of remedies promoted by a "wellness company" named Flourish added one for diabetes. Its claimed features cannot be endorsed in any degree. Unfortunately, testimonials rather than clinical trial data are offered to convince the reader of the product's value. This is not to deny the components' having actions that may be relevant to diabetes, but rather to insist that diabetes therapy is too critical to health and life for using remedies unproven by appropriate clinical research.

PART VI: The Future of Dietary Supplements

The major limitation of alternative medicine is that it is based on theory, hearsay, and hope, but not fact. The "scientific" studies that support many alternative therapies are observational and do not stand up to scientific rigor . . . Alternative medicine is seductive, however, in that it promises empowerment of the individual, an approach that is even more attractive as our health care systems become more expensive, more technological, and more impersonal . . . Prevention is too important not to be under the auspices of the scientific medical profession.

Gordon A. Ewy, MD (1999)

A senior executive with Britain's biggest drugs company has admitted that most prescription medicines do not work on most people who take them. Allen Roses, worldwide vice-president of genetics at Glaxo SmithKline, said fewer than half of the patients prescribed some of the most expensive drugs actually derived any benefit from them. It is an open secret within the drugs industry that most of its products are ineffective in most patients, but this is the first time that such a senior drugs boss has gone public.

Steve Connor (2003)

Chapter 32

Accreditation, Validation, Standardization, Assimilation, and Attrition

Never make forecasts, especially about the future.

Samuel Goldwyn
Hollywood movie producer

Natural medicine, therapeutic practices that avoid using synthetic pharmaceuticals whenever a natural product is available as an alternative, was a remarkable mushrooming phenomenon in the last decades of the twentieth century. Although it does not comprise all of CAM, it is surely a major component. The question of where we go from here is an important one. Some of that natural medicine is self-prescribed, but MDs (or DOs) who embrace a holistic or natural practice model are becoming more commonplace. Of course, naturopathic physicians (NDs) are an increasingly significant part of the picture. Some natural physicians have the same motivation as many consumers, that of looking to natural agents as being less toxic and thus a less risky mode of therapy.

If adequate efficacy were to be established for many CAM remedies it would surely provide great impetus to this trend. The outcomes of the NCCAM-sponsored projects described later in this chapter could contribute greatly to answering the uncertainties about efficacy that prevail all too broadly at present. However, many are preliminary investigations of the phases I and II varieties, whereas phase III testing would be more fruitful in obtaining such answers.

VALIDATION OF DIETARY SUPPLEMENTS' THERAPEUTIC ABILITIES

Because of the paucity of clinical trials in support of the efficacy and safety of many widely used dietary supplements the federal government has

Consumer's Guide to Dietary Supplements and Alternative Medicines

doi:10.1300/5698_32

begun a testing program through the NCCAM of NIH. Table 32.1 provides a summary of such clinical research on supplements as of July 10, 2003, to illustrate topics being pursued; some having passed their completion date (See www.nccam.nih.gov/clinicaltrials/treatmenttherapy.htm).

In 2004 the National Institute On Aging initiated a multicenter trial on the ability to improve patients with Alzheimer's disease by use of huperzine A, a natural moss extract used in used in China to treat Alzheimer's disease (AD). Researchers will conduct a Phase II study to test whether huperzine A slows or prevents Alzheimer's symptoms in patients showing mild-to-moderate disease effects (www.clinicaltrials.gov/show/NCT/00083590). The project was enrolling patients who could no tolerate commonly used Alzheimer's drugs such as Aricept, even though huperzine A may act similarly by blocking the enzyme that breaks down the neurotransmitter acetylcholine in the brain. Raj Shah, MD, principal investigator at the Rush University Medical Center study site (www.rush.edu/webapps/MEDREV/servlet/NewsRelease?ID=583) believes that huperzine A may provide benefits to AD patients similar to those derived from antioxidants such as Vitamin E in addition to sparing the levels of acetylcholine. Phase III-type studies in China have shown that the efficacy of huperzine A may be comparable to that of currently approved drugs for Alzheimer's while reducing the severe side effects, such as gastrointestinal upset, that are commonly seen with established Alzheimer's medications.

In light of these and more efforts yet to occur, it should be noted that the alternative to a successful validation of these supplements is a failure to validate. Rightly, the latter outcome should put a quietus to remedies that fall short; in such instances should include *attrition,* such as the stamp of "unworthy" appropriately being wielded by a federal agency other than the FDA. On the other hand, if worthiness is to be demonstrated in some proportion of the investigations, *assimilation* of those agents into mainline medical usage should occur. Most practitioners among those oriented to natural medicine will suspect that this process will not thrive because of the implicit or explicit opposition of "Big Pharma" toward competition from alternative therapies. Won't it be interesting to see what transpires?

MORE THOUGHTS ON VALIDATION

Evidence-Based Medicine versus Dietary Supplements As CAM

The trend of recent decades in medicine toward evidence-based therapeutics has brought conflict with various CAM therapies. This is seen in no

TABLE 32.1. Natural agents undergoing human research with NCCAM support

Test agent	Research objective(s)
Alpha-lipoic acid	For immune restoration in AIDS patients; test for treatment of multiple sclerosis (along with essential fatty acids).
Black cohosh	For reduction of menopausal hot flashes, osteoporosis, or memory and other cognitive problems.
Borage oil	As a nontoxic alternative against bronchial inflammation in asthma.
Chamomile tea	Relief of abdominal pain of functional bowel disorders in children.
Chondroitin	Test if chondroitin, glucosamine, and/or their combination are more active than placebo, and if the combination is more effective than the components alone in treating knee pain experienced with osteoarthritis.
Creatine	Test safety and tolerability in patients with Huntington's disease, and collect data on how it impacts disease symptoms and progression.
Echinacea	For the prevention of acute otitis media in children with recurrent otitis media; assess efficacy for prevention or treatment of the common cold; test against upper respiratory infections in childhood.
Essential fatty acids	For potential therapy in multiple sclerosis patients.
Flaxseed	Test its safety and efficacy in reducing excessive blood cholesterol levels.
Garlic	For lowering cholesterol or triglycerides in HIV-infected persons.
Ginkgo biloba	For action against the insulin resistance via alteration of efficacy of three classes of antidiabetic drugs (Actose, Glucotrol, Glucophage); for benefit to patients with intermittent claudication of peripheral vascular disease; as an alternative therapy (with dietary borage oil) for opposing bronchial changes in patients with asthma; for treatment of multiple sclerosis; for changes in pharmacokinetics of probe drugs and enzymes implicated in chemoprevention of cancer; effect of *Ginkgo biloba,* sex therapy, or their joint use on subjective and physiological measures of sexual function in women who experience sexual disorders secondary to antidepressants; to determine ability to decrease the incidence of Alzheimer's disease, to slow cognitive decline and disability, or to reduce cardiovascular disease and decrease total mortality.

TABLE 32.1. *(continued)*

Test agent	Research objective(s)
Ginseng	Test for effects on pharmacokinetic disposition of probe drugs, on cognitive function, and on enzymes that are implicated in chemoprevention of cancer; test for an ability to reverse the impacts of bacterial and psychosocial stressors as a means for improving the management of periodontitis.
Glucosamine	As for CHONDROITIN.
"Herbs"	Testing beta-carotene, vitamin C, zinc, flavonoids, primrose oil, echinacea, golden seal, and licorice for treating children with recurrent otitis media.
L-carnitine	Test whether it can oppose fatigue in terminal cancer patients.
Lutein	Determine safety and effective dose of lutein for therapy in retinitis pigmentosa.
Magnesium	Test the effect of oral Mg supplement on clinical markers of asthma, biomarkers of inflammation, bronchial hyperreactivity, and indices of oxidative defense or damage in persistent mild-to-moderate asthma; a component of naturopathic connective tissue nutrient formula for management of periodontitis.
Milk thistle	Assess silymarin derived from milk thistle in preventing or reversing complications of chronic hepatitis C virus infection or clearing hepatitis C infection.
Mistletoe	Test antineoplastic activity in persons with inoperable or metastatic breast, pancreatic, colorectal, or lung cancer.
Noni	Find maximum tolerated dose of noni fruit extract, define toxicities by mouth, get preliminary data on efficacy for anti-tumor and symptom-control properties in cancer patients; identify constituents of the extract useful to characterize the bioavailability and pharmacokinetic properties of food supplement products.
NPI-028 (a Chinese herbal medicine)	Manage withdrawal and prevent relapse in persons diagnosed with alcoholism.
Omega-3 fatty acids	Compare prophylactic efficacy vs. placebo in bipolar I patients.
Pancreatic enzyme therapy	Phase III trial comparing gemcitabine with pancreatic enzyme therapy plus specialized diet (Gonzalez regimen) in patients who have stage II, III, or IV pancreatic cancer.

Test agent	Research objective(s)
Phytoestrogens	Test natural sources of estrogenic substances for preventing metabolic changes leading to bone loss after menopause; determine if soy phytoestrogens taken as supplements improve memory in women who have early memory decline.
Red clover	Assess reduction of menopausal and postmenopausal symptoms (includes memory and cognition problems) in healthy menopausal-postmenopausal women.
Saw palmetto	Test an extract of the plant for relief of benign prostatic hyperplasia.
Selenium	Test for potential (along with vitamin E) as a therapy for multiple sclerosis.
Shark cartilage	Phase III test of the efficacy of chemotherapy plus radiation with or without shark cartilage to treat patients having inoperable stage III non-small-cell lung cancer; a randomized phase III trial testing the efficacy of shark cartilage in patients with advanced colorectal or breast cancer.
Siliphos (oral silybin-phosphatidylcholine phytosome)	Test safety and tolerability of 3 doses in patients with hepatitis C not responding to or who are poor candidates for interferon.
Soy isoflavones	Dietary intervention in hemodialysis (kidney failure) patients to test possible clinical-metabolic effects on disease, e.g., reduction of blood markers for inflammation and for metabolic bone disease.
St. John's wort	Test efficacy and safety in comparison with citalopram (Celexa) and placebo in minor depression; compare to placebo in treating outpatients with obsessive compulsive disorder; determine efficacy versus placebo in treating social phobia; test for alteration of oral contraceptive efficacy in terms of risk of ovulation while taking an oral contraceptive before or with St. John's Wort; assess potential adverse interaction (to lower efficacy) with two pain medications, oxycodone and fentanyl; detect herb-drug interactions in human volunteers receiving one dose of the Rx drug alprazolam and the OTC cough suppressant dextromethorphan on two occasions before and during SJW for 2 weeks.
Traditional Chinese medicine	Evaluate holistic treatment of temporomandibular joint disorders (often associated with depression, anxiety, sleep disturbances, alimentary tract symptoms, frequent infections, etc.) via three different approaches, naturopathic medicine, traditional Chinese medicine, and usual conventional care.

TABLE 32.1. *(continued)*

Test agent	Research objective(s)
Vitamin C	Test effects of oral vitamin C on insulin sensitivity and vascular reactivity in persons with type 2 diabetes.
Vitamin E	For reducing the progression of carotid atherosclerosis in persons with coronary artery disease; for action (with selenium) against multiple sclerosis.

area more clearly than for treatments hypothesized to oppose various adverse states correlated to aging. Clinical trials are difficult and expensive when oriented toward even short-term efficacy of a new medication. Obtaining human data to provide scientific validation for a treatment that would extend life span and/or improve health through old age would require such complex research designs and lengthy intervals of study that the expenses would likely be of overwhelming magnitude. Thus, it seems improbable that clinical research will ever happen to validate many of the dietary supplement treatments that have been proposed to oppose aging and improve health in old age.

Much more circumscribed research objectives, e.g., treatment of a particular disease of old age, such as Alzheimer's disease, are within the realm of possibility as pharmaceutical-development projects, and are currently ongoing. These must produce a patentable product for the industry to invest the many millions of dollars required to develop and market a new drug. Thus, it is significant that a variety of substances that are now being touted as extenders of good health into older years of life are by their nature unpatentable. This means that little or no economic motivation exists for research that *might* validate benefits or prove the long-term safety of such dietary supplements. In light of these considerations, we face a situation in which claims for benefits from certain diets, natural metabolites, enzymes, herbs, food factors, and hormones against the ravages of aging will continue unabated but also untested.

Thus, a discussion of "the marketplace" of agents for aging and its problems cannot now be, and will not in the foreseeable future become, truly "evidence-based." The best to hope for is availability of relevant laboratory animal data, but these too are lacking in many instances. In this situation a physician or pharmacist can only advise the enquirer that the use of many such agents is at the user's own risk, a calculated gamble as to whether any return for the cost will be entailed. Although many products may seem on the face of it to be safe, no assurance can be given of this when long-term use is likely at levels of intake for which there is little or no foundation of evidence.

ACCREDITATION: WHO IS LOOKING AFTER JOHN/JANE Q. PUBLIC?

If the FDA is not monitoring the reliability of supposed contents of food supplement products (as we've seen in Chapter 8), and the producers' labels are commonly found to be unreliable, to whom can the consumer turn for help? A few answers to this question have been emerging. However, they are all based on voluntary submission to a validation and certification process. Unless or until a sufficiently strong financial incentive exists, such voluntarism seems unlikely to gain more than a minority participation. Consumer pressure must function to encourage the broad acceptance of a certification process for this approach to achieve the needed upgrade of the quality control standards in the supplement manufacturing industry.

ConsumerLab Product Validation Program

The first source of analytical findings to appear outside the technical publication literature is provided to consumers by an Internet-based analytical service known as ConsumerLab. This organization was founded to supply a validation program for dietary supplements. As their analytical data are copyrighted proprietary information, we cannot cite directly their reports of analytical findings. However, their data are similar to those described in Chapter 10 supporting the conclusion that all products supposedly providing the same biochemical ingredient(s) are not created equal when it comes to dietary supplements. The reader may consult the ConsumerLab program's general outcomes for no cost, and detailed data on a brand-name basis are provided on a fee-for-subscription basis also via this Web site: http://www.consumerlab.com/index.asp.

The United States Pharmacopoeia (USP)

In January 2002 the USP Convention announced their launching of a verification program for dietary supplements. The USP offers a seal or "mark of approval" to denote products marketed by qualifying manufacturers for the information of retail vendors, health care practitioners, and consumers. Qualifying for the mark will assure the consumer that a supplement has passed five important quality tests under USP's Dietary Supplement Verification Program. It means that the supplement does the following:

- Contains the ingredients listed on the label
- Has the declared amount and strength of ingredients
- Will break down easily in stomach fluids so the body can effectively absorb the nutrients in the supplement
- Has been screened for harmful contaminants such as heavy metals, microbes, and pesticides
- Has been manufactured in safe, sanitary, and controlled conditions

In order to qualify, a manufacturer will be required to sign a licensing agreement with the USP Convention and to supply documentation of their quality assurance standards and processes for each product to be certified, showing that they are in compliance with published standards. After certification is granted all products will be subject to random, off-the-shelf sampling and analysis to make sure that the criteria of quality are being maintained.

NSF International Certified

A separate development to promote certification has been launched by an alliance of two groups, the National Nutritional Foods Association (NNFA) and National Sanitation Foundation International (NSFI), which is a not-for-profit organization known for the development of standards, product testing, and certification services in public health and safety and environmental protection. Based upon NNFA's GMP (good manufacturing practices) standards and audits, NSFI will review and approve qualifying applicants. Upon approval, the product may bear a seal, "NSF Independently Certified," which indicates verification of contaminant testing, manufacturing consistency/accuracy, validation of labeled quantity of ingredients, absence of undeclared ingredients, and a demonstrated conformity with industrial GMPs for dietary supplements.

FDA-Initiated GMPs

The DSHEA legislation spoke of good manufacturing practices regulations to be promulgated by FDA over the production of dietary supplements. This assignment was neglected and failed to be carried forward for nearly nine years. In March 2003 the FDA issued a set of proposed GMP regulations with a call for public (i.e., industry) comments. As of September 2004 about 1,500 pages of "substantive" comments (protests) were received to which the agency needed to prepare its responses. Some hope, but no assurances, of finalizing the process before 2005 existed. Whenever the promised GMPs should indeed be put into effect, the question would shift to obtaining compliance. It seems likely that more companies that have a more conscientious leadership will "do what is right." On the other hand, it seems likely that less conscientious ones will attempt to delay and evade new restrictions. The FDA's bringing a vigorous action against some of the latter, to demonstrate early on that the agency intends to ensure compliance with the regulations, would seem to be needful.

Scientists Collaborate for Greater Quality-Assurance in Supplement Products

The AOAC International, the Association of Official Analytical Chemists is a scientific organization that is seeking to push forward with efforts toward science-based characterization of nonnutrient dietary supplements. This group represents the scientists in industry, government, and academia who are the source of new methods for standardization of various chemical products. Their attention to the matter of raising the standardization and quality standards for botanicals is a welcome development. Their Web site on the subject points out that,

> Unfair competition is a major concern in the dietary supplements industry. Reputable manufacturers who pride themselves on quality must compete with those whose products may not meet label claims. In order to level the playing field, validated methods are needed for quality assurance, regulation, safety and efficacy testing, and building public confidence. (www.aoac.org/ILM/level_field.htm)

Work progressing toward these goals will be helpful to the consumer as well as to the supplier of supplements.

Summary

Optimistically speaking, a movement toward providing consumers with a basis for judging whether or not a particular product can be trusted to be what it is labeled to be is now occurring. However, the pessimistic view is that, despite these options for voluntary standardization and certification, response from the whole supplement producing industry will not be adequate. Until the FDA requires that the long-delayed good manufacturing practice standards be met, voluntary approaches are the only protective resources for consumers. Industry-based self-regulation has been discussed, but without enforcement mechanisms any voluntary approach to quality control can and will be ignored by the unscrupulous few.

AN ALTERNATIVE ROUTE FOR ALTERNATIVE REMEDIES

The question may be put forth, "must the U.S. citizenry continue to tolerate the current situation? Cannot a modification be made to the DSHEA legislation that would constitute an improvement over the prevailing situation?" Indeed, the late Professor Varro Tyler, one of the twentieth century's leading experts on herbal medicines urged that the United States begin regulating herbal products much the way Germany does (Tyler, 1993). There, a "reasonable" level of evidence is accepted as efficacy for plant-based medications. These products are an integral part of mainstream medicine, distributed as a special OTC class or, where indicated, as prescription drugs. He advocated that satisfactory evidence for the efficacy of each herb could be obtained through two well-designed, placebo-controlled studies—costing at most a few million dollars instead of hundreds of millions.

Efforts from the supplement industry, via its various supporters, are being made to mobilize a public outcry against the prospect of legislative that would move toward stiffening of quality control aspects of DSHEA. This stems from a fear that the FDA would add substantial restrictions to the availability of supplements compared to their prevailing status. A paranoid outlook exists toward any FDA action based upon some past history and upon a fixed view that the FDA is a servant of "Big Pharma," and toward the pharmaceutical industry's behind-the-scenes promoting actions that would reduce competition from supplements for the U.S. public's health dollars. This paranoia is fueled by the 2004 action by FDA against ephedra-containing products.

Reintegration via Integrative Medicine?

Integrative medicine may be seen as a merging of two (formerly and still) conflicting beliefs or philosophies. Some of those viewing from inside conventional medicine see a merger as occurring when those CAM therapies that "prove out" (i.e., are found to be validated by the standards of evidenced-based medicine) are accepted into conventional or mainline medical practice. Those who are stoutly entrenched in the unconventional CAM camp likely feel that no organic reunion will occur because of the estrangement by philosophical differences that they have experienced, along with years of denigration of what they see as their innovative approaches to health care practice. For example, members of the 30-year-old ACAM (American College for Advancement of Medicine) have gone their way without leave from mainline medicine and likely will continue to do so regardless of whatever "enlightenment" may be entering the curricula and clinical services of medical colleges and cancer centers.

It is noteworthy that an organization known as the International College of Integrative Medicine has formed and is operating to provide educational short-courses in conjunction with scientific meetings that resemble those of ACAM topicwise more than those of the AMA (American Medical Association. Healing the breach between these conventional and unconventional wings of medical practice probably will require the advent of another generation of physicians "brought up" to have more respect and acceptance toward CAM and natural medicine.

LEGISLATION REQUIRING STANDARDIZATION

Congressional Action for Change?

An official statement from the American Society for Pharmacology and Experimental Therapeutics in the context of the ephedra controversy called for a major change to cause dietary supplements no longer to go unregulated. A most practical step that was suggested would be to require monitoring by a product's marketer of the occurrence of adverse events and the reporting of such events to the FDA. Despite the congressional hearings associated with the ephedra tumult, it seems likely that nothing significant will ensue in terms of legislation. The U.S. Congress seems incapable of dealing with such controversial topics as alteration of DSHEA when it cannot handle matters of much more weighty consequence. Thus, substantive changes cannot be foreseen unless or until a major disaster—a catastrophic, scene-changing event of the sort seen in 1938 following a toxic disaster from "sulfanilamide elixir" that brought legislation for an enlarged role of the FDA in drug-safety regulations—occurs. Another case was the 1962 changes precipitated by the thalidomide disaster in western Europe.

Voices from the natural medicine contingent were raised against legislative responses to the ephedra controversy with the anticipation that it would be a broad-scale change covering a whole spectrum of dietary ingredients so as to destroy the DSHEA exemption for supplements by bringing them under the prior-review status of drugs. The issues heightened by the ephedra problem were somewhat muted by the early 2004 action of the FDA to declare a ban on ephedra-containing products. However, a U.S. Senate subcommittee held a hearing in summer 2004 at which strong disfavor was expressed at the long delay of positive action by the FDA to provide better consumer protection.

GLOBALIZATION EFFECTS ON THE DIETARY SUPPLEMENT SCENE

A major factor that might precipitate changes to DSHEA could come from abroad. A United Nations (UN) movement toward a set of internationally-uniform guidelines, Codex Alimentarius, exists for growing and producing, processing, labeling, and trading in food materials. Its goal is for improving consumer safety and for improving fairness of trade practice with respect to foods. The project stems from the World Health Organization (WHO), and the program would be binding upon all UN and WHO signatory nations. Such international regulations as should be issued would apply also to dietary supplements in the United States as long as they are classified under our system as foods rather than drugs. This contrasts with some countries in which botanicals are and long have been treated as prescription drugs; thus, they would not be affected.

The currently proposed Codex Alimentarius Guidelines for Vitamins and Mineral Supplements would establish maximum ceilings on potency. It is not clear how this would be applied to metabolites or botanicals. However, this restriction is being perceived as potentially hindering the currently existing practice of natural/nutritional medicine. The seriousness is not obvious to an outsider if it were to affect only vitamins and minerals, for which daily needs are defined. The protests being voiced suggest that it would have a revolutionary influence.

Chapter 33

Would You Bet Your Life on Good Advice?

> . . . a consistently higher intake of fruits, vegetables, whole grains and plant proteins such as soy—in comparison with the typical American diet—is associated with a markedly reduced risk of cancer, heart disease and some chronic diseases of ageing.
>
> David Heber, MD, PhD (2004)

Life is full of risks and gambles. In the summer of 2002 across the eastern half of the United States a major outbreak of an invasive new viral encephalitis occurred. Borne to its human victim by a seemingly unimportant mosquito bite, it put a different light on outdoor activities. One older gentleman in Louisiana was the only member at a family picnic on an Independence-Day outing who refused the offer of a mosquito repellant, betting that it would not matter. He may have been the only one present who experienced a mosquito bite that day. He most certainly was the only one of the group who died because of it a matter of days later in July from encephalitis caused by West Nile virus (WNV).

It is statistically more likely to be involved in a car crash than it is to be stricken with WNV. However, because the risk is disproportionately high for older persons, some of us choose to avoid chances for incurring a mosquito bite while also continuing to drive our automobiles.

For the "post-mature" reader an option is not likely available to avoid risks that can be encountered by use of either Rx drugs, OTC drugs, or dietary supplements. With the onslaught of advancing age more and more people make use of such products in their attempts to attain an acceptable or tolerable level of health. Where does one at any age encounter the greater level of risk, with materials from the Rx, OTC, or supplement group of products? Of course, it matters little to the victim whether a terminal incident arises from an unfortunate response to an agent from one group or the

Consumer's Guide to Dietary Supplements and Alternative Medicines

doi:10.1300/5698_33

other. On the whole, as we best can tell from a very faulty and very likely incomplete database, the greatest risk would be for Rx drugs, less for OTCs, and least for supplements. Among supplements it clearly may be said that products containing only vitamins are safest of all, hardly ever causing life-threatening adverse reactions, and very seldom causing illness of any sort.

When statements are made about the odds of an adverse response they address the population in general, which may not apply to any one person. Whether the odds of a fatal occurrence are merely one in one million, one in 100,000 or one in 1,000, the person who comes to be that "one" is equally dead. No comfort may be found in the fact that death or permanent injury to an organ was "a highly improbable event."

ADVERSE REACTIONS

Sometimes the concern is not for a fatal adverse event but rather for a nonfatal but incapacitating one. Examples abound. A "young" 45-year-old fellow may need a kidney transplant, and in lieu of one he must undergo dialysis for several hours on three days of every week. The chances are that he lost his kidney function from taking a nonsteroidal anti-inflammatory drug (NSAID) despite his poorly controlled hypertension, which should have dictated against NSAID use. By 20-20 hindsight, a physician should not have prescribed an NSAID for this patient, but the fellow might have chosen to take one anyway from among several possible OTC analgesic choices, which might have brought on the same injury to his kidneys.

A loss of one's kidneys owing to toxicity of herbal products has also happened to many unsuspecting victims of a nephrotoxic herbal agent in the major European disaster that was described in Chapter 29. Despite the many reported instances of this tragic occurrence in western Europe, the causative herbal was still available in some herbal shops in the United States for several years after recognition of the nature and causes for the Chinese herbal nephropathy. Action by the FDA to ban the class of plants incriminated in the disaster was *entirely too slow* to give us confidence that such a disaster could never occur in the United States. To feel safe we would need to assume that they have "learned a lesson," but that often would be too generous an assumption in human affairs.

Therefore, it can be assumed that an unknown level of risk, albeit a small one, is associated with a use of some of the many "new" botanicals being sold in multiple component combinations. As Chapter 30 described, the United States has experienced one disaster from toxic effects of even a single-component nutrient supplement. Has a lesson been learned well enough the first time, or might there be a rerun? It seems clear that conditions are not in place to ensure against a similar event occurring. Therefore, we must accept the uncertainty (as in Chapter 3) about not *whether* but rather *how much* we are at risk from the use of chemicals foreign to our bodies. (Remember how we were assured that mechanisms were in place to prevent BSE [bovine spongiform encephalopathy, or mad cow disease] from ever entering the United States?) Whether they be Rx, OTC, or dietary supplement agents, we must accept the proposition that there is no such thing as absolute safety, just as we accept that there is no such thing as a free lunch—someone must and will pay.

Thus, we should understand and apply the principle of *benefit-to-risk ratio.* When one expects to receive a large benefit (as from a life-sustaining drug) a considerable risk is likely to be accepted. But the same type or level of risk may be deemed unacceptable and intolerable when the benefit is relatively small, short-term, and/or trivial in nature. Some supplement products may contribute significantly to our living more comfortably with a serious health problem. On the other hand, many uses for supplements are now associated only with "lifestyle benefits."

Especially questionable is the use of a supplement to avoid a healthful practice. A reprehensible case is the advertising of a product as constituting a "fat sponge." It urges people to eat all the fat you desire, but avoid the consequences by taking a dose of a "fat sponge," called chitosan. This is not a worthy illustration of either responsible self-medication behavior, or responsible product promotion.

HOW CAN THE BUYER BEWARE?

L. L. Augsburger, a distinguished professor of industrial pharmacy at the University of Maryland School of Pharmacy, in a forum on nutriceuticals at the 2000 meeting of the American Academy of Pharmaceutical Sciences recommended that consumers know the answers to the following questions before they use any dietary supplement:

- Could the product have a negative interaction with prescription medicines that you are taking? Example: A highly marketed energy bar for women does not warn against excessive doses of vitamin K that could interfere with certain blood clotting medicines.
- Is the product absorbable in its purchased form? People assume that anything in a capsule or tablet will be absorbed into the body. Reality is that substances added to botanicals to permit the dosage form to be manufactured can oppose the efficiency of absorption, as has occurred for Rx drugs.

- Could additional warnings or cautions about the category of dietary supplements exist that the manufacturer chose to omit? For example, a popular OTC memory concentrate containing *Ginkgo biloba* has potential drug interactions with medicines that prevent blood clotting, yet the label has no warnings.
- Has the product's usage been cited in clinical trials with favorable outcomes? If so, copies of this information may by obtained via the Internet or through the study's author.
- Consumers should not choose products on the basis of price. Comparative product studies show that quality is not clearly related to price (www.aapspharmaceutica.com/about/press/newsreleases/2000/062900_1.asp).

More Advice from a Toxicology Professor

Ryan J. Huxtable did considerable research in regard to hepatotoxic botanicals during the earlier years of recognition of the hazards of pyrrolizidine alkaloids. Huxtable (1992) suggested the following guidelines for reducing the risk of using botanical remedies or teas:

- Do not take herbs if pregnant or attempting to become pregnant.
- Do not take herbs if you are nursing.
- Do not give herbs to your baby.
- Do not take a large quantity of any one herbal preparation.
- Do not take any herb on a daily basis.
- Buy only preparations when the plants are listed on the packet (no guarantee of safety or correctness, but better than nothing).
- Do not take anything containing comfrey.

Watch for "Weasel Words"

Attention was called earlier to the supplement promotional material that uses many flowing, glowing, and "snowing" words and phrases. One example of a "snow-job" may be instructive. A recent "health bulletin" described, among others, a new dietary ingredient, cruciferous vegetables, about which it was stated that "there is no known instance in the medical record of ill effects from too much (name deleted)." A computer search using PubMed revealed no references to this compound in that database! This supports the accuracy of the quoted statement, but it reveals how far from telling the truth it was. If the compound is (as suspected) a brand-new dietary supplement ingredient, and nothing about it at all exists in the medical literature, then certainly no record of ill effects or favorable effects will exist.

Scientists have a dictum that applies to this situation: "An absence of evidence is not equal to evidence of absence!" Or, one could say, "Surely you can have found no evidence before you begin to look for it!" When it is used to argue for the safety of an ingredient, "absence of evidence" likely comprises a specious argument—meaning the argument seems to be plausible but actually is not genuine. It is indeed a shame when advertisements for dietary supplements lay a verbal trap for the consumer to fall into, or to change the metaphor, when they bait a hook and seek to make a "sucker" of the consumer who swallows their "line," as it is said, "hook, line and sinker!"

Where to Go for Help?

Few independent sources exist with the purpose of ensuring the quality of dietary supplements. The following sources may be helpful to consumers researching the more popular dietary supplements:

- ConsumerLab.com: Does comparative studies across brands especially for reliability of labeling for ingredients. A whopping seven out of nine *Gingko biloba* products didn't pass, and five of 14 Saw Palmetto products failed. (See more about this source in Chapter 33.)
- Quackwatch.org: Focuses with great fervor on what they deem to be irrational or unvalidated remedies being widely promoted.
- Local pharmacists having special expertise on supplements
- Nearby universities with pharmacy schools
- Local and/or regional poison control centers

In short, learn considerably more than a bare minimum about the supplement you may be considering using.

CAN WE EAT OUR WAY TO BETTER HEALTH?

One way to be less concerned about our usage of supplements is to increase our confidence in the diet that we eat. Some sources would have us to believe that all of the nutrients have been lost from the foods before they reach us. Perhaps one should first consider the "ax being ground" by such preachers of doom before we give up on the available food supply. Granted, breeding for better shelf life rather than better nutrition has led to loss of good consistency and sometimes even flavor—an example being the over-blown red imitations of fresh "homegrown" strawberries now being sold. They have a consistency reminiscent of a plastic or paper imitation of a strawberry, and the flavor is no better that if they were cardboard! However, folks living in many areas can with a little extra effort locate local or nearby sources that have not yet gone down the road to commercialized imitation fruits and vegetables.

The regular eating of 400 to 600 grams per day (13 to 20 ounces) of vegetables and fruits is associated with a significant reduction of the rates of many common forms of cancer. Moreover, such diets rich in plant foods are also associated with a reduced risk of heart disease and many chronic diseases of ageing. That is because those foods contain phytochemicals that have antioxidant and anti-inflammatory properties and thus confer various health benefits. A recently devised scheme to simplify one's strategy for a more healthful pattern of eating has been published in 2002 by nutritionist and physician, Dr. Heber David, MD, PhD, *What Color Is Your Diet?* A 2003 book by James A. Joseph, PhD seconding the motion is *The Color Code: A Revolutionary Eating Plan Your Life.* Dr. David has further presented his strategy in a summer 2004 review article, "Vegetables, fruits and phytoestrogens in the prevention of diseases."

This approach arises from the many health-promoting phytochemicals being colorful. Thus, by choosing a diet to include a wide array of colored vegetables and fruits a person can easily increased their ingestion of a diverse array of desirable food components. For example, foods that are colored red contain lycopene, very familiar for its supplying the pigment in tomatoes. Lycopene may localize in the prostate gland, and data indicate that it reduces the risk for diseases of that gland, and also of cardiovascular disease. Cherries are another fruit and red beets are a vegetable supplying lycopene.

Green vegetables such as broccoli, brussels sprouts, and kale supply glucosinolates, which have been associated with a decreased risk of cancer. Moreover, a further constituent of these vegetables, indole-3-carbinol, has shown chemopreventive effects in mouse models of colon cancer. In addition, isothiocyanates have an enzyme-enhancing effect to favor a higher level of glutathione production. Persons who display a very common genetic mutation causing a deficit of an enzyme normally producing glutathione respond to the isothiocyanates by activation of alternative enzymes. In population-level studies, such persons show a significant reduction in their risk of colon cancer if they eat broccoli or other cruciferous vegetables regularly.

Garlic as well as other white-to-green foods from the onion family contain allyl sulfides, which laboratory data have shown to inhibit the growth of cancer cells. Allicin, the major ingredient in crushed garlic, has been shown to inhibit cell division in vitro of human mammary, endometrial, and colon cancer cells. Gold color, as for carrots, is an indicator of carotenoids, which are necessary for optimal eye health and vision (as is described in Chapter 27). Consumers are advised to eat one serving of each of the seven color groups per day; this puts one within the guidelines of five to nine servings per day promoted by the National Cancer Institute and American Institute for Cancer Research.

PERSONAL ADVICE TO CONSUMERS OF DIETARY SUPPLEMENTS

Consider basic changes favoring better health suggested by these question: *What is needed in your life for better health?*

- Weight loss and maintenance?
- Better nutrition as an alternative to medications, now or later?
- Avoidance of "poisons"—tobacco, overindulgence in alcohol, sugar, calories?
- Avoidance of other risky behaviors (e.g., sexual promiscuity leading to STDs)?
- Better cardiovascular conditioning and perhaps other benefits from exercise?
- Lowering of emotional stress, plus pursuit of positive emotions?
- Making room for the spiritual aspects of life?
- Becoming willing and able to adopt new ways, reexamine critically the old ways?

Great advice was put succinctly by William Faulkner: "Don't bother just to be better than your contemporaries or predecessors. Try to be better than yourself."

Choosing not to make lifestyle changes now may mean missing out on better health later. Not choosing to make lifestyle changes means nothing will get better later. For example, "No one consciously chooses to become an alcoholic" (Sidney Cohen, MD, 1910-1987, a prominent researcher on dependence-producing behaviors). Rather, alcoholism happens from a process of *not* choosing to moderate one's behavior, or to abstain, while instead choosing to indulge one's impulses—"one more time, just for today"—and postponing the choice for change, betting one's life on a known loser!

> While we are postponing, life speeds by. (Seneca, 3 BC to AD 65)

> But because we still think in terms of magic bullets, the consequences of diet, exercise, and smoking are not really taken seriously because they are seen to be nonscientific. (Golub, 1997)

LAUGHTER IS THE BEST MEDICINE

The Association for Applied and Therapeutic Humor (www.aath.org/) founded in 1988 states that

> Therapeutic humor is defined to be: any intervention that promotes health and wellness by stimulating a playful discovery, expression, or appreciation of the absurdity or incongruity of life's situations. This intervention may enhance work performance, support learning, improve health, or be used as a complementary treatment of illness to facilitate healing or coping, whether physical, emotional, cognitive, social, or spiritual.

Many members of this group are health care professionals actively involved in the use of humor in a therapeutic context (see for example McGuire et al., 1992).

Attesting to the seriousness of the subject is another organization pertaining to this subject, the International Society for Humor Studies, which sponsors and publishes the journal *Humor*:

> Here are some tips to help you put more laughter in your life:
>
> - Figure out what makes you laugh and do it (or read it or watch it) more often.
> - Surround yourself with funny people—be with them every chance you get.
> - Develop your own sense of humor. Maybe even take a class to learn how to be a better comic—or at least a better joke-teller at that next party. Be funny every chance you get—as long as it's not at someone else's expense! (Brian, 2006)

One physician, Michael Miller, MD, Center for Preventive Cardiology at the University of Maryland Medical Center suggested that:

> It may be possible to incorporate laughter into daily activities, just as is done with other heart-healthy activities, such as taking the stairs instead of the elevator. The recommendation for a healthy heart may one day be exercise, eat right and laugh a few times a day (Miller, 2000).

Others within and outside of medicine have recognized the potential value of this feature of life—humor. The writer Norman Cousins (1983) directed much attention to this by writing books describing how he adopted an active plan to bring laughter into his efforts to get pain relief and to overcome a serious chronic illness. Proverbs (17:22, New King James Version) said many centuries before Cousins: A merry heart does good like a medicine, but a broken spirit dries the bones.

Someone calling themselves the "The AntiAging and Longevity Project" sponsors a Web site espousing the motto, "Laughter Is the Best Medicine," which supplies many one-liner jokes to dispense that remedy, can be found at www.csmngt.com/laughter_the_best_medicine.htm.

One research observation about the physiological basis for such benefit is that during a hearty laugh a slight increase in heart rate and blood pressure occurs, followed by an immediate recoil as muscles relax and blood pressure sinks below prelaugh levels (Fry and Savin, 1988). The obvious changes from the usual breathing pattern during laughter being predominantly an expiratory exercise was described in research conducted as early as 1938. However, the oxygen level in the blood does not fall appreciably (Fry and Stoft, 1971). The work of Dr. Fry and others reached publication in *JAMA* in an April 1, 1992, issue that featured laughter as a theme of the journal's occasional special medical student section (Fry, 1992). Some students of humor suggest that it causes the brain to release endorphins and enkephalins, endogenous pain-relieving hormonal peptides, which would explain how Cousins' "laughter therapy" provided relief for his pain.

As for some other aspects of CAM related in Chapter 32, a federally funded project is submitting humor therapy to validation.[1] According to a spring 2004 Associated Press report, the National Cancer Institute has approved a two million dollar grant for a three-pronged, five-year study of 282 juvenile patients who continue to deal with leukemia and other cancers after stem cell transplants (www.wholehealtheducation.com/resources/articles/article14.shtml). Besides a group receiving the humor therapy, another segment of the total participant pool will test the healing influence of massage therapy, and a third will receive both humor and massage. All of these will be in addition to standard chemotherapy regimens.

WHERE ARE MEDICINE AND HEALTH CARE GOING?

J. Neuberger of the King's Fund, London, United Kingdom, at the onset of the new century and millennium (in the *Journal of Internal Medicine*) looked forward to a new challenges for the medical profession saw as one of them, The Educated Patient. His thoughts were summarized as follows:

> The medical profession is facing significant changes in the way the rest of society relates to it. . . . They [doctors] will have to be more accountable for the quality of care they provide and work with a wider range of health and non-health professionals to meet patients' needs. . . . They can work to ensure that the benefits of the information revolution are felt by people excluded from consumerism because of poverty and social isolation, working to create an empowered, informed public whose members are given the best opportunity to look after their own health. (Neuberger, 2000, p. 6)

The Internet is not explicitly cited in this excerpt from Neuberger's analysis, but it is surely a major factor in the new equation that he discussed.

Professor Edward S. Golub (1997, p. 214) poses a highly cogent question: "What is it we really want from scientific medicine in a century when science has been elevated to the level of religion and the scientific healer has become the custodian of knowledge about our most personal and intimate selves?"

Many would say that where medical practice *must* be reoriented is toward a much greater emphasis on maintaining health and preventing illness, which could reduce the amount of effort and money spent on treatment of preventable disease (putting out fires that shouldn't have been lighted!). At this moment the problem of epidemic obesity and consequent type 2 diabetes, atherosclerosis, and heart attack or stroke constitutes a prime case for severely needed but dearly expensive firefighting. Prevention is a major theme of natural-holistic-nutritional medicine. Physicians in that camp avow that there has been, or is now underway, a paradigm shift through their practices that concentrate on methods of health maintenance and prevention of illness rather than merely treating the symptoms of illness and hoping that the underlying causes will go away.

Indeed, an area of study and emphasis that is known as "salutogenesis" is newly arising, which is approximately the opposite of "pathogenesis."

Whereas the latter focuses on the factors and processes that result in illness and disease, salutogenesis instead focuses on the factors and processes that result in our maintaining a state of health. This shows promise of becoming a fruitful direction of research in support of so-called preventive medicine, which is generally not a major (or even minor) focus of contemporary medical practice, with an important exception of (mainly) childhood vaccines for active immunization against infectious diseases.

Nutritional physicians say that a change in people's eating patterns and habits is necessary for enabling the body to heal itself after nutritional deficits have been corrected and cumulative poisons have been removed. Obviously, they also emphasize diet in preventing illnesses. Such practitioners may not pass a test for their practicing evidence-based medicine (nor would any but a very small proportion of all the physicians who have gone before them), but the sincerity of their efforts should not be denigrated. Improvements in medical practice will occur, and nutritional physicians will be seen to have made significant, positive contributions toward accomplishing that goal.

It should be considered seriously whether the preventive emphasis that is so strongly associated with nutritive treatments may point to a solution to the rising concern about the economics of U.S. health care. The prevention of obesity and its highly expensive pathologic consequences is at this writing a superb example of the need for greatly increased prevention efforts with the resulting cost savings of successful programming.

Another potential area for cost savings seems significant if dietary supplements could be shown to be feasible, effective therapeutic alternatives for expensive prescription pharmaceuticals. Some examples might be the several therapeutic interventions via magnesium salts and the many applications of ascorbate as described in Chapter 24, e.g., its serving as both anti-infective and anticancer chemotherapies as well as preventive for illnesses related to oxidative stress.

FINAL THOUGHTS

Andrew Saul (2003), emphasizes the need for patients to take charge of their health and health care, as it is "too important to leave in the hands of physicians." Sounding a similar note is the proclamation by W. C. Douglas, MD, that the four most dangerous words are "You are the doctor" (Douglas, 2003). This viewpoint advocates an actively informed position as a *safer* one than a passive acceptance of the physician's every thought and action. (Even if your physician would have you believe that he or she knows it all, be fully assured that it is not true.)

Chapter 34

Epilogue: Spiritual Aspects of Health and Healing

> God heals and the doctor takes the fee.
>
> Benjamin Franklin

> Spirituality, which pertains to meaning in life, has clinical relevance.
>
> Post et al. (2000)

> Although our medical and surgical procedures have become more powerful and more sophisticated, we still must rely heavily on the patient's own recuperative powers, which can be enhanced by hope and faith.
>
> Sir William Osler, MD
> (quoted in Frank [1975])

The important theme of *hope* has been emphasized explicitly from the preface of this book to its ending. The importance to medicine of hope and faith on the part of patients for helping them recover from illness was stated by a medical giant of a century ago, Sir William Osler (see above quote). Hope has a close association with faith and matters of the spiritual realm. "Now faith is the substance of things hoped for, the evidence of things not seen" (Hebrews 11:1, NKJV). Moreover, it seemed fitting to close this writing with a consideration of the close companion of hope—prayer—which is

---

Quotations from the Holy Bible are from either the New King James Version (NKJV) or the New International Version (NIV).

Consumer's Guide to Dietary Supplements and Alternative Medicines

doi:10.1300/5698_34

the most-used aspect of complementary and alternative medicine today, with the highest rate of practice (45 percent) reported in a 2002 federal survey of the U.S. population (Barnes et al. 2004). Thus, use of prayer exceeds the rate of usage for the natural products (19 percent) that comprise dietary supplements, our primary focus herein.

THE NATURE OF US ALL

Much of the thought about human nature recognizes a principle of dualism or duality of our nature—body and soul (as a mid-twentieth century ballad described it). However, the Holy Scriptures provide a basis for perceiving our nature instead as being threefold. The Apostle Paul stated (1 Thessalonians 5:23, NKJV), "May your whole spirit, soul, and body be preserved blameless at the coming of our Lord Jesus Christ." This is in accord with the Christian understanding of the godhead as existing in three persons, a doctrine of the Holy Trinity—Father, Son, and Holy Spirit—as well as the Genesis account of human creation: "So God created man in his own image; in the image of God he created him" (Genesis 1:27, NKJV). With the nature of the Creator being a Trinity, so also the human species created in his image has a threefold nature. The soul (psyche), some prefer to say "mind," is best understood, as also in the concept of dualism, to encompass will plus all mental and emotional features of our personality.[1]

What then do we understand about the spirit of humankind? It is that aspect of the human being that imparts a capacity for the knowledge of, and a relationship with, the Divine. (Note that *soul* may include this characteristic for many who hold a dualistic position.) In this respect the spirit of humankind is regarded as comprising the fundamental distinction between our species and all other forms of life. The spirit for the unregenerate person has been described as "a godshaped vacuum" awaiting fulfillment of the capacity that the spirit imparts for being in relationship to the Creator. It is helpful to make a physical analogy with the conventional (*not* the wireless) telephone receiver and speaker. We are likely to describe a disconnected telephone as being "dead" when it is nonfunctional because of not being "plugged in" to the telephone system. In an unregenerate state a person is "dead" to God—not prepared for receiving intimate communication and spiritual knowledge because of the person not being "plugged in" to him.

The Apostle Paul addressed the Christian converts at Ephesus: "You were dead in your trespasses and sins . . . God who is rich in mercy made us alive with Christ . . ." (Ephesians 2:1, 4, 5, NKJV). Thus, a "saving," regenerating relationship with Jesus establishes a connection with God and an enlivening of the human spirit. Clearly the Apostle Paul was addressing a state of spiritual deadness rather than a bodily one. The spirit of man being in contact with Divinity is reflected by a verse from one of the most ancient books of the Hebrew Scriptures, Job, which says that: "Age should speak and multitude of years should teach wisdom but there is a spirit in man, and the breath [Spirit] of the Almighty gives him understanding" (Job 32:7). These thoughts about the spiritual aspect of human beings should convey the idea of the vital importance of spiritual "aliveness" and well-being for a person to experience the maximal fulfillment of human capacity for life and health, versus the state of deprivation associated with spiritual alienation from the Creator.

MAINTAINING HEALTH: WHAT WE NEED TO AVOID

Worry: An Enemy of Health

Worry robs the one who practices it—robs not only physically and mentally but also spiritually. Most analysts would say that worry is a mental activity, and it is. But even so one also can say that it involves a spiritual activity, because it is the opposite of trust or faith that one may rely on providence to be fulfilling our needs. In every case it represents a negative condition that acts adversely against physical health. Among the results of worry are loss of sleep, both in quantity and quality, which in turn serves as a mechanism for various adverse physical and mental consequences. As insomnia settles upon a worrier, he or she adds ever more reasons to worry. Most worrisome is concern for one's ability to perform as is necessary in tomorrow's duties. A vicious cycle can quickly arise when one is thus afflicted, and it points the route to depression.

Lest we be thought to oversimplify, all insomnia problems do not originate in worry. Various physical conditions, especially those of chronic discomfort, as results from musculoskeletal inflammations (arthritis, fibromyalgia), exist that can greatly hinder sleep. However, though the origins of insomnia may be physical, the perpetuation of it through worrisome thoughts becomes a likely consequence. Worry is listed as one of the foremost manifestations of anxiety, along with fears and nervousness. Finding a positive response to its attack is better than submitting to it. One Internet physician suggests reading, and more specifically reading the Scriptures or other materials having a positive spiritual impact. Similar advice from a pioneer of personal development and public speaking, "It is worrying about the insomnia that does the damage—not the insomnia" (Dale Carnegie, 1884, p. 231).

In what way does a spiritual aspect of worrying exist? It is in opposition to living in a mode of faith. It comprises a deficit or a lack of reliance on God's care and provision for us. The New Testament clearly teaches against worrying and in favor of reliance on God (*anxious* is the usual term for worry in most translations); from a letter of Paul: "Be anxious for nothing, but in everything by prayer and supplication with thanksgiving, let your requests be made known to God" (Philippians 4:6, NKJV).

In Jesus' own teaching He challenged his followers:

> Therefore I tell you, do not worry about your life, what you will eat or drink, or about your body, what you will wear. . . . Who of you by worrying can add a single hour to his life? . . . . But seek His kingdom and His righteousness, and all these things will be given to you as well. Therefore, do not worry about tomorrow, for tomorrow will worry about itself. Each day has enough trouble of its own. (Matthew 6:25, 27, 33-34, NIV)

He promised the care and provision of a loving Father. Avoidance of worry is not to be regarded as possible through human effort alone, but rather is to be seen as a grace gift received by faith from Jehovah, the Lord God Almighty, who is named as the source of all good and perfect gifts, and is described as desiring to give gifts freely.

Excessive Stress Can Be Very Health Damaging

Chronic anxiety can become one important type of stressful experience, among many. The biomedical concept of stress was pioneered by a Viennese-born researcher, Hans Selye (1907-1982) who conducted his research for more that 50 years in Montreal, Canada. He took a medical degree before becoming a medical physiologist, more especially a renowned endocrinologist. While still in his second year of medical school in 1926 he began to develop his later-to-be-famous theories about the influence of stress on our human capacity to cope and adapt physiologically when under the pressures of injury and disease. Dr. Selye discovered that patients with a variety of ailments manifested a pattern that included many similar symptoms. This pattern he ultimately came to interpret as the efforts of our bodies to respond to the negative influences of being ill. This collection of symptoms that characterize a distinct "stress disease" or "stress syndrome" he named the general adaptation syndrome (GAS).

Dr. Selye spent his lifetime in research on GAS about which he wrote some 30 books and more than 1,500 articles dealing with stress and related problems. Among those books were *The Stress of Life* (1956) and *Stress without Distress* (1975). The latter points to a failed response to stress, *distress,* as the damaging aspect of our encountering stress. Some of his contemporaries were so impressed by the impact of his research findings and theories that they have called him the Einstein of medicine, and he is unquestionably known as the father of research on stress.

More than any other scientist Selye demonstrated the role of negative physical, mental, and emotional responses in causing much of the wear and tear experienced by human beings throughout their lives. Thus, coping with life's adverse events so as to minimize negative mental-emotional responses is a very healthful strategy of life. When a person lacks spiritual resources that enable turning negative situations into a positive response they may fail to combat effectively and successfully their encounters with the universal stresses of life. Thus, circumstances and stimuli that serve to trigger bodily stress responses may overwhelm the defensive adaptations. One of the major findings concerning long-term stress is that it exerts a negative effect on the needed functions of the immune system, which lowers our defenses against infections, cancer, and probably other serious diseases.

Damage from Stress Demonstrated by Aftereffects of 9/11

Within certain limits the adrenocortical activation response to stress is an adaptive one. However, beyond a limit of intensity and duration that activation can become damaging; a sustained activation will interfere with immune system activities. It has been recognized for some time that long-continuing exposure to stress can be a significant factor contributing to heart attacks and underlying cardiovascular disease. A dramatic example was reported in the September 15, 2004, issue of the *Journal of the American College of Cardiology* by Jonathan S. Steinberg, MD, a cardiologist at the St. Luke's-Roosevelt Hospital and Columbia University College of Physicians and Surgeons in New York City (Steinberg et al., 2004).

In the days after the World Trade Center was destroyed on September 11, 2001, Dr. Steinberg and colleagues who serve heart patients in the area of greater New York and New Jersey realized that automatic recorders in implantable cardioverter defibrillators (ICDs), or intracardiac echocardiographs (ICE) offered a treasure store of data on heart rhythms before and after the attack. The devices are designed to deliver corrective shocks to the heart if they detect potentially dangerous arrhythmias. They store data on each event, which is later downloaded during regular checkups with their cardiologist. They found that over the 30 days after 9/11, 16 patients (8 percent of 200 consecutive patients) experienced tachyarrhythmias, contrasting with only seven (3.5 percent) over the preceding 30 days. This represents a 2.3-fold increase in risk (95 percent confidence interval, 1.1 to 4.9; probability = 0.03).

These are the first results documenting such a direct link between a traumatic event and an increase in cardiac arrhythmias. Although all these patients survived, that might not have been the case if they had not been equipped with the defibrillator devices! The researchers say of their findings that arrhythmias may play a role in the underlying causes of increased cardiac death rates previously observed after natural disasters. However, in contrast to prior reports of cardiac deaths spiking upward immediately after some natural disasters and then quickly subsiding, the first arrhythmic events from this group did not occur for three days after 9/11, and the data showed less a spike than a swell, with excess arrhythmias lasting about a month. The events were not concentrated merely in Manhattan, but across the metropolitan region. Moreover, the scope of this effect went far beyond the immediate area.

Suspecting that the stress may have been felt by heart patients around the country, Dr. Steinberg contacted Anne B. Curtis, MD, Omer L. Shedd, MD, and others of their colleagues at the University of Florida and the Veterans Affairs Medical Center in Gainesville, Florida, to find out whether their ICD patients were also affected.

The findings of the Florida group were almost identical (Shedd et al., 2004). Dr. Shedd did not expect to see such effects in the patients almost a thousand miles from the 9/11 attack.

> I was surprised. I actually did not feel that we would see an effect when we first began to think about the study. At the time, I knew of the results of the original New York study, but I thought patients were not likely to experience these same problems if they were not physically near the attacks. I think this says a lot about the power of our media. When events such as 9/11 are brought into our homes by television, the Internet or newspapers people are clearly moved by what they are seeing, and they physically share in the experience just as if they were near the event. (Shedd et al., 2004)

Among 132 consecutive Florida patients with ICEs, 14 patients (11 percent) had ventricular tachyarrhythmias in the 30 days following the World Trade Center attack compared with five (3.8 percent) in the preceding 30 days (95 percent confidence interval was 0.4 to 13.3 and probability was 0.0389). Although this represents a 2.8-fold risk increase, Dr. Shedd said he would not conclude the effect was larger in Florida than in New York. However, the multitude of persons across the whole United States who saw the planes impact the towers as well as the fall of the towers either live or on later news received quite a strong dose of stress in addition to the persons in and near Manhattan on that ghastly day. (www.acc.org/media/releases/highlights/2004/sept04/arrhythmias.htm)

Broader Aspects of Stress-Related Injury

Besides injurious effects on the structure and function of the heart and blood vessels, other systems and organs of our body may also be harmed by sustained stress that goes beyond our capacity for coping. The digestive tract and all its functions is another major site for stress to manifest its injurious influences. Moreover, stress can affect also our mental activities and health. Chronic severe stress is believed by some authorities to be a cause of major depression. Granted, it is also believed that inborn genetic factors make some persons more susceptible than others to develop depression via individual characteristics of our brain chemistry. With severe stress a state of hyperactivity of the adrenal cortex, the gland that secretes cortisol (or hydrocortisone), the major corticosteroid in human beings is to be found. This is the gland and the secretion that Hans Selye found to constitute the most prominent mechanism for the response to stress—adrenal cortex hyperactivity became known as the primary indicator that an animal or a person is undergoing stress.

Depression is one variety of mental disruption that is often associated with abnormal adrenocortical activity, and it may be accompanied by memory retrieval difficulties. Among younger people in recent years one hears of memory problems that have long been associated more typically with old age. Some would suggest that people generally in the United States live under more stressful circumstances than was true in much of our prior history. Thus, stress-dependent memory impairment can be attributed to the ability of excess quantities of our normal corticosteroid secretion to be especially damaging to brain cells in that area of the brain thought to be critical for memory, the hippocampus. One line of supporting evidence for this is derived from persons suffering the extreme chronic stress of torture or from concentration camp survival over the last half of the twentieth century. Study of such persons' brains and cognition shows that the survivors carry with them a shrinkage of the brain substance (prominently so in the hippocampus) as well as showing deficits of memory and/or other cognitive activities. That the physical change is responsible for the mental ones, and that both are consequences of severe chronic stress, are very attractive inferences to be drawn from such observations.

Avoidance of Stress-Related Illness

Dr. Selye has been credited with this on our outlook to the consequences of stress: "Adopting the right attitude can convert a negative stress into a positive one" (www.giga-usa.com/quotes/authors/hans_selye_a001.htm). Providing the means for coping with the stressful aspects of our lives is a basic aspect of the spiritual life that makes it significant to maintaining health. In the New Testament we find the injunction (cited previously) not to live our life in worry, which will sooner or later make us subject to damage from stress. Instead, persons may walk through life and all its negative phases in relationship with a loving Creator who wishes to supply us with the means to cope with all circumstances so as to avoid succumbing to stress: "Be joyful always; pray continually; give thanks in all circumstances, for this is God's will for you in Christ Jesus" (1 Thessalonians 5:16-18, NIV).

A positive attitude of joyfulness along with thanksgiving for our daily benefits enables a person to rise above the adverse situations of life and makes it possible to defeat stress. By this manner of living it is possible to blunt the damaging effects of too-long-sustained stress, which otherwise may overwhelm the capacity of our protective physiological responses.

Spiritual Readiness for Surviving Stress

Living in freedom from stress when one's life conditions are very stressful requires a walk of faith that enables the believer to draw on supernatural provision. One person most epitomizing such a walk is a man about whom Jehovah said to Satan, "Have you considered my servant Job? There is no one on earth like him; he is blameless and upright, a man who fears God and shuns evil" (Job 1:8, NIV). There followed a testing as to whether Job's uprightness would continue through the loss of all of his many material advantages, as well as that of all of his children. The immediate outcome after a series of catastrophes was that despite such severely testing stress Job was able by faith to say "Naked I came from my mother's womb and naked I will depart. The Lord gave and the Lord has taken away; may the name of the Lord be praised" (Job 1:21, NIV).

But Job had a long session of "advising" from his so-called friends during which he said many good things about God, but yet was shown to be imperfect in self-righteous attitudes and by his words. So God gave Job a new level of revelation of himself, as a result of which Job was driven to say "my ears had heard of you but now my eyes have seen you. Therefore I despise myself and repent in dust and ashes" (Job 42:5-6, NIV). And the final result of Job's testing time was that, "The LORD blessed the latter part of Job's life more than the first" (Job 42:12, NIV). This ancient story exemplifies the recent saying that catastrophe will make a person bitter or better, depending upon one's response to it.

Care of the Body

The Hebrews in the time of Moses received, besides the Ten Commandments and other specific behavioral prohibitions, a set of dietary laws or regulations that were to set them apart from other peoples, and also to protect them from certain infectious disease that might more likely have been contracted through eating of the creatures forbidden to them. In parallel would stand several proscriptions against sexual impurity or deviance that were seemingly intended in part for their avoidance of sexually transmitted diseases as well as adverse nonbodily effects.

The dietary laws were set aside in New Testament times through a revelation to the Apostle Peter. However, the commandments against sexual impurity and/or deviance were not changed, but rather were reinforced. Indeed, sexual impurity (premarital sex, adultery, or homosexual intercourse) was established at a renewed degree of significance—for example, that for a believer, joining oneself to a prostitute was equivalent to a defiling of the Temple of God. New Testament teaching describes the conversion to faith in Jesus as the Christ (the Messiah, the prophesied Savior) as accomplishing a spiritual rebirth by which the believer's being is indwelt by the Holy Spirit, the Spirit of Christ, and thus becomes a temple (dwelling-place) of God. For the Jewish people, among whom the New Testament Church came into being, a reference to defiling the Temple of God had extreme importance because of the very strict Old Testament regulations in the Torah about ceremonial cleansing required before a Israelite could enter even the outer court of the Tabernacle of Moses, or later the Temple of Solomon, lest their entry cause defilement of those sacred surroundings.

Twentieth-century U.S. evangelical Christianity was prone to extend the injunction against "profaning of the believer's body as the temple of God" to any use of chemicals having an injurious and/or dependence-producing potential (and thus desired for "recreational use" in contemporary terms). Abstinence from tobacco usage to avoid injury of a medical nature was endorsed, although this was not a popular concept in tobacco-growing regions. By the end of the twentieth century not a slightest doubt was left of the multiplicity of seriously injurious outcomes from habitual use of tobacco products—to the lungs, cardiovascular system, and other organs—which continue to be responsible for a considerable annual death toll. Eventually, addictiveness (dependence-producing capacity) of tobacco use became recognized (for some but not all persons) to rival that seen with so-called "hard drugs" such as opiates and stimulants. Preservation of health entails not only avoidance of smoking, but even avoiding habitual second-hand exposure to tobacco smoke.

Alcoholic beverage use was strongly attacked in the nineteenth century by such organizations as the Woman's Christian Temperance Union, formally founded in 1874 after women conducted prohibitionist crusade activities in the prior summer in Ohio and New York. As early as 1875 there was a beginning of the members' concern also about tobacco. Although the death toll from alcohol-related events is tabulated as lower than that for tobacco, the degree to which deaths are induced by alcohol use in innocent bystanders is considerably greater leading to the development of efforts such as that of Mothers Against Drunk Driving (MADD). Certainly the Bible cannot easily be read to endorse total abstinence or social prohibition, but the Book of Proverbs and the Book of Isaiah soundly condemn drunkenness and every degree of immoderation, "alcohol abuse" in today's parlance.

Besides the clear Old Testament condemnations of drunkenness, a prominent New Testament position-statement exists from the Apostle Paul: "Be not drunk with wine wherein is excess, but be filled with the Spirit, speaking to yourself in psalms and hymns and spiritual songs, singing and making melody in your heart to the LORD" (Ephesians 5:18-19, NKJV). This passage indicates that a "spiritual high" is available that does not carry the damaging potential associated with various states of chemically induced highs. This passage can be extrapolated to support the prohibition of nonmedical, recreational, self-administration of other natural or synthetic drugs affecting the brain and nervous system broadly—stimulants, hallucinogens, opiates, tranquilizers, or sleeping-aid medicines.

Current-Day Dietary Matters

What we take into our body needs to be of concern in other ways than the avoidance of injurious or dependence-producing substances such as excess refined sugar, pollutants, or additives (e.g., the artificial sweeteners). "You are what you eat" is a touchstone among aphorisms on dietary habits that expresses much truth. In an era when "grossly overweight" is a state now having its onset all too often in childhood, it is certainly clear that too many children are eating badly to acquire a condition that is a serious threat to health and even survival past middle age.

Our society's current search for desirable, healthful patterns of food consumption have come to the attention of not only the secular populace and writers but also to Christians and their teachers about nutrition. A currently notable example is a new book and regimen titled *The Maker's Diet* by a naturopathic physician trained also in nutrition, Jordan N. Rubin (2004), which promises, "In as little as 40 days, 'The Maker's Diet' can transform the way you eat and live." (An eDiets news story on Rubin's system can be found at http://www.ediets.com/news/article.cfm?cmi=552186&cid=1&code=24565.) The author presents as his basic credentials a remarkable personal story of health restoration from severe gastrointestinal illness. He describes his survival and recovery as hinging on his making dietary/nutritional changes that stemmed from biblical wisdom and example. His program is described as focusing "on the four pillars of health (physical, spiritual, mental, and emotional) to help readers achieve optimum energy and wellness." However, the validation of his program is based on testimonials rather than designed experiments. The regimen that Rubin has supplied requires very drastic changes that many will not likely succeed in following, and hardly lend themselves to clinical-trial validation. Other recent diet-spirituality books are *Body by God: The Owners Manual for Maximized Living* by Dr. Ben Lerner (2003), and Don Colbert's (2001) *Toxic Relief: Restore Health and Energy Through Fasting and Detoxification.*

HEALINGS: FROM ILLNESS TO RECOVERY

The outstanding evidence to his contemporaries that Jesus of Nazareth had a very special ministry from God was the extremely frequent occurrence of instantaneous miraculous recoveries from sickness to those he touched or those who in faith touched even "the hem of his garment." In several recorded instances, his healing power and authority were exerted despite the sick person being quite a distance removed from his presence. Even more miraculous were healings of incurable diseases or afflictions (the blind, the deaf, the speechless) that caused many to raise the question as to whether Jesus was indeed the prophesied Messiah, Redeemer, Savior, Incarnation of God, whose coming had been long-promised in the Old Testament, from the Book of Genesis to the Book of Malachi. Indeed, many believed in his messiahship because of the miraculous signs, which included even resurrections of the dead.

Moreover, he sent forth disciples who were to preach, heal, and perform miracles as he not only enjoined them but also empowered them to do: "He called the twelve disciples to him and gave them authority to drive out evil spirits and to cure every kind of disease and sickness" (Matthew 10:1, NIV). These events all can be seen as a divine validation of Jesus being indeed the Son of God and Savior as John the Baptist acknowledged Him to be: "Behold, the Lamb of God who takes away the sin of the world!" (John 1:29, NKJV).

But some argue that the gifts for healing to the early Christians had the purpose of supporting the founding of the Church, and that such gifts "expired" upon the death of the twelve apostles before the end of the first century. Unquestionably, such gifts were ordained by Jesus before his crucifixion and resurrection, but it is not at all clear that this impartation was limited to the Twelve to whom these words were addressed:

> Believe me when I say that I am in the Father and the Father is in Me, or at least believe on the evidence of the miracles themselves. I tell you the truth, anyone who has faith in me will do what I have been doing. He will do even greater things than these, because I am going to the Father. (John 14:11-12, NIV)

Indeed, Scripture states that the gifts of God, once truly given, are not withdrawn ("For the gifts and the calling of God are irrevocable," Romans 11:29, NKJV). Thus it is that Bible-focused segments of Christendom have continued to believe for divine healing benefits down through the centuries. Moreover, in modern times a renewal of emphasis upon healing through supernatural gifts occurred in early pentecostalism shortly after the beginning of the twentieth century, and again with the 1970s era of neopentecostal charismatic renewal. For this reason a restoration of the early New Testament style of ministry, including "sign gifts" such as healings by prayer and laying on of hands prevails into the twenty-first century among a significant portion of evangelical believers.

In a 2002 book on prayer, R. B. Cherry (2002) emphasizes that prayer should be the first recourse for healing, rather than our last resort.

This exhortation is indeed consistent with the practice followed by a significant, though undefinable, fraction of contemporary Christian believers. Surveys by Gallup indicate that a majority of the U.S. citizenry observes private nonritual prayer on a regular basis, but that only 42 percent claimed to ever pray for material things such as physical healing or health (Poloma, 1993). However, survey data reported by Poloma and Gallup (1991) showed that 89 percent of those who prayed experienced either rarely, occasionally, or regularly "a deep sense of peace and well-being" in their mental-emotional realm.

In the mental health arena, alcoholism and other chemical dependencies have been most successfully overcome for those persons who can commit to a wholehearted participation in Twelve Step programs that began with Alcoholics Anonymous. The terminology of Alcoholics Anonymous is that its approach emphasizes spirituality, not religion, but some will reject its quasi-religious mode and not accept the whole program, as Peteet (1993) observed.

Can Spiritual Factors in Healing Be Verified by Scientific Analysis?

Efforts to obtain documentation for validating spiritual healing have arisen in parallel to the search for evidence-based medicine. A search of PubMed from 1966 to 2004 (accessed June 6, 2004) using the term "prayer" yielded 544 hits from articles in the medical and allied literature; "faith healing" received 206 hits, and "divine healing" had five hits, but "spiritual healing" had none.[2] Thus, the relationship of spirituality, faith, and prayer to medicine, health care, and healing is hardly being ignored or overlooked. A U.S. survey published in 2004 found that 35 percent of adults used prayer for health concerns in 1998. Only 11 percent of those using prayer discussed it with their physician. Prayer was used frequently for common medical conditions, and users reported high levels of perceived helpfulness.

An expert panel of the National Institute for Healthcare Research (www.nihr.org) prepared a report in 1997 on an evaluation of scientific evidence for any association between spirituality or religious practices and health. Their conclusion was that indeed a positive association has been found between spirituality/religious practices and health benefits across a wide variety of health areas (Larson, 1997).

A review published in 2000 attempted to analyze trials of several forms of "distant healing" (prayer, mental healing, therapeutic touch, or spiritual healing) as therapies for any medical condition, but was unable to find sufficient similarity of 23 published studies to perform a meta-analysis (Astin et al., 2000). However, because 17 of the 23 trials (57 percent) showed a positive treatment effect, they concluded that currently available evidence warrants additional studies regarding "distant healing."

Results of a 2004 study on patient preference regarding spiritual discussions and practices supported the authors' recommendation that physicians should realize that a substantial minority of patients desire spiritual interaction in routine office visits (McCord et al., 2004). When asked about specific prayer behaviors across a range of clinical scenarios, the patients' desire for such spiritual interaction increased with the greater severity of their illnesses.

CONCLUSION

The pursuit of continued good health and/or healing of illness and disease is one that involves body, soul (mind, emotions), and spirit. Finding hope in various approaches to that pursuit is a basic essential to a positive outlook on life. Having faith in a higher power, as Alcoholics Anonymous expresses it, and in whatever approach(es) one chooses to pursue, is another closely allied essential.

Above all, an active rather than passive attitude toward one's goal of good health is necessary if a person is to access and utilize all that is being made available—both the remedies and the important information resources about those remedies, about illnesses, and about methods for our health maintenance. It is my hope that the readers' efforts in this worthy pursuit will be aided significantly by their time devoted to materials encompassed by this source.

Appendix

Book-Length Resources

Basara LR and Montagne M. *Searching for Magic Bullets: Orphan Drugs, Consumer Activism, and Pharmaceutical Development.* Binghamton, NY: Pharmaceutical Products Press, 1994. A broad but compact insight into the drug development process and its history, evolving regulations, and economic and social aspects.

Berkson B. *The Alpha Lipoic Acid Breakthrough.* New York: Prima Publishing, 1998. Dr. Berkson was appointed by the FDA as U.S. principal investigator for therapy with intravenous alpha-lipoic acid (alpha-LA) of acute liver failure from poisoning by eating *Amanita* mushrooms, which has produced "marvelous" recoveries. He deals with the use of oral alpha-LA supplementation as a superior antioxidant tool for health.

Blaylock RL. *Excitotoxins: The Taste That Kills.* Santa Fe, NM: Health Press, 1997. A consideration of the neurotoxic effects of excitatory compounds such as glutamic acid/glutamate and aspartic acid/aspartate.

Braverman E. *The Healing Nutrients Within: Facts, Findings and New Research on Amino Acids.* New Canaan, CT: Keats Publishing, 1997. A broad treatment of amino acids, both normal functions and their value as therapeutic agents.

Chan K, Dhabi A, and Cheung L. *Interactions Between Chinese Herbal Medicines and Orthodox Drugs.* Harwood Academic, 1999. Its 166 pages show that the topic has been receiving some still-needed attention.

Cheraskin E and Ringsdorf, WM, Jr. *The Vitamin C Connection.* New York: Harper and Row, 1983. A classic analysis on ascorbate.

Coats BC and Ahola R. *Aloe Vera the New Millennium: The Future of Wellness in the 21st Century.* New York: iUniverse, Inc., 2003. Coats is the developer of patented processes for retaining the healing properties of fresh aloe vera in a stabilized form for internal or external indications.

Crook TH, III and Adderly B. *The Memory Cure: The Safe, Scientifically Proven Breakthrough That Can Slow, Halt or Even Reverse Memory Loss.* New York: Pocket Books, 1998. Phosphatidyl serine is greatly emphasized as an answer for many persons with a failing memory.

Diamond J. *Snake Oil and Other Preoccupations.* London: Vintage, 2001. A broad but succinct analysis of the CAM movement that was undertaken by a British writer as he underwent conventional treatment for cancer, resisting unconven-

Consumer's Guide to Dietary Supplements and Alternative Medicines

doi:10.1300/5698_35

tional treatments urged upon him by friends, and which was published after his death.

Fetrow CW and Avila JR. *Professional's Handbook of Complementary and Alternative Medicines.* Springhouse, PA: Springhouse Corp., 2001.

Foster S and Tyler VE. *Tyler's Honest Herbal: A Sensible Guide to the Use of Herbs and Related Remedies,* Fourth edition. Binghamton, NY: The Haworth Press, Inc., 1999.

Golub ES. *The Limits of Medicine: How Science Shapes Our Hope for the Cure.* Chicago: University of Chicago Press, 1997.

Heber D and Bowerman S. *What Color Is Your Diet?* New York: Regan Books, 2002. Add some color to your diet to attain a higher level of health and energy. Details his unique "7 Colors of Health" food-selection system, which groups vegetables and fruits by the colorful and beneficial chemical substances they supply.

Jacob SW and Appleton J. *MSM The Definitive Guide.* Topanga, CA: Freedom Press, 2003. The physician who discovered DMSO and "son of DMSO," MSM, describes limited animal research and many clinical experiences with the anti-inflammatory uses of MSM, which qualifies as a dietary supplement, unlike DMSO.

Levy TE. *Vitamin C, Infectious Diseases, and Toxins.* Princeton, NJ: Xlibris Corp, 2002. A thorough review of the literature and history of vitamin C employed as a pharmacologic, antidotal, and anti-infective chemotherapeutic agent.

Pauling L. *How to Live Longer and Feel Better.* Freeman, 1986. A pioneer of the concept of orthomolecular medicine expounds on this "megavitamin therapy."

Ross J. *The Mood Cure.* New York: Viking, 2002. The use of nutritional "repair tools" to complement conventional medical care, psychotherapy, and spiritual counseling.

Saul A. *Doctor Yourself: Natural Healing That Works.* North Bergen, NJ: Basic Health Publications, 2003. Natural medicine approaches to particular illnesses from a major advocate.

Senneff, JA. *Numb Toes and Burning Soles: Coping with Peripheral Neuropathy,* 1999; *Numb Toes and Other Woes,* 2001, and *Nutrients for Neuropathy,* 2002; all from San Antonio, TX: MedPress. A series of three books by a nonphysician sufferer on coping with the chronic pain of peripheral neuropathy (PN). Senneff provides a broad consideration of both conventional, nutritional and various other alternative therapies for PN.

Stoll AL. *The Omega-3 Connection: The Groundbreaking Antidepression Diet and Brain Program.* New York: Simon and Schuster, 2001. Contains many details concerning the value of omega-3 fats in medical and neuropsychiatric problems.

Stone I. *The Healing Factor: Vitamin C Against Disease.* New York: Putnam, 1972. One of the earlier sources expounding benefits of elevated intake of ascorbate.

Notes

Chapter 1

1. The patient's name and biographical information were obtained at www.horror-wood.com/hayes.htm (article copyright Jackrandall Earles).

Chapter 2

1. For a broad directory to such Web sites, see www.ksu.edu/english/nelp/rowling/.
2. For background on the philosophy, nature, and mode of research, see: Geoffrey Stokes (1998). *Popper: Philosophy, Politics, and Scientific Method.* Malden, MA: Blackwell Publishers.
3. Premature publicity issued with "puffery" or "spin" is found commonly to occur in media coverage of both laboratory and clinical research. Blame for it often lies with the researcher's egoism that expresses outcomes in the most favorable light possible, but journalists actively seek statements that lend themselves to such headlines even when it requires hyperbole.
4. For a more elaborate discussion of drug testing for FDA approval, see Basara and Montagne (1994), page 44.

Chapter 4

1. The instance alluded to involved Neurontin (gabapentin). The cases of sudden, unexplained death occurred in early studies of the compound as an adjunct antiepileptic in persons having a diagnosis of epilepsy; therefore, it may not be applicable to persons taking the drug for one of the many "off-label" uses such as peripheral neuropathy.

Chapter 5

1. Quotes of Dr. Johann Hartmann and Dr. Velpeauwere are from Cerf C and Navasky V. (1998). *The Experts Speak, Expanded and Updated.* New York: Villard, p. 34.

Consumer's Guide to Dietary Supplements and Alternative Medicines

doi:10.1300/5698_36

Chapter 6

1. A safety debate concerning COX-2 inhibitors for osteoarthritis was heightened in Fall 2004 by question of their safety and the withdrawal of one, Vioxx, because of a *doubling* of the users' risk for cardiac deaths. Bextra was withdrawn in April 2005 because of its association with serious dermatologic reactions.

Chapter 13

1. Ponce de Leon may have been maligned by his contemporaries. Current-day sources deny the "fountain of youth" explanation for his explorations as entirely a myth made up to sully his name.

Chapter 15

1. An actual example of a disaster resulting from a soy-based infant formula that lacked sufficient vitamin B1 supplementation is detailed in Chapter 21.

2. The source cited by Julia Ross (2002) was an Internet site that became no longer available by 2003. Inquiring minds became highly suspicious about the reason or motive for this removal from public notice.

Chapter 16

1. Although it can hardly match the nomenclature tour de force of horny goat weed!

Chapter 18

1. This chapter relates to established, diagnosed cancers, not to attempted reduction of the risk for cancer, i.e., cancer chemoprevention, which is covered in Chapter 24.

2. This characterization is not based on hard data, but it is supported by survey findings about the patients' reports of interactions with physicians (Boon et al., 2000).

3. Because of a predetermined conclusion that supplements are not significant, no justification would exist for "wasting" valuable time to become well-informed on those subjects.

4. A similar accusation has been made of "a massive conspiracy" by "the medical establishment"—the multinational pharmaceutical giants, the AMA, and the FDA—to suppress "wondrous cancer cures" for venal reasons. It may well qualify to be classed as an urban legend.

5. On October 12, 2004, zero hits were obtained from a PubMed search of the National Library of Medicine database, 1966 to 2004, for both proxeronine and xeronine. Sixty hits were found for *Morinda citrifolia* itself.

6. The source for this section was material presented at the May 2003 meeting of the American College for Advancement of Medicine in Washington, DC.

Chapter 31

1. Recent reports indicate that former usage of "adult-onset" for NIDDM is clearly no longer a correct description as the U.S. epidemic of juvenile obesity is tending to bring with it an epidemic of type 2 diabetes beginning in adolescence or even before!

Chapter 34

1. Dr. Fry had an NIH research grant for study of humor physiology around 1970.

Chapter 35

1. I am qualified to approach this topic from the viewpoint of only the Judeo-Christian teachings, and not of those of other world religions, because I am a follower of the Christian faith. Persons with qualifications regarding other bodies of religious teachings that recognize spiritual aspects of health and healing might agree with some of these thoughts and differ from others. In faith matters one must write from where one has walked and wherein one resides.

2. Many of these citations were from nursing practice journals (e.g., *Journal of Holistic Nursing, Holistic Nursing Practice*), more so than from journals of medical practice.

Glossary

In addition to this resource, please note the availability of an online medical dictionary at www.nlm.nih.gov/medlineplus/mplusdictionary.html on the National Library of Medicine Web site.

acute: Having an early or rapid onset, as in early-developing symptoms in response to a toxic chemical exposure, or an occurrence of a pathological state. The timescale is usually minutes to hours.

adducts: Combined form of a large endogenous molecule—protein or nucleic acid—with a smaller exogenous chemical. Such firm chemical interactions are responsible for some types of delayed toxicity such as induction of cancers, mutations, or birth defects.

alkaloid: The class of basic (alkaline) chemicals found in various families of plants, many of which are pharmacologically active and important both as poisons and potential drugs.

anaphylaxis: A type of acute, severe allergic reaction that may cause life-threatening hindrances to respiration and/or circulation.

antibodies: The specific proteins produced by special immune cells (B-lymphocytes) to act against the foreign proteins of invaders, which provoked their production. This is a fundamental aspect of acquired immunity.

antineoplastic: Acting against cancer, usually applied regarding drugs used for cancer chemotherapy.

atherogenic diet: A diet fed to laboratory animals to provoke the blood vessel lesions typical of human atherosclerosis in order to obtain an animal model for research dealing with atherosclerosis.

atherosclerosis: An arterial blood vessel disorder in which fatty deposits (known as atheroma) develop in the lining wall of the vessel and gradually fill it, thus reducing the ability of the vessel to carry the normal, needed flow of blood. When the oxygen supply becomes greatly deficient it may lead to an acute heart attack, or possibly a stroke. It is an especial hazard for persons with diabetes.

Consumer's Guide to Dietary Supplements and Alternative Medicines

doi:10.1300/5698_37

bioavailability: The quantitative measures of the ability of a therapeutic agent when administered (usually by mouth) into a person's body to be able to be absorbed into the circulation and to reach the intended site of action in some tissue or organ of the body.

body mass index: A measure of obesity calculated as the person's weight in kilograms divided by the square of their height in meters. An index from 25 upward earns a state of "overweight," and 30 or higher is the criterion for outright "obesity."

carcinogens: Chemical agents that have a capacity to provoke cancer development.

cardiac arrhythmia: A condition in which the internal impulse-conducting system of the heart malfunctions, which results in an abnormal pattern of excitation and contraction of that muscle (the myocardium).

chronic: A long-continuing or sometimes indefinitely continuing disease state. The timescale is weeks to years. Regarding toxicity, it describes a late-developing response to exposures over a long time interval, continuously or in often-repeated fashion.

Cochrane reviews: A phrase describing reviews of clinical trials employing an extensive database (Cochrane Library) maintained by the Cochrane Collaboration, an international not-for-profit organization. The Cochrane Library contains regularly updated health care databases providing up-to-date information about the effects of the health care practices used for making systematic reviews of drugs, procedures, and supplements.

cognition/cognitive: Pertaining to intellectual functions of the brain—one's perceiving, thinking, remembering, and knowing.

colitis: An inflammatory state of the colon, as in *ulcerative colitis* if ulcers and bleeding are present; or it may be *ischemic colitis,* which occurs when the blood supply is cut off, possibly leading to a major injury to the colon. The latter, but not the former, is an emergency usually requiring prompt surgical intervention to prevent death.

complement: A group of serum proteins that are part of the intrinsic or innate immunity system. They attract phagocytes to the needed site and enhance their activity, some of which directly attack invading microbes. This is a basic aspect of intrinsic immunity.

compound: A chemical that consists of a stable combination of two or more elements, e.g., carbon and oxygen forming, carbon dioxide (CO_2).

confounding: An experimental situation in which inadequacy of control designs allows another factor to potentially be responsible for a difference between groups other than the factor on which the research was focused. It prevents drawing of valid conclusions.

contraindication: A condition that dictates that a certain drug or supplement should not be used because of excess hazard for a dangerous adverse response.

cytokines: A diverse family of important peptides secreted by cells of the immune system to exert varied important biological activities; for example, some are pro-inflammatory but others are anti-inflammatory.

echocardiography (echocardiogram): An imaging method for visualizing the heart muscle, chambers, and valves in operation to check for abnormalities (resulting image).

efficacy: Concerning a remedy, it regards the remedy's effectiveness in achieving the claimed health benefit.

element: A chemical substance that comprises one of the nearly 200 basic units of matter (e.g., carbon, hydrogen, oxygen, nitrogen, sulfur, calcium, aluminum, iron, etc.).

elixir: An oral, liquid pharmaceutical product that is sweetened, usually flavored, and commonly consists mainly of a mixture of water and alcohol (ethanol). The term is also used metaphorically as in "the elixir of life."

emesis: Vomiting.

emetic: A chemical or other stimulus provoking vomiting.

encephalopathy: A nervous system pathology consisting of an impairment of brain function.

endogenous: From within, as in an the case of an internally produced biochemical that acts as a neurotransmitter, enzyme, or hormone.

enteral feeding/nutritional therapy: The process of providing nourishment to a patient in the hospital by way of an enteral tube, one that goes via the nose, esophagus, and stomach into the upper intestine.

enteric coated: A tablet form that has special coating to avoid exposure to gastric juices so that it doesn't disintegrate until arriving in the intestine.

exogenous: From without, as in a substance ingested, injected, or applied to the body surfaces.

fibrillation: A deranged state of the heartbeat that diminishes or prevents normal pumping of the blood *Atrial f.* occurs when only the upper chambers are involved, and *ventricular f.* when the more essential lower chambers are affected, which will shortly be fatal if not reversed.

gastroesophageal reflux disease (GERD): A problem arising from failure of the sphincter at the junction of esophagus and stomach to prevent the gastric secretions (especially hydrochloric acid) from rising (refluxing, flowing backward) into the esophagus. If it occurs chronically it may cause a dangerous injury to the lower part of the esophagus and may cause severe pain that can be mistaken for cardiac pain.

hepatic: Pertaining to the liver.

hepatotoxicity: Causing or constituting injury to the liver and impairment of its functions.

HRT (hormone replacement therapy): Therapy given when a hormonal deficiency is diagnosed and an exogenous source of the hormone is provided.

hyperesthesia: Abnormality of sensations (a type of paresthesia), which are intensified so as to cause discomfort or severe pain from a mild stimulus.

hypospadias: A congenital (present at birth) malformation in which structural development of the penis is deranged.

idiosyncratic: Showing a response to an externally supplied chemical that is different from that shown by the vast majority of persons because of a preexisting deviation, such as a genetically determined level of an enzyme activity.

incidence: The rate of occurrence, especially for a disease condition or an adverse response to a pharmaceutical or other remedy.

indication: A disease state or condition of a person that calls for the use of a particular therapeutic action.

leukocytes: All the white blood cells (WBCs), mainly including lymphocytes and neutrophils or monocytes that are transposed into macrophages, that direct their attacks against invading microorganisms and may be provoked to secrete cytokines by certain chemical messengers (known as lymphokines) that are secreted by T-lymphocytes in response to needs occurring.

lipid peroxidation: A state in which a reactive oxygen species (ROS) causes oxidation of fatty acids, either in the blood (e.g., LDL) or in cell membranes, both of which may contribute to the pathological processes of important diseases.

lymphocytes: A major family of immune system cells, white blood cells, broadly divided between B- and T-lymphocytes. The former are responsible for antibody functions, and the latter provide cell-mediated attacks against invaders and regulate the action of B-lymphocytes in generating antibodies.

meta-analysis: A methodology of statistical analysis employed to combine and together evaluate multiple clinical trials on a pharmaceutical, supplement, or other therapy.

methylation: A biochemical process by which a methyl group ($-CH_3$) is added by action of an enzyme (a "methylase") to any product (nucleic acid, amino acid, etc.).

microflora: The microbial population of the gastrointestinal tract, especially the colon.

mitochondria: The microscopic-sized compartments within all cells (except for the red blood cells) that contain the enzymes that are fundamental to energy release from foods in their terminal metabolism.

molecule: The smallest amount of a chemical compound that can exist alone as a distinctive combination of atoms.

morbidity: Occurrence of a state of disease, illness, or injury (as by poisoning); any sickness short of death.

myocardial infarction (MI): Commonly known as a heart attack, it is the occurrence of an acute blockage of the circulation to the heart muscle, causing insufficiency of the oxygen supply for normal operation and leading to acute death of some amount of the muscle fibers, which may bring an early or delayed fatality or a continuing state of cardiac failure.

natural killer cells: Lymphocyte-like cells that have a major role in eliminating invading foreign cells (including cancer cells). They perform "search and destroy" missions, as do also certain T-lymphocytes, the "cytotoxic T-cells."

necrosis: A state of such extensive injury that considerable death of cells in an organ occurs, possibly leading to organ failure and perhaps to death of the individual.

neoplastic: Literally a "new growth," namely one that differs significantly from normal in its uncontrolled mode of growth so as to constitute a "malignant neoplasm" or a cancerous growth.

neurotransmitter: An endogenous compound that acts in the nervous system to aid the passage of neural messages between adjacent nerve cells, or from a neuron to cells of muscles or glands. They are usually fairly small molecules.

oncology: The medical science specialty concerning cancer, its diagnosis, and therapies.

organic compound: All compounds that have a basic structure consisting of atoms of the element carbon.

orphan drug: A drug useful for a rare "orphan disease" that may be given FDA approval through relaxed procedures that demand less research data.

palliative: A treatment for cancer that relieves pain and/or other symptoms but will not be expected to eradicate the cancerous growth or to prolong life.

parenteral feeding (or nutritional therapy): The process of providing nourishment to a hospitalized patient by way of an intravenous tube, or via a portal device surgically implanted under the skin.

paresthesia: Abnormal sensations resulting from a deranged state of the peripheral nerves resulting from a neuropathy, often as a result of diabetes; there may be numbness or other uncomfortable—often a burning of the bottoms of the feet.

peer review: The process of review by which medical or science journals gather at least two reviews by qualified researchers on submitted research reports on which the decision to accept or reject the report for publication is based.

phagocytes: White blood cells that act aggressively against foreign cells to engulf and destroy them.

phytochemicals: Purified chemical substances obtained from a plant source, usually for its use as a "dietary ingredient" in supplement products (e.g., lycopene from tomatoes).

precursor: A molecule that is necessary because of its being converted into another important molecule (e.g., a hormone or neurotransmitter).

prevention trials: (Primary or secondary) Referring especially to cardiovascular disease, if a treatment is directed to preventing an event (e.g., a heart attack) after the person has already experienced it once, it becomes secondary prevention. If an intervention is aimed to avoid a first event, it is called primary prevention.

prognosis: The projection by a physician of the likely outcome of a person's illness.

replication: repetition of an experimental design with an intent to determine whether the results will be the same as the original results (i.e., reproducible). If such is found to occur, it will tend to strengthen and confirm the prior outcomes.

signs and symptoms: Whereas *symptoms* are those problems/complaints that a patient feels or otherwise notices subjectively (e.g., malaise, nausea, dizziness, pain), *signs* are conditions that a physician (or another person) can detect, and often measure, objectively (e.g., blood pressure, heart rate, body temperature) for comparison to norms.

solvent: The liquid used to dissolve a chemical, as in a medicine that is an injectable solution or an oral liquid.

steroid(s): A name for a basic chemical structure that occurs widely in nature, both in plant and animal species, the biological properties of which may be quite varied. The most familiar of these are the mammalian hormones from the ovaries, testes, or adrenal cortex. Thus, the word *steroids* is ambiguous without an adjective to specify to which class of steroids the agent belongs (e.g., estrogenic steroid, anabolic-androgenic steroid, adrenocortical steroid, or cardioactive plant steroid).

stroke: A "brain attack" in which blood flow to or within the brain is blocked, which quickly leads to at least temporary (and often permanent) malfunctions. It may be either *hemorrhagic,* caused by rupture of a blood vessel and consequent bleeding within the skull, or *ischemic,* caused by a blockage of a major blood vessel, as by a thrombus (clot) that prevents blood and oxygen from being delivered to certain parts of the brain.

subclinical: The occurrence of illness, deficiency, or injury that is below the threshold of being easily detectable; i.e., clinical signs are not yet apparent.

synergism: The combined action of two (or more) chemical compounds leading to a greater biological effect than would be achieved by either (any) one acting singly.

synergistic: The property of one compound being capable of entering into a synergism with another one.

teratogen/teratogenic agent: A substance that can act during pregnancy to disorder the developmental process so that congenital malformations occur.

ventricular fibrillation: An abnormal desynchronized state of the contractility of the heart in which the muscular action of the ventricles (the main lower chambers of the heart) is no longer coordinated; this arises from a state of hyperirritability that often occurs following occlusion of the coronary arteries or from a progression from atrial fibrillation or ventricular tachycardia. It is rapidly fatal if not reversed immediately by means of a defibrillator device.

Bibliography

Foreword

Enerson OD. (2001). Alexis Carrel. Available at: http://www.whonamedit.com/doctor.cfm/445.html.

Preface

Cousins N. (1989). *Head First: The Biology of Hope*. New York: E. Dutton.

Crosby WH. (1977). Lead-contaminated health food: Association with lead poisoning and leukemia. *Journal of the American Medical Association 237:* 2627-2629.

Davis M. (2001). Dietary supplements: Are they safe and reliable? *Drug Topics 8:* 61.

Eisenberg DM, Davis RB, Ettner SL, Appel S, Wilkey S, Van Rompay M, Kessler RC. (1998). Trends in alternative medicine use in the United States, 1990-1997: Results of a follow-up national survey. *Journal of the American Medical Association 280:* 1566-1575.

Ewy GA. (1999). Antioxidant therapy for coronary artery disease: Don't paint the walls without treating the termites! *Archives of Internal Medicine 1999 159:* 1279-1280.

Sampson W. (1996). Antiscience trends in the rise of the "alternative medicine" movement. In PR Gross, N Levitt, and MW Lewis (eds.), *The Flight from Science and Reason*. New York: The New York Academy of Sciences, pp. 188-197.

Chapter 1

Earles J. (2000). The real Allison Hayes. *Horror-Wood Webzine*. March. Available at: http://www.horror-wood.com/allison.htm.

Chapter 2

Als-Nielsen B, Chen W, Gluud C, Kjaergard LL. (2003). Association of funding and conclusions in randomized drug trials: A reflection of treatment effects or adverse events? *Journal of the American Medical Association 290:* 921-928.

Angell M. (2004). *The Truth About Drug Companies: How They Deceive Us and What to Do About It*. New York: Random House.

Consumer's Guide to Dietary Supplements and Alternative Medicines

doi:10.1300/5698_38

Anonymous [Evidence-Based Medicine Working Group]. (1992). Evidence-based medicine: A new approach to teaching the practice of medicine. *Journal of the American Medical Association 268:* 2420-2425.

Barrett S. (2004). Some notes on Jeffrey Bland. Available at: quackwatch.org/04ConsumerEducation/Bland.html.

Basara LR, Montagne M. (1994). *Searching for Magic Bullets: Orphan Drugs, Consumer Activism, and Pharmaceutical Development.* Binghamton, NY: Pharmaceutical Products Press.

Bodenheimer T. (2000a). Conflict of interest in clinical drug trials: A risk factor for scientific misconduct. Available at: www.hsph.harvard.edu/bioethics/uae/BodenheimerCOI.htm.

Bodenheimer T. (2000b). Uneasy alliance—Clinical investigators and the pharmaceutical industry. *New England Journal of Medicine 342:* 1539-1544.

Davidson F, DeAngelis CD, Drazen JM, et al. (2001). Sponsorship, authorship, and accountability. *Journal of the American Medical Association 286:* 1232-1235.

Davis SR, Briganti EM, Chen RQ, Dalais FS, Bailey M, Burger HG. (2001). The effects of Chinese medicinal herbs on postmenopausal vasomotor symptoms of Australian women: A randomised controlled trial. *Medical Journal of Australia 174:* 68-71.

Egan ME, Pearson M, Weiner SA, Rajendran V, Rubin R, Glockner-Paget J, Canny S, Du K, Lukacs GL, Caplan MJ. (2004). Curcumin, a major constituent of turmeric, corrects cystic fibrosis defects. *Science 304:* 600-601.

Frank JD. (1975). The faith that heals. *The Johns Hopkins Medical Journal 137:* 127-131.

Golub ES. (1975). *The Limits of Medicine: How Science Shapes Our Hope for the Cure.* Chicago: University of Chicago Press.

Golub ES. (1997). *The Limits of Medicine: How Science Shapes Our Hope for the Cure.* Chicago: University of Chicago Press.

Goodwin JS, Tangum MR. (1998). Battling quackery: Attitudes about micronutrient supplements in American academic medicine. *Archives of Internal Medicine 158:* 2187-2191.

Holden C. (2002). Drugs and placebos look alike to the brain. *Science 295:* 947-948.

Johnson J. (2004). Outing the conflicted: Et tu NIH? *Science 303:* 1610.

Karlawish JH, Whitehouse PJ. (1998). Is the placebo control obsolete in a world after donepezil and vitamin E? *Archives of Neurology 55:* 1420-1424.

Levi-Strauss C. (1983). *The Raw and the Cooked: Mythologiques.* Reprint, Chicago: University of Chicago Press.

Petrovic P, Kalso E, Petersson KM, Ingvar M. (2002). Placebo and opioid analgesia—Imaging a shared neuronal network. *Science 295:* 1737-1740.

Rowling JK. (1999). *Harry Potter and the Chamber of Secrets.* New York: Arthur A. Levine Books.

Spiro HM. (1998). *The Power of Hope: A Doctor's Perspective.* New Haven, CT: Yale University Press.

Sweet M. (2003). Website launched to expose "tricks" of drug ads. *British Medical Journal 327:* 936.

Szasz T. (1973). *The Second Sin.* Nelson, New Zealand: The Anchor Press.

Tyler V. (1999). *The Honest Herbal,* Fourth edition. Binghamton, NY: The Haworth Press.

Warner S. (2004). On ethics, goals of post-marketing trials. *The Scientist 18:* 22-23.

Chapter 3

Cameron E, Pauling L. (1973). Ascorbic acid and the glycosaminoglycans: An orthomolecular approach to cancer and other diseases. *Oncology 27:* 181-192.

Cameron E, Pauling L. (1976). Supplemental ascorbate in the supportive treatment of cancer: Prolongation of survival times in terminal human cancer. *Proceedings of the National Academy of Sciences USA 73:* 3685-3689.

Hlatky MA, Boothroyd D, Vittinghoff E, Sharp P, Whooley MA, for the HERS Research Group. (2002). Quality-of-life and depressive symptoms in postmenopausal women after receiving hormone therapy. *Journal of the American Medical Association 287:* 591-597.

Hulley S, Grady D, Bush T, Furberg C, Herrington D, Riggs B, Vittinghoff E, for the Heart and Estrogen/Progestin Replacement Study (HERS) Research Group. (1998). Randomized trial of estrogen plus progestin for secondary prevention of coronary heart disease in postmenopausal women. *Journal of the American Medical Association 280:* 605-613.

Levy TE. (2002). *Vitamin C, Infectious Diseases, and Toxins: Curing the Incurable.* Philadelphia: Xlibris Corp.

Petitti DB. (1998). Hormone replacement therapy and heart disease prevention. Experiment trumps observation. *Journal of the American Medical Association 280:* 650-651.

Thiessen M. (2005). Judge rules against FDA ban on ephedra. *Washington Post,* April 15, p. E05. Available at: http://www.washingtonpost.com/wp-dyn/articles/A53586-2005Apr14.html.

Vastag B. (2002). Hormone therapy falls out of favor with expert committee. *Journal of the American Medical Association 287:* 1923-1924.

Writing Group [for the Women's Health Initiative Investigators] (2002). Risks and benefits of estrogen plus progestin in healthy postmenopausal women. *Journal of the American Medical Association 288:* 321-333.

Yaroch AL. (2001). Low-dose DHEA has beneficial effects in women with low androgens. Available at: www.pslgroup.com/dg/1FF046.htm. Accessed May 2, 2005.

Chapter 4

Baron S. (2001). Living on the edge. *British Medical Journal 323:* 291.

Barraclough K. (2001). An afternoon of alternative medicine. *British Medical Journal 323:* 1011.

Bouldin AS, Smith MC, Garner DD, Szeinbach SL, Frate DA, Croom EM. (1999). Pharmacy and herbal medicine in the US. *Social Science & Medicine 49:* 279-289.

Crawford LM. (2005). Remarks of the acting FDA commissioner: FDLI's 48th annual conference. *Food and Drug Law Journal 60:* 99-102.

Eisenberg DM, Davis RB, Erner SL, Appel S, Wilkey S, Van Rompay M, Kessler RC. (1998). Trends in alternative medicine use in the United States, 1990-1997: Results of a follow-up national survey. *Journal of the American Medical Association 280:* 1569-1575.

Fontanarosa PB, Drummond R, DeAngelis CD. (2004). Post-marketing surveillance: Lack of vigilance, lack of trust. *Journal of the American Medical Association 292*: 2647-2650.

Jarvis WT. (1999). Quackery: The National Council Against Health Fraud perspective. *Rheumatic Disease Clinics of North America 25:* 805-814.

Kurtzweil P. (1998). An FDA guide to dietary supplements. *FDA Consumer,* September-October. Available at: www.fda.gov/fdac/default.htm.

Mertens G. (1999). *From Quackery to Credibility: Unconventional Healthcare in the Era of High-Tech Medicine.* London: The Financial Times Business Ltd.

Mukherjee D, Nissen SE, Topol EJ. (2001). Risk of cardiovascular events associated with selective COX-2 inhibitors. *Journal of the American Medical Association 286:* 954-959.

Theodosakis J. (2004) Should our current treatment for osteoarthritis be considered malpractice? Available at drtheo.com/editorial.html. Accessed April 28, 2005.

Therapeutics Initiative (2002). COX-2 inhibitors update: Do journal publications tell the full story? *Therapeutics Letter 43.* Available at: http://www.ti.ubc.ca/pages/letter43.htm.

Tyler VE. (1981). *The Honest Herbal,* First Edition. Philadelphia: G.F. Stickley Co.

Wolfe MM, Lichtenstein DR, Singh G. (1999). Gastrointestinal toxicity of nonsteroidal antiinflammatory drugs. *New England Journal of Medicine 340:* 1888-1899.

Chapter 5

Cerf C, Navasky V. (1998). *The Experts Speak, Expanded and Updated.* New York: Pantheon Books.

Fabricant DS, Farnsworth NR. (2001). The value of plants used in traditional medicine for drug discovery. *Environmental Health Perspectives 109* (Suppl. 1): 69-75.

Smith CF. (1992). *Lenny, Lefty, and the Chancellor: The Len Bias Tragedy and the Search for Reform in Big-Time College Basketball.* Baltimore, MD: Bancroft Press.

Chapter 6

DeAngelis CD, Fontanarosa PB. (2003). Drugs alias dietary supplements. *Journal of the American Medical Association 290:* 1519-1520.

Etminan M, Gill S, Samii A. (2003). Effect of non-steroidal anti-inflammatory drugs on risk of Alzheimer's disease: Systematic review and meta-analysis of observational studies. *British Medical Journal 327:* 128-131.

Vainio H, Morgan G. (1998). Cyclo-oxygenase 2 and breast cancer prevention. Non-steroidal anti-inflammatory agents are worth testing in breast cancer. *British Medical Journal 317:* 828-830.

Chapter 7

Ames BN, Profet M, Gold LS. (1990). Nature's chemicals and synthetic chemicals: Comparative toxicology. *Proceeding of the National Academy of Sciences USA 87:* 7782-7786.

Basara LR and Montagne M. (1994). *Searching for Magic Bullets: Orphan Drugs, Consumer Activism and Pharmaceutical Development.* Binghamton, NY: Pharmaceutical Products Press.

Bent S, Avins AL. (1999). An herb for every illness? *American Journal of Medicine 106:* 259-260.

Borins M. (1998). The dangers of using herbs. What your patients need to know. *Postgraduate Medicine 104:* 91-95, 99-100.

Ernst E. (2003). Herbal medicines put into context: Their use entails risks, but probably fewer than with synthetic drugs. *British Medical Journal 327:* 881-882.

Hardy ML. (2000). Herbs of special interest to women. *Journal of the American Pharmaceutical Association NS40:* 234-242.

Huxtable RJ. (1992) The myth of beneficent nature: The risks of herbal preparations. *Annals of Internal Medicine 117:* 165-166.

Kinnell HG. (2001). Serial homicide by physicians: Shipman in perspective. *British Medical Journal 321:* 1594-1597.

MacGregor FB, Abernethy VE, Duhabra S, Cobden I, Hayes PC. (1989). Hepatotoxicity of herbal remedies. *British Medical Journal 299:* 1156-1157.

Noah ND, Bender AE, Readil GB, Gilbert RJ. (1980). Food poisoning from red kidney beans. *British Medical Journal 281:* 236-237.

Norton SA. (2000). Raw animal tissues and dietary supplements. *New England Journal of Medicine 343:* 304-305.

Pillan, PI. (1995). Toxicity of herbal products. *New Zealand Medical Journal 108:* 469-471.

ProMED. (2004). Toxic ingestion, tung oil—China (Hunan). *ProMED Digest, 174,* May 4. Available at: www.promedmail.org/pls/askus/. Accessed June 5, 2004.

Purdue University. (2002) School of Veterinary Sciences. Available at: vet.purdue .edu/depts/addl/toxic/plant40.htm. Accessed April 8, 2002.

Sekercioglu CH. (2004). Prion disease and a penchant for brains. *Science 305:* 343-344.

Stickel F, Egerer G, Seitz HK. (2000). Hepatotoxicity of botanicals. *Public Health Nutrition 3:* 113-124.

Tomlinson B, Chan TYK, Chan JCN, Critchley JAJH But PP. (2000). Toxicity of complementary therapies: An Eastern perspective. *Journal of Clinical Pharmacology 40:* 451-456.

Williamson BL, Klarskov K, Tomlinson AJ, Gleich GJ, Naylor S. (1998). Problems with over-the-counter 5-hydroxy-L-tryptophan. *Nature Medicine 4:* 983.

Williamson D. (2000). Expert calls for common sense, science in national response to medicinal herbs. Available at: www.eurekalert.org/pub_releases/200003/U.NC.

Chapter 8

Centers for Disease Control and Prevention (CDC). (1996). Adverse events associated with ephedrine-containing products: Texas, December 1993-September 1995. *Morbidity and Mortality Weekly 45*(32): 689-692.

Connell PH. (1958). *Amphetamine Psychosis* (Maudsley Monographs No. 5). London: Oxford University Press.

Davis WM, Pinkerton JT, III. (1972). Synergism by atropine of central stimulant properties of phenylpropanolamine. *Toxicology and Applied Pharmacology 22:* 138-145.

Enders JM, Dobesh PP, Ellison JN. (2003). Acute myocardial infarction induced by ephedrine alkaloids. *Pharmacotherapy 23:* 1645-1651.

Haller CA, Benowitz NL. (2000). Adverse cardiovasculare and central nervous system events associated with dietary supplements containing ephedra alkaloids. *New England Journal of Medicine 343:* 1833-1838.

Pentel P. (1984). Toxicity of over-the-counter stimulants. *Journal of the American Medical Association 252:* 1898-1903.

Powell T, Hsu FF, Turk J, Hruska K. (1998). Ma-huang strikes again: Ephedrine nephrolithiasis. *American Journal of Kidney Diseases 32:* 153-159.

Shekelle PG, Hardy ML, Morton SC, Maglione M, Mojica WA, Suttorp MJ, Rhodes SL, Jungvig L, Gagne J. (2003). Efficacy and safety of ephedra and ephedrine for weight loss and athletic performance: A meta-analysis. *Journal of the American Medical Association 289:* 1537-1545.

Traboulsi AS, Viswahathan R, Coplan J. (2002). Suicide attempt after use of a herbal diet pill. *American Journal of Psychiatry 159:* 318-319.

Wolfe SM. (2003). Ephedra—Scientific evidence versus money/politics. *Science 300:* 905.

Zahn KA, Li RL, Purssell RA. (1999). Cardiovascular toxicity after ingestion of "herbal ecstasy." *Journal of Emergency Medicine 17:* 289-291.

Chapter 9

Ang-Lee MK, Moss J, Yuan C-S. (2001). Herbal medicines and postoperative care. *Journal of the American Medical Association 286:* 208-216.

Barone GW, Gurley BJ, Ketel BL, Abul-Ezz SR. (2001). Herbal dietary supplements: A source for drug interactions in transplant recipients. *Transplantation 71:* 239-241.

Barone GW, Gurley BJ, Ketel BL, Lightfoot ML, Abul-Ezz SR. (2000). Drug interaction between St. John's wort and cyclosporine. *Annals of Pharmacotherapy 34:* 1013-1016.

Breidenbach T, Kliem V, Burg M, Radermacher J, Hoffmann MW, Klempnauer J. (2000). Profound drop of cyclosporine A whole blood trough levels caused by St. John's wort *(Hypericum perforatum). Transplantation 69:* 2229-2230.

Fugh-Berman A. (2000). Herb-drug interactions. *Lancet 355:* 134-138.

Gordon JB. (1998). SSRIs and St. John's wort: Possible toxicity? *American Family Physician 57:* 950, 953.

Heck AM, DeWitt BA, Lukes AL. (2000). Potential interactions between alternative therapies and warfarin. *American Journal of Health Systems Pharmacy 57:* 1221-1227.

Hirata JD, Swiersz LM, Zell B, Small R, Ettinger B. (1997). Does dong quai have estrogenic effects in postmenopausal women? A double-blind, placebo-controlled trial. *Fertility and Sterility 68:* 981-986.

Izzat MB, Yim APC, El-Zufari MH. (1998). A taste of Chinese medicine! *Annals of Thoracic Surgery 66:* 941-942.

Lantz MS, Buchalter E, Giambanco V. (1999). St. John's wort and antidepressant drug interactions in the elderly. *Journal of Geriatric Psychiatry and Neurology 12:* 7-10.

Mathijssen RH, Verweig J, de Bruijn , Loos WJ, Sparreboom A. (2002). Effects of St. John's wort on irinotecan metabolism. *Journal of the National Cancer Institute 94:* 124749.

Nierenberg AA, Burt T, Matthews J, Weiss AP. (1999). Mania associated with St. John's wort. *Biological Psychiatry 46:* 1707-1708.

Norred CL, Zamudio S, Palmer SK. (2000). Use of complementary and alternative medicine by surgical patients. *American Association of Nurse Anesthetists Journal 68:* 13-18.

Parker V, Wong AHC, Boon HS, Seeman MV. (2001). Adverse reaction to St. John's wort. *Canadian Journal of Psychiatry 46:* 77-79.

Turton-Weeks S, Barone G, Gurley BJ, Ketel BL, Lightfoot ML, Abdul-Ezz SR. (2001). St. John's wort: A hidden risk for transplant patients. *Progress in Transplantation 11:* 116-120.

Chapter 10

Abourashed EA, Khan IA. (2000) Determination of parthenolide in selected feverfew products by liquid chromatography. *Journal of the Association of Official Agricultural Chemists International 83:* 789-792.

Abourashed EA, Khan IA. (2001). GC determination of parthenolides in feverfew products. *Die Pharmazie 56:* 971-972.

Abourashed EA, El-Alfy AT, Khan IA, Walker L. (2003). Ephedra in perspective—A current review. *Phytotherapy Research 17:* 703-712.

Bensoussan A, Talley NJ, Hing M, Menzies R, Guo A, Ngu M. (1998). Treatment of irritable bowel syndrome with a Chinese herbal medicine. *Journal of the American Medical Association 280:* 1585-1589.

California Department of Health Services. (2000). News release: State health director warns consumers about prescription drugs in herbal products. February 15. Available at: http://www.fda.gov/oc/po/firmrecalls/Herbal.html.

ConsumerLab.com. (2004). Product review: St. John's wort. Available at: http://www.consumerlab.com/results/sjw.asp.

FDA. (1991). Dietary supplement/herbal products: Chuifong toukuwan IA #66-10—Revised 2/21/91, Chinese Herbal Medicines. Available at: www.fda.gov/ora/fiars/ora_import_ia6610.html.

FDA. (199X). Dietary supplement/herbal products: Tongyi tang. Available at: www.fda.gov/ora/fiars/ora_import_ia6610.html.

FDA. (2000). New warning on diabetes and Chinese herbs: Zhen qi, yongyitang, and others. Available at: www.fda.gov/womens/owhupdate/march2000.html.

FDA. (2002a). Dietary supplement/herbal products: On SPES and PC-SPE. Available at: www.fda.gov/medwatch/safety/2002/safety02.htm#spes.

FDA. (2002b). FDA warns public about chinese diet pills containing fenfluramine. August 13. Available at: www.fda.gov/bbs/topics/NEWS/2002/NEW00826.html.

FDA. (2004). Available at: fda.gov/medwatch/SAFETY/2003/vinarol.htm.

FDA. (2005). 2004 safety alerts for drugs, biologics, medical devices, and dietary supplements. Available at: http://www.fda.gov/medwatch/SAFETY/2004/safety04.htm.

Gugliotta G. (2001). Women wins $13.3 million against dietary company. Washington Post, February 8, p. A08. Available at: http://jameshoyer.com/ephedra_wp2.pdf.

Gurley BJ, Gardner SF, Hubbard MA. (2000). Content versus label claims in ephedra-containing dietary supplements. *American Journal of Health System Pharmacy 57:* 963-969.

Gurley BJ, Gardner SF, White LM, Wang PL. (1998). Ephedrine pharmacokinetics after the ingestion of nutritional supplements containing ephedra sinica (ma huang). *Therapeutic Drug Monitoring 20:* 439-445.

Haller CA, Benowitz NL. (2000). Adverse cardiovascular and central nervous system events associated with dietary supplements containing ephedra alkaloids. *New England Journal of Medicine 343:* 1833-1838.

Heck AM, DeWitt BA, Lukes AL. (2000). Potential interactions between alternative therapies and warfarin. *American Journal of Health-System Pharmacy 57:* 1221-1227.

Huggett DB, Block DS, Khan IA, Allgood JC, Benson WH. (2000). Environmental contaminants in the botanical dietary supplement ginseng and potential human risk. *Human and Ecological Risk Assessment 6:* 767-776.

Larsen TM, Toubro S, Astrup A. (2003). Efficacy and safety of dietary supplements containing CLA for the treatment of obesity: Evidence from animal and human studies. *Journal of Lipid Research 44:* 2234-2241.

Lasso de la Vega R, Gupta MP, Cedeno JE. (1982). Corticoid activity of chuifong toukuwan pills and detection of indomethacin. (In Spanish.) *Revue Medicina Panama 13:* 62-65.

Lau KK, Lia CK, Chan AYW. (2000). Phenytoin poisoning after using Chinese proprietary medicines. *Human and Experimental Toxicology 19:* 385-386.

Levy S. (2002). Watch for new seals of approval on dietary supplements. *Drug Topics 1:* 29. Available at: www.drugtopics.com/drugtopics/article/articleDetail.jsp?id=116519.

Metcalf K, Corns C, Fahie-Wilson M, Mackenzie P. (2002). Chinese medicines for slimming still cause health problems. *British Journal of Medicine 324:* 679.

Mirand PP, Arnal-Bagnard MA, Mosoni L, Faulconnier Y, Chardigny JM, Chilliard Y. (2004). Cis-9,trans-11 and trans-10,cis-12 conjugated linoleic acid isomers do not modify body composition in adult sedentary or exercised rats. *Journal of Nutrition 134:* 2263-2269.

National Center for Complementary and Alternative Medicine (NCCAM). (2003). Vinarol and Viga tablets contaminated with sildenafil (Viagara). June 6. Available at: http://nccam.nih.gov/health/alerts/viagra/viagra.htm.

Raloff J. (2001). The good trans fat. Will one family of animal fats become a medicine? *Science News 159:* 136-138.

Rubin BK, LeGatt DF, Audette RJ. (1990). The Mexican asthma cure: Systemic steroids for gullible gringos. *Chest 97:* 959-961.

Tricon S, Burdge GC, Kew S, Banerjee T, Russell JJ, Jones EL, Grimble RF, Williams CM, Yaqoob P, Calder PC. (2004). Opposing effects of cis-9,trans-11 and trans-10,cis-12 conjugated linoleic acid on blood lipids in healthy humans. *American Journal of Clinical Nutrition 80:* 614-620.

Wang YW, Jones PJ. (2004). Conjugated linoleic acid and obesity control: Efficacy and mechanisms. *International Journal of Obesity & Related Metabolic Disorders 28:* 941-955.

Whigham LD, O'Shea M, Mohede IC, Walaski HP, Atkinson RL. (2004). Safety profile of conjugated linoleic acid in a 12-month trial in obese humans. *Food & Chemical Toxicology 42:* 1701-1709.

Yarney G. (2000). Inquiry discovers fraudulent skin treatments. *British Medical Journal 320:* 76.

Chapter 11

Armanini D, Bonanni G, Palermo M. (1999). Reduction of serum testosterone in men by licorice. *New England Journal of Medicine 341:* 1158.

Blachley JD, Knochel JP. (1980). Tobacco chewer's hypokalemia: Licorice revisited. *New England Journal of Medicine 302:* 784-785.

Epstein MT, Espiner EA, Donald RA, Hughes H. (1997). Effects of eating liquorice on the renin-angiotensin-aldosterone axis in normal subjects. *British Medical Journal* 488-490.

Eriksson JW, Carlberg B, Hillörn V. (1999). Life-threatening ventricular tachycardia due to liquorice-induced hypokalaemia. *Journal of Internal Medicine 245:* 307-310.

Harries K, Shute K, Edwards D. (1998). Hazards of a "healthy" diet. *Annals of the Royal College of Surgeons of England 80:* 72.

Jarmon PR, Kehley AM, Mather HM. (2001). Hyperkalemia and apple juice. *Lancet 358:* 841-842.
Luchon L, Meyrier A, Paillard F. (1993). Hypokalemia without arterial hypertension by licorice poisoning. (In French.) *Nephrologie 14:* 177-181.
McGuire JK, Kulkarni MS, Baden HP. (2000). Fatal hypermagnesemia in a child treated with megavitamin/megamineral therapy. *Pediatrics 105:* e18.
Mueller BA, Scott MK, Sowinski KM, Prag KA. (2000). Noni juice *(Morinda citrifolia):* Hidden potential for hyperkalemia? *American Journal of Kidney Disease 35:* 310-312.
Suvarna S, Pirmohamed M, Henderson, L. (2003). Possible interaction between warfarin and cranberry juice. *British Medical Journal 327:* 1454.
Visvanathan R. (1998). Hazards of a "healthy" diet. *Annals of the Royal College of Surgery England 80:* 302.

Chapter 12

Australian Adverse Drug Reactions Advisory Committee. (1999). An adverse reaction to the herbal medicine milk thistle *(Silybum marianum). Medical Journal of Australia 170:* 218-219.
Bass NM. (1999). Is there any use for traditional or alternative therapies in patients with chronic liver disease? *Current Gastroenterology Reports 1:* 50-56.
Berkson BM. (1999). A conservative triple antioxidant approach to the treatment of hepatitis C. Combination of alpha lipoic acid (thioctic acid), silymarin, and selenium: Three case histories. *Medizinische Klinik 94* (Suppl. III): 84-89.
Bunout D, Hirsch S, Petermann M, De la Maza MP, Silva G, Kelly M, Ugarte G, Iturriaga H. (1992). Estudio controlado sobre el efecto de la silimarina en la enfermedad hepática alcohólica [Effects of sylimarin on alcoholic liver disease: A controlled trial]. *Revista Medica de Chile 120:* 1370-1375.
Escher M, Desmeules J, Giostra E, Mentha G. (2001). Hepatitis associated with kava: A herbal remedy for anxiety. *British Medical Journal 322:* 139.
Estes JD, Stolpman D, Olyaei A, Corless CL, Ham JM, Schwartz JM, Orloff SL. (2003). High prevalence of potentially hepatotoxic herbal supplement use in patients with fulminant hepatic failure. *Archives of Surgery 138:* 852-858.
Favreau JT, Ryu ML, Braunstein G, Orshansky G, Park SS, Coody GL, Love LA, Fong TL. (2002). Severe hepatotoxicity associated with the dietary supplement LipoKinetix. *Annals of Internal Medicine 136:* 590-595.
Food and Drug Administration (FDA). (2001). FDA warns consumers not to use the dietary supplement LipoKinetix. Available at: http://www.cfsan.fda.gov/~dms/ds-lipo.html.
FDA. (2002). Consumer advisory: Kava-containing dietary supplements may be associated with severe liver injury. Available at: www.cfsan.fda.gov/~dms/addskava.html.
Fetrow CW, Avila JR. (1999) *Professional's Handbook of Complementary & Alternative Medicines,* Second Edition. Springhouse, PA: Springhouse Publishing.

Flora K, Hahn M, Rosen H, Benner K. (1998). Milk thistle *(Silybum marianum)* for the therapy of liver disease. *American Journal of Gastroenterology 93:* 139-143.

Humberston CL, Akhtar J, Krenzelok EP. (2003). Acute hepatitis induced by kava kava. *Journal of Toxicology-Clinical Toxicology 41:* 109-113.

Huxtable RJ. (1989). Herbal teas and toxins: Novel aspects of pyrrolizidine poisoning in the United States. *Perspectives in Biology and Medicine 24:* 1-14.

Huxtable RJ. (1990). The harmful potential of herbals and other plant products. *Drug Safety 5* (Suppl. 1): 126-136.

Huxtable RJ. (1992). The myth of beneficent nature: The risks of herbal preparations. *Annals of Internal Medicine 117:* 165-166.

Katz M, Saibil F. (1990). Herbal hepatitis: Subacute hepatic necrosis secondary to chaparral leaf. *Journal of Clinical Gastroenterology 12:* 203-206.

Larrey D, Pageaux GP. (1995). Hepatotoxicity of herbal remedies and mushrooms. *Seminars in Liver Disease 15:* 183-188.

Larrey D, Vial T, Pauwels A, Vastot A, Biour M, David M, Michel H. (1992) Hepatitis after germander *(Teucrium chamaedrys)* administration: Another instance of herbal medicine hepatotoxicity. *Annals of Internal Medicine 117:* 129-132.

MacGregor FB, Abernethy VE, Dahabra S, Cobden I, Hayes PC. (1989). Hepatotoxicity of herbal remedies. *British Medical Journal 299:* 1156-1157.

Mato JM, Camara J, Fernandez de Paz J, Caballeria L, Coll S, Caballero A, Garcia-Buey L, Beltran J, Benita V, Caballeria J, Sola R, et al. (1999). S-adenosylmethionine in alcoholic liver cirrhosis: a randomized, placebo-controlled, double-blind, multicenter clinical trial. *Journal of Hepatology 30*(6): 1081-1089.

Mills E, Singh R, Ross C, Ernst E, Ray JG. (2003). Sale of kava extract in some health food stores. *Canadian Medical Association Journal 169:* 1158-1159.

National Institute on Alcohol Abuse and Alcoholism (NIAAA). (2005). Alcoholic liver disease. *Alcohol Alert,* no. 64, January. Available at: http://pubs.niaaa.nih.gov/publications/aa64/AA64.pdf.

Stickel F, Egerer G, Seitz HK. (2000). Hepatotoxicity of botanicals. *Public Health Nutrition 3:* 113-124.

Sullivan JB, Rumack BH, Thomas H Jr, Peterson RG, Bryson P. (1979). Pennyroyal poisoning and hepatotoxicity. *Journal of the American Medical Association 242:* 2873-2874.

Woolf GM, Petrovic LM, Roitjer SE, Wainwright S, Villamil FG, Katkov WN, Michieletti P, Wanless IR, Stermitz FR, Beck JJ, Vierling JM. (1994). Acute hepatitis associated with the Chinese herbal product jin bu huan. *Annals of Internal Medicine 121:* 729-735.

Chapter 13

Arendt J. (1997). Safety of melatonin in long-term use. *Journal of Biological Rhythms 12:* 673-681.

Bunk, S. (2002). The molecular face of aging. *The Scientist 16:* 16-18.

Di WL, Kadva A, Johnston A, Silman R. (1997). Variable bioavailability of oral melatonin. *New England Journal of Medicine 336:* 1028-1029.

Institute of Medicine. (2003). *Testosterone and Aging.* Washington, DC: National Academies Press.

Jockovich M, Cosentino D, Cosentino L, Wears RL, Seaberg DC. (2000). Effect of exogenous melatonin on mood and sleep efficiency in emergency medicine residents working night shifts. *Academic Emergency Medicine 7:* 955-958.

Juengst ET, Binstock RH, Mehlman MJ, Post SG. Antiaging research and the need for public dialogue. *Science 299*(5611): 1323

Lamberg L. (1996). Melatonin potentially useful but safety, efficacy remain uncertain. *Journal of the American Medical Association 276:* 1011-1014.

Liverman CT and Blazer DG (Eds.). (2004). *Testosterone and Aging.* Washington, DC: The National Academies Press.

Markowitz JS, Carson WH, Jackson CW. (1999). Possible dihydroepiandrosterone-induced mania. *Biological Psychiatry 45:* 241-242.

Planter HA. (1964). Precocious pubescence—Iatrogenic. *New England Journal of Medicine 270:* 141-142.

Sack RL, Lewy AJ, Hughes RJ. (1998). Use of melatonin for sleep and circadian rhythm disorders. *Annals of Medicine 30:* 115-121.

Sahelian R. (2002). Caution urged with high dose DHEA and pregnenolone. Available at: www.tldp.com/issue/175-6/Caution.html.

Satoh K, Mishima K. (2001). Hypothermic action of exogenously administered melatonin is dose-dependent in humans. *Clinical Neuropharmacology 24:* 334-340.

Scheer FA, Van Montfrans GA, van Someren EJ, Mairuhu G, Buijs RM. (2004). Daily nighttime melatonin reduces blood pressure in male patients with essential hypertension. *Hypertension 43:* 192-197.

Taaffe DR, Pruitt L, Reim J, Hintz RL, Butterfield G, Hoffman AR, Marcus R. (1994). Effect of recombinant human growth hormone on the muscle strength response to resistance exercise in elderly men. *Journal of Clinical Endocrinology and Metabolism 79:* 1361-1366.

Tailleux A, Torpier G, Bonnefont-Rousselot D, Lestavel S, Lemdani M, Caudeville B, Furman C, Foricher R, Gardes-Albert M, Lesieur D, et al. (2002). Daily melatonin supplementation in mice increases atherosclerosis in proximal aorta. *Biochemical and Biophysical Research Communications 293:* 1114-1123.

Testosterone and Aging: Clinical Research Directions, http://www.nap.edu or http://national-academies.org.

Vance ML. (2003). Can growth hormone prevent aging? *New England Journal of Medicine 348*(9): 779-780.

Whitten PL, Patisaul HB. (2001). Cross-species and interassay comparisons of phytoestrogen action. *Environmental Health Perspectives 109* (Suppl. 1): 5-20.

Yaroch AL. (2001) Low-dose DHEA has beneficial effects in women with low androgens. Available at: www.pslgroup.com/dg/1FF046.htm. Accessed May 2, 2005.

Zeitzer JM, Daniels JE, Duffy JF, Klerman EB, Shanahan TL, Dijk DJ, Czeisler CA. (1999). Do plasma melatonin concentrations decline with age? *American Journal of Medicine 107:* 432-436.

Zwain IH, Yen SS. (1999). Dehydroepiandrosterone: Biosynthesis and metabolism in the brain. *Endocrinology 140:* 880-887.

Chapter 14

Alzheimer's Research Forum. (2004). News: Gingko goes on trial again . . . this time in London. Available at: http://www.alzforum.org/new/detail.asp?id=1067.

Bagis S, Tamer L, Sahin G, Bilgin R, Guler H, Ercan B, Erdogan C. (2003). Free radicals and antioxidants in primary fibromyalgia: An oxidative stress disorder? *Rheumatology International.* December 20. ePublication. Available at: www .ImmuneSupport.com.

Block G. (1990). Epidemiologic data on the role of ascorbic acid in cancer prevention. Paper presented at National Institutes of Health conference "Vitamin C: Biologic Functions and Relation to Cancer", September 10-12, 1990, Bethesda, MD.

Conklin KA. (2000). Dietary antioxidants during cancer chemotherapy: Impact on chemotherapeutic effectiveness and development of side effects. *Nutrition and Cancer 7:* 1-18.

Crook, TH, III, Adderly B. (1998). *The Memory Cure: The Safe, Scientifically Proven Breakthrough That Can Slow, Halt or Even Reverse Memory Loss.* New York: Pocket Books.

Delanty N, Dichter MA. (2000). Antioxidant therapy in neurologic disease. *Archives of Neurology 57:* 1265-1270.

DiBenedetto P, Iona LG, Zidarich V. (1993). Clinical evaluation of S-adenosyl-L-methionine versus transcutaneous electrical nerve stimulation in primary fibromyalgia. *Current Therapeutic Research 53:* 222-229.

Grundman M, Petersen RC, Ferris SH, Thomas RG, Aisen PS, Bennett DA, Foster NL, Jack CR, Jr, Galasko DR, Doody R, et al. [Alzheimer's Disease Cooperative Study Group]. (2004). Mild cognitive impairment can be distinguished from Alzheimer disease and normal aging for clinical trials. *Archives of Neurology 61:* 59-66.

Haynes RB, McKibbon KA, Fitzgerald D, Guyatt GH, Walker CJ, Sackett DL. (1986). How to keep up with the medical literature: How to store and retrieve articles worth keeping. *Annals of Internal Medicine105:* 976-984.

Hercberg S, Preziosi P, Galan P, Faure H, Arnaud J, Duport N, Malvy D, Roussel AM, Briancon S, Favier A. "The SU.VI.MAX Study": A primary prevention trial using nutritional doses of antioxidant vitamins and minerals in cardiovascular diseases and cancers. Supplementation on VItamines et Mineraux AntioXydants. *Food and Chemical Toxicology 37*(9-10): 925-930.

Jorissen BL, Brouns F, Van Boxtel MP, Riedel WJ. (2002). Safety of soy-derived phosphatidylserine in elderly people. *Nutritional Neuroscience 5:* 337-343.

Joseph JA, Denisova NA, Bielinski D, Fisher DR, Shukitt-Hale B. (2000). Oxidative stress protection and vulnerability in aging: Putative nutritional implications for intervention. *Mechanisms of Ageing and Development 116:* 141-153.

Joseph JA, Shukitt-Hale B, Denisova NA, Bielinski D, Martin A, McEwen JJ, Bickford PC. (1999). Reversals of age-related declines in the neuronal signal transduction, cognitive, and motor behavioral deficits with blueberry, spinach, or strawberry dietary supplementation. *Journal of Neuroscience 19:* 8114-8121.

Karlawish JH, Whitehouse PJ. (1998). Is the placebo control obsolete in a world after donepezil and vitamin E? *Archives of Neurology 55:* 1420-1424.

Kaufman W. (1992). Vitamin deficiency, megadoses, and some supplemental history. Available at: www.doctoryourself.com/kaufman2.html.

Knopman D, Kahn J, Miles S. (1998). Clinical research designs for emerging treatments for Alzheimer disease: Moving beyond placebo-controlled trials. *Archives of Neurology 55:* 1425-1429.

Lim GP, Chu T, Yang F, Beech W, Frautschy SA, Cole GM. (2001). The curry spice curcumin reduces oxidative damage and amyloid pathology in an Alzheimer transgenic mouse. *Journal of Neuroscience 21:* 8370-8377.

Luchsinger JA, Tang MX, Shea S, Mayeux R. (2003). Antioxidant vitamin intake and risk of Alzheimer disease. *Archives of Neurology 60:* 203-208.

Martin A, Cherubini A, Andres-Lacueva C, Paniagua M, Joseph J. (2002). Effects of fruits and vegetables on levels of vitamins E and C in the brain and their association with cognitive performance. *Journal of Nutrition, Health & Aging 6:* 392-404.

Melov S, Ravenscroft J, Malik S, Gill MS, Walker DW, Clayton PE, Wallace DC, Malfroy B, Doctrow SR, Lithgow GJ. (2000). Extension of life-span with superoxide dismutase/catalase mimetics. *Science 289:* 1567-1569.

Morris MC, Evans DA, Bienias JL, Tangney CC, Bennett DA, Wilson RS, Aggarwal N, Schneider J. (2003). Consumption of fish and n-3 fatty acids and risk of incident Alzheimer disease. *Archives of Neurology 60:* 940-946.

Morris MC, Evans DA, Bienias JL, Tangney CC, Wilson RS. (2002). Vitamin E and cognitive decline in older persons. *Archives of Neurology 59:* 1125-1132.

Peretz A, Siderova V, Neve J. (2001). Selenium supplementation in rheumatoid arthritis investigated in a double blind, placebo-controlled trial. *Scandinavian Journal of Rheumatology 30:* 208-212.

Rimando AM, Cuendet M, Desmarchelier C, Mehta RG, Pezzuto JM, Duke SO. (2002). Cancer chemopreventive and antioxidant activities of pterostilbene, a naturally occurring analogue of resveratrol. *Journal of Agricultural & Food Chemistry 50:* 3453- 3457.

Rimando AM, Kalt W, Magee JB, Dewey J, Ballington JR. (2004). Resveratrol, pterostilbene, and piceatannol in vaccinium berries. *Journal of Agricultural & Food Chemistry 52:* 4713-4719.

Suzuki S, Yamatoya H, Sakai M, Kataoka A, Furushiro M, Kudo S. (2001). Oral administration of soybean lecithin transphosphatidylated phosphatidylserine improves memory impairment in aged rats. *Journal of Nutrition 131:* 2951-2956.

Wardle EN. (1999). Antioxidants in the prevention of renal disease. *Renal Failure 21:* 581-591.

Wu X, Beecher GR, Holden JM, Haytowitz DB, Gebhardt SE, Prior RL. (2004). Lipophilic and hydrophilic antioxidant capacities of common foods in the United States. *Journal of Agricultural and Food Chemistry 52:* 4026-4037.

Zandi PP, Anthony JC, Khachaturian AS, Stone SV, Gustafson D, Tschanz JT, Norton MC, Welsh-Bohmer KA, Breitner JC [Cache County Study Group].

(2004): Reduced risk of Alzheimer disease in users of antioxidant vitamin supplements: The Cache County Study. *Archives of Neurology 61:* 82-88.

Chapter 15

Belobrajdic DP, McIntosh GH, Owens JA. (2004). A high-whey-protein diet reduces body weight gain and alters insulin sensitivity relative to red meat in Wistar rats. *Journal of Nutrition 134:* 1454-1458.

Borsheim E, Aarsland A, Wolfe RR. (2004). Effect of an amino acid, protein, and carbohydrate mixture on net muscle protein balance after resistance exercise. *International Journal of Sport Nutrition & Exercise Metabolism 14:* 255-271.

Engelman HM, Alekel DL, Hanson LN, Kanthasamy, AG, Reddy MB. (2005). Blood lipid and oxidative stress responses to soy protein with isoflavones and phytic acid in postmenopausal women. *American Journal of Clinical Nutrition 81:* 590-596.

Fallon S, Enig M. (2000). Soy alert—tragedy and hype: The third international soy symposium. *Nexus Magazine 7*(3), April-May. Available at: www.ratical.com/ratville/soydangers.html#p2,WestonAPrice.org/soy/tragedy.html.

Huntley AL, Ernst E. (2004). Soy for the treatment of perimenopausal symptoms—a systematic review. *Maturitas 47:* 1-9.

Murkies AL, Teede HJ, Davis SR. (2000). What is the role of phytoestrogens in treating menopausal symptoms? *Medical Journal of Australia 173* (Suppl): S97-98.

North K, Golding J. (2000). A maternal vegetarian diet in pregnancy is associated with hypospadias. The ALSPAC study team. Avon longitudinal study of pregnancy and childhood. *BJU International 85:* 107-113.

Roberts J. (2003). Biotech in agriculture huge and growing. *The Memphis Commercial Appeal,* November 30.

Ross J. (2002). *The Mood Cure.* New York: Viking Penguin.

Whitehead SA, Cross JE, Burden C, Lacey M. (2002). Acute and chronic effects of genistein, tyrphostin and lavendustin A on steroid synthesis in luteinized human granulosa cells. *Human Reproduction 7:* 589-594.

Yellayi S, Naaz A, Szewczykowski MA, Sato T, Woods JA, Chang J, Segre M, Allred CD, Helferich WG, Cooke PS. (2002). The phytoestrogen genistein induces thymic and immune changes: A human health concern? *Proceedings of the National Academy of Sciences of the United States of America 99:* 7616-7621.

Chapter 16

Brubacher J, Hoffman RS, Bania T, Ravikumar P, Heller M, Reimer S, Smiddy M, Mojica B. (1995). Death associated with a purported aphrodisiac—New York City, February 1993-May 1995. *Journal of the American Medical Association 274:* 1828-1829.

Buster J. (2004). Large phase III study confirms that transdermal testosterone patch 300 mcg/day significantly improves sexual function with minimal side effects in surgically menopausal women. Paper presented at the 86th Annual Meeting of The Endocrine Society, June 17, 2004, New Orleans, LA.

Centers for Disease Control (CDC). (1995). Deaths associated with a purported aphrodisiac: New York City, February 1993-May 1995. *Morbidity and Mortality Weekly Report 44* (46): 853-855, 861. Available at: http://www.cdc.gov/mmwr/preview/mmwrhtml/00039633.htm.

Cohen AJ, Bartlik B. (1998). *Ginkgo biloba* for antidepressant-induced sexual dysfunction. *Sex and Marital Therapy 24:* 139-143.

Davis WM. (1994). Health problems of aging. *Drug Topics 138* (17): 96-105.

Gauthaman K, Ganesan AP, Prasad RN. (2003). Sexual effects of puncturevine *(Tribulus terrestris)* extract (protodioscin): An evaluation using a rat model. *Journal of Alternative and Complementary Medicine 9:* 257-265.

Gearon, C. (2006). The search for a female Viagra. Available at: http://health.discovery.com/centers/womens/viagra/viagra.html.

Karras DJ, Farrell SE, Harrigan RA, Henretig FM, Gealt L. (1996). Poisoning from "Spanish fly" (cantharidin). *American Journal of Emergency Medicine 14:* 478-483.

Klaasen, CD, Amdur MO, Doull J. (eds.). (1996). *Casarett and Doull's Toxicology, The Basic Science of Poisons,* Fifth Edition. New York: McGraw-Hill.

Kohut ML, Thompson JR, Campbell J, Brown GA, Vukovich MD, Jackson DA, King DS. (2003). Ingestion of a dietary supplement containing dehydroepiandrosterone (DHEA) and androstenedione has minimal effect on immune function in middle-aged men. *Journal of the American College of Nutrition 22:* 363-371.

McKay D. (2004). Nutrients and botanicals for erectile dysfunction: Examining the evidence. *Alternative Medicine Review 9:* 4-16.

Polettini A, Crippa O, Ravagli A, Saragoni A. (1992). A fatal case of poisoning with cantharidin. *Forensic Science International 56:* 37-43.

Reiter WJ, Pycha A. (1999). Placebo-controlled dihydroepiandrosterone substitution in elderly men. (In German.) *Gynakologie Geburtshilfliche Rundsch 39:* 208-209.

Silvestri A, Galetta P, Cerquetani E, Marazzi G, Patrizi R, Fini M, Rosano GM. (2003). Report of erectile dysfunction after therapy with beta-blockers is related to patient knowledge of side effects and is reversed by placebo. *European Heart Journal 24:* 1928-1932.

Chapter 17

Cho SH, Jung YB, Seong SC, Park HB, Byun KY, Lee DC, Song EK, Son JH. (2003). Clinical efficacy and safety of Lyprinol®, a patented extract from New Zealand green-lipped mussel *(Perna Canaliculus)* in patients with osteoarthritis of the hip and knee: A multicenter 2-month clinical trial. *Allergie et Immunologie 35:* 212-216.

ConsumerLab.com. (2004). Product review: Omega-3 fatty acids (EPA and DHA) from fish/marine oils. Available at: http://consumerlab.com/results/omega3.asp.

Darlington LG, Stone TW. (2001). Antioxidants and fatty acids in the amelioration of rheumatoid arthritis and related disorders. *British Journal of Nutrition 85:* 251-269.

Food and Drug Administration (FDA). (2003a). FDA acts to provide better information to consumers on trans fats. Available at: http://www.fda.gov/oc/initiatives/transfat/.

Food and Drug Administration (FDA). (2003b). Revealing *trans* fats. *FDA Consumer Magazine,* September-October. Pub no. FDA04-1329C. Available at: http://www.fda.gov/fdac/features/2003/503_fats.html.

Food and Drug Administration (FDA). (2004). FDA news: FDA announces qualified health claims for omega-3 fatty acids. Available at: http://www.fda.gov/bbs/topics/news/2004/NEW01115.html.

Food and Drug Administration (FDA). (2006). General information on qualified health claims. Available at: http://www.cfsan.fda.gov/~dms/lab-qhc.html.

Halpern GM. (2000). Anti-inflammatory effects of a stabilized lipid extract of Perna canaliculus (Lyprinol). *Allergie et Immunologie 32:* 272-278.

Hauswirth CB, Scheeder MR, Beer JH. (2004). High omega-3 fatty acid content in alpine cheese: The basis for an alpine paradox. *Circulation 109:* 103-107.

Kris-Etherton PM, Taylor DS, Yu-Poth S, Huth P, Moriarty K, Fishell V, Hargrove RL, Zhao G, Etherton TD. (2000). Polyunsaturated fatty acids in the food chain in the United States. *American Journal of Clinical Nutrition 71* (Suppl): 179S-188S.

Phillips J. (1995). *Wild Edibles of Missouri,* Second Edition, Jefferson City, MO: Missouri Department of Conservation.

Raloff J. (2001). The good fat. Will one family of animal fats become a medicine? *Science News Online 150:* 1-7. Available at: www.sciencenews.org/printthis.asp?clip+%2Farticles%2F.

Sinclair AJ, Murphy KJ, Li D. (2000). Marine lipids: Overview "news insights and lipid composition of Lyprinol. *Allergie et Immunologie 32:* 261-271.

Steinberg D, Parthasarath S, Carew TE, Witztum JL. (1989). Beyond cholesterol: Modification of low-density lipoprotein that increases its atherogenicity. *New England Journal of Medicine 320:* 915-924.

Steinberg D, Witztum JL. (1990). Lipoproteins and atherogenesis. Current concepts. *Journal of the American Medical Association 264:* 3047-3052.

Stoll AL (2001). *The Omega-3 Connection: The Groundbreaking Antidepression Diet and Brain Program.* New York: Simon and Schuster.

Chapter 18

Anonymous [FDA]. (2003). Laetrile promoter convicted of contempt, July 23, 2003. Available at: consumeraffairs.com/news03/laetrile.html. Accessed September 14, 2003.

Anonymous (2004). Desert shrub may help some cancer patients. August 10, 2004. Reuters News Service. Available at: www.reuters.co.uk/newsArticle.jhtml?type=healthNews&storyID= 5928053§ion=news.

Atanackovic D. (2004). Vaccination strategies for solid tumors—Fundamentals, limitations, and recent results. (In German.) *Therapeutische Umschau 61:* 389-396.

Black M, Hussain H. (2000). Hydrazine, cancer, the Internet, and the liver. *Annals of Internal Medicine 133:* 911-913.

Boon H, Brown JB, Gavin A. (2000). What are the experiences of women with breast cancer as they decide whether to use complementary/alternative medicine? *Western Journal of Medicine 173:* 39.

Burzynski SR, Janicki TJ, Weaver RA, Burzynski B. (2006). Targeted therapy with antineoplastons A10 and AS2-2 of high-grade, recurrent, and progressive brainstem glioma. *Integrative Cancer Therapies* 5(1): 40-47.

Calabresi P, Parks RE, Jr. (1985). Chemotherapy of neoplastic diseases: Introduction. In AG Gilman, LS Goodman, TW Rall, and F Murad (eds.), *Goodman and Gilman's The Pharmacological Basis of Therapeutics,* Seventh Edition. New York: Macmillan Publishing Co., pp. 1240-1246.

The Cancer Letter. (1998). The antineoplaston anomaly: How a drug was used for decades in thousands of patients, with no safety, efficacy data. *The Cancer Letter 24* (36). Available at: http://www.cancerletter.com/vol24n36.html.

Center for Drug Evaluation and Research (CDER). (2002). Cyber letter. Available at: http://www.fda.gov/cder/warn/cyber/2002/CFSANoptimal.htm.

Chernyshov VP, Heusser P, Omelchenko LI, Chernyshova LI, Vodyanik MA, Vykhovanets EV, Galazyuk LV, Pochinok TV, Gaiday NV, Gumenyuk ME, et al. (2000). Immunomodulatory and clinical effects of Viscum album (Iscador M and Iscador P) in children with recurrent respiratory infections as a result of the Chernobyl nuclear accident. *American Journal of Therapeutics 7:* 195-203.

Davis JN, Muqim N, Bhuiyan M, et al. (2000). Inhibition of prostate specific antigen expression by genistein in prostate cancer cells. *International Journal of Oncology 16:* 1091-1097.

DiPaola RS, Zhang H, Lambert GH, Meeker R, Licitra E, Rafi MM, Zhu BT, Spaulding H, Goodin S, Toledano MB, et al. (1998). Clinical and biologic activity of an estrogenic herbal combination (PC-SPES) in prostate cancer. *New England Journal of Medicine 339:* 785-791.

Doctor's Guide (2000). FDA grants orphan drug status to Wobe-mugos for multiple myeloma. August 10. Available at: www.pslgroup.com/dg/1DCC36.htm.

Dunn GP, Old LJ, Schreiber RD. (2004a). The immunobiology of cancer immunosurveillance and immunoediting. *Immunity 21:* 137-148.

Dunn GP, Old LJ, Schreiber RD. (2004b). The three Es of cancer immunoediting. *Annual Review of Immunology 22:* 329-360.

Dunphy FR, Dukelow KK, Provenzal J, Crawford J. (2004). Phase I clinical results of intralesional injection of tetra-O-methynordihydroguaiaretic acid (M4N) in refractory head and neck cancer. American Society of Clinical Oncology Annual Meeting proceedings, *Journal of Clinical Oncology* 22(Suppl. 14): 5614.

Fuchs NK. (2003). *Modified Citrus Pectin 9MCP, A Super Nutraceutical.* North Bergen, NJ: Basic Health Publications.

Goldberg B. (2000). If it were any good, my doctor would know about it. In J Diamond and WL Cowden (eds.), *Cancer Diagnosis: What to Do Next.* Tiburon, CA: Alternative Medicine.com Books, pp. 13-17.

Gorter RW, van Wely M, Reif M, Stoss M. (1999). Tolerability of an extract of European mistletoe among immunocompromised and healthy individuals. *Alternative Therapies in Health & Medicine 5:* 37-44, 47-8.

Gotay CC, Dumitriu D. (2000). Health food store recommendations for breast cancer patients. *Archives of Family Medicine 9:* 692-699.

Green S. (1993). Immunoaugmentative therapy: An unproven cancer treatment. *Journal of the American Medical Association 270:* 1719-1723.

Grossarth-Maticek R, Kiene H, Baumgartner SM, Ziegler R. (2001). Use of Iscador, an extract of European mistletoe (Viscum album), in cancer treatment: Prospective nonrandomized and randomized matched-pair studies nested within a cohort study. *Alternative Therapies in Health & Medicine 7:* 57-66, 68-72, 74-76.

Guess BW, Scholz MC, Strum SB, Lam RY, Johnson HJ, Jennrich RI. Modified citrus pectin (MCP) increases the prostate-specific antigen doubling time in men with prostate cancer: a phase II pilot study. *Prostate Cancer and Prostatic Diseases 6*(4): 301-304.

Hainer MI, Tsai N, Komura ST, Chin CL. (2000). Fatal hepatorenal failure associated with hydrazine sulfate. *Annals of Internal Medicine 133:* 877-880.

Hercberg S, Galan P, Preziosi P, Bertrais S, Mennen L, Malvy D, Roussel AM, Favier A, Briancon S. (2004). The SU.VI.MAX Study: A randomized, placebo-controlled trial of the health effects of antioxidant vitamins and minerals. *Archives of Internal Medicine 164:* 2335-2342.

Hirazumi, A., Furusawa, E. (1999). An immunomodulatory polysaccharide-rich substance from the fruit juice of *Morinda citrifolia* (noni) with antitumour activity. *Phytotherapy Research 13:* 380-387.

Kaegi E. (1998a). Unconventional therapies for cancer: 2. Green tea. *Canadian Medical Association Journal 158:* 1033-1035.

Kaegi E. (1998b). Unconventional therapies for cancer: 3. Iscador. *Canadian Medical Association Journal 158*: 1157-1159.

Kaegi E. (1998c). Unconventional therapies for cancer: 5. Vitamins A, C and E. *Canadian Medical Association Journal 158:* 1483-1488.

Kucuk O, Sakr W, Sarkar F, et al. (1999). Lycopene supplementation decreases serum PSA, PIN and tumor volume in early stage prostate cancer. Paper presented at the Proceedings of the American Association for Cancer Research 40, April, 1999, Philadelphia, PA.

McClatchey W. (2002). From polynesian healers to health food stores: Changing perspectives of *Morinda citrifolia* (Rubiaceae). *Integrative Cancer Therapies 1:* 110-120.

MedlinePlus. (2005). Essiac. Available at: http://www.nlm.nih.gov/medlineplus/druginfo/natural/patient-essiac.html.

Moss RW. (1994). Immunoaugmentative therapy. *Journal of the American Medical Association 271:* 1319.

Mueller B, Scott MK, Sowinski KM, Prag KA. (2000). Noni juice *(Morinda citrifolia):* Hidden potential for hyperkalemia? *American Journal of Kidney Disease 35:* 310-312.

Nam RK, Fleshner N, Rakovitch E, Klotz L, Trachtenberg J, Choo R, Morton G, Danjoux C. (1999). Prevalence and patterns of the use of complementary therapies among prostate cancer patients: An epidemiological analysis. *Journal of Urology 161:* 1521-1524.

National Cancer Institute (NCI). (2005). Questions and answers about laetrile/amygdalin. Available at: http://www.cancer.gov/cancertopics/pdq/cam/laetrile/Patient/page2.

National Center for Complementary and Alternative Medicine (NCCAM). (2006). All NCCAM clinical trials. Available at: http://nccam.nih.gov/clinicaltrials/alltrials.htm.

Oberlies NH, Chang C, McLaughlin JL. (1997a). Structure-activity relationships of diverse annonaceous acetogenins against multidrug-resistant human mammary adenocarcinoma (MCF-7/Adr) cells. *Journal of Medicinal Chemistry 40:* 2102-2106.

Oberlies NH, Croy VL, Harrison ML, McLaughlin JL. (1997b). The annonaceous acetogenin bullatacin is cytotoxic against multidrug-resistant human mammary adenocarcinoma cells. *Cancer Letters 115:* 73-79.

Olajide OA, Awe SO, Makinde JM, Morebise O. (1999). Evaluation of the antidiabetic property of *Morinda lucida* leaves in streptozotocin-diabetic rats. *Journal of Pharmacy and Pharmacology 51:* 1321-1324.

Richardson MA, Sanders T, Palmer JL, Greisinger A, Singletary, SE. (2000). Complementary/alternative medicine use in a comprehensive cancer center and the implications for oncology. *Journal of Clinical Oncology 18:* 2505-2514.

Sahelian R. (2002). Noni juice: Is it a cure all or just a healthy drink? Available at: www.raysahelian.com/noni.html.

Schmidt K, Ernst E. (2004). Assessing websites on complementary and alternative medicine for cancer. *Annals of Oncology 15:* 733-742.

Sheikh NM, Philen RM, Love LA. (1997). Chaparral-associated hepatotoxicity. *Archives of Internal Medicine 157:* 913-919.

Solomon N. (1998). *Noni: Nature's Amazing Healer.* Pleasant Grove, UT: Woodland Publishing, Inc.

Solomon N. (2006). Dr. Neil Soloman's view on Noni Juice from Tahiti. Available at: http://www.healthwizz.com/Dr.%20Solomon's%20Noni%20Testimony.htm.

van Wely M, Stoss M, Gorter RW. (1999). Toxicity of a standardized mistletoe extract in immunocompromised and healthy individuals. *American Journal of Therapeutics 6:* 37-43.

Wang MY, Su C. (2001). Cancer preventive effect of *Morinda citrifolia* (Noni). *Annals of the New York Academy of Sciences 952:* 161-168.

Chapter 19

Alvarez-Olmos MI, Oberhelman RA. (2001). Probiotic agents and infectious diseases: A modern perspective on a traditional therapy. *Clinical Infectious Diseases 32:* 1567-1576.

Anonymous. (2000). Larch arabinogalactan. *Alternative Medicine Review 5:* 463-466.

Bhaskaram P. (2002). Micronutrient malnutrition, infection, and immunity: An overview. *Nutrition Reviews 60* (suppl. 5 Pt 2): S40-45.

Bogden JD. (2004). Influence of zinc on immunity in the elderly. *Journal of Nutrition, Health & Aging 8:* 48-54.

Calder PC. (2003). Immunonutrition. *British Medical Journal 327:* 117-118.

Calder PC, Kew S. (2002). The immune system: A target for functional foods? *British Journal of Nutrition 88* (Suppl. 2): S165-177.

Cameron E, Pauling L. (1973). Ascorbic acid and the glycosaminoglycans: An orthomolecular approach to cancer and other diseases. *Oncology 27:* 181-192.

Capek P, Hribalova V, Svandova E, Ebringerova A, Sasinkova V, Masarova J. (2003). Characterization of immunomodulatory polysaccharides from *Salvia officinalis* L. *International Journal of Biological Macromolecules 33:* 113-119.

CDC. (1999). Workshop on micronutrients and infectious diseases: Cellular and molecular immunomodulatory mechanisms. Available at: www.cdc.gov/ncidod/eid/vol16no1/newsnotes.htm#workshop.

Chandra RK. (1997). Graying of the immune system. Can nutrient supplements improve immunity in the elderly? *Journal of the American Medical Association 277:* 1398- 1399.

Chandra RK. (2002). Nutrition and the immune system from birth to old age. *European Journal of Clinical Nutrition 56* (Suppl 3): S73-S76.

Croom E. (2004). Presented at the Workshop on Scientific Approaches to Quality Assessment of Botanical Products, National Center for Natural Products Research, The University of Mississippi School of Pharmacy, September 7-9, 2004, University, MS.

de Pablo MA, Alvarez de Cienfuegos G. (2000). Modulatory effects of dietary lipids on immune system functions. *Immunology & Cell Biology 78:* 31-39.

Di Benedetto, Iona LG, Zidarich AV. (1993). Clinical evaluation of S-adenosyl-L-methionine versus transcutaneous electrical nerve stimulation in primary fibromyalgia. *Current Therapeutic Research 53:* 222-229.

Erickson KL, Hubbard NE. (2000). Probiotic immunomodulation in health and disease. *Journal of Nutrition 130* (Suppl. 2): S403-S409.

Erickson KL, Medina EA, Hubbard NE. (2000). Micronutrients and innate immunity. *Journal of Infectious Diseases 182* (Suppl 1): S5-S10.

Grimm H, Calder PC. (2002). Immunonutrition. *British Journal of Nutrition 87* (Suppl. 1): S1.

Hamilton-Miller JM. (2004). Probiotics and prebiotics in the elderly. *Postgraduate Medical Journal 80:* 447-451.

Herraiz LA, Hsieh WC, Parker RS, Swanson JE, Bendich A, Roe DA. (1998). Effect of UV exposure and beta-carotene supplementation on delayed-type hypersensitivity response in healthy older men. *Journal of the American College of Nutrition 17:* 617-624.

Hinds A. (1991). Nutrients as modulators of immune function. *Canadian Medical Association Journal 145:* 35.

Houssay BA. (1956). Trends in physiology as seen from South America. *Annual Review of Physiology 18:* 1-13.

Jenkins DJ, Kendall CW, Axelsen M, Augustin LS, Vuksan V. (2000). Viscous and nonviscous fibres, nonabsorbable and low glycaemic index carbohydrates, blood lipids and coronary heart disease. *Current Opinion in Lipidology 11:* 49-56.

Manning TS, Gibson GR. (2004). Microbial-gut interactions in health and disease. Prebiotics. *Best Practice & Research in Clinical Gastroenterology 18:* 287-298.

Marteau PR, de Vrese M, Cellier CJ, Schrezenmeir J. (2001). Protection from gastrointestinal diseases with the use of probiotics. *American Journal of Clinical Nutrition 73* (Suppl): 430S-436S.

Marteau P, Seksik P. (2004). Tolerance of probiotics and prebiotics. *Journal of Clinical Gastroenterology 38* (Suppl. 6): S67-S69.

Rivera MT, De Souza AP, Araujo-Jorge TC, De Castro SL, Vanderpas J. (2003). Trace elements, innate immune response and parasites. *Clinical Chemistry & Laboratory Medicine 41:* 1020-1025.

Tharanathan RN. (2002). Food-derived carbohydrates—Structural complexity and functional diversity. *Critical Reviews in Biotechnology 22:* 65-84.

Van Loo JA. (2004). Prebiotics promote good health: The basis, the potential, and the emerging evidence. *Journal of Clinical Gastroenterology 38* (Suppl. 6): S70-S75.

Walker M. (2001). Medical journalist report of innovative biologics. *Townsend Letter for Doctors & Patients 211:* 58-63.

Wilasrusmee C, Siddiqui J, Bruch D, Wilasrusmee S, Kittur S, Kittur DS. (2002). In vitro immunomodulatory effects of herbal products. *American Journal of Surgery 68:* 860-864.

Chapter 20

Bose A, Vahistha K, O'Loughlin BJ. (1983). *Azarcón por empacho*—Another cause of lead toxicity. *Pediatrics 72:* 106-108.

Chan H, Billmeier GJ, Evans WE, Chan H. (1977). Lead poisoning from ingestion of Chinese herbal medicine. *Clinical Toxicology 10:* 273-281.

Crosby WH. (1977). Lead-contaminated health food. *Journal of the American Medical Association 237:* 2627-2629.

Edden MD, Torre MS. (1997). Physician's guide to herbs. *Practical Diabetology 10:* 10, 12-13, 16-17, 20.

Espinoza EO, Mann M-J, Bleasdell, B. (1995). Arsenic and mercury in traditional Chinese herbal balls. *New England Journal of Medicine 333:* 803-804.

Food and Drug Administration (FDA) (2004). Import alert #66-10. Available at: http://www.fda.gov/ora/fiars/ora_import_ia6610.html.

Huggett DB, Khan IA, Allgood JC, Block DS, Schetz D. (2001). Organochlorine pesticides and metals in select botanical dietary supplements. *Bulletin of Environmental Contamination and Toxicology 66:* 150-155.

Keen RW, Deacon AC, Delves HT, Moreton JA, Frost PG. (1994). Indian herbal remedies for diabetes as a cause of lead poisoning. *Postgraduate Medical Journal 70:* 113-114.

Kew J, Morris C, Aihie A, Fysh R, Jones S, Brooks D. (1993). Arsenic and mercury intoxication due to Indian ethnic remedies. *British Medical Journal 306:* 506-507.

Lightfoot J, Blair HJ, Cohen JR. (1977). Lead intoxication in an adult caused by Chinese herbal medication. *Journal of the American Medical Association 238:* 1539.

McRill C, Boyer LV, Flood TJ, Ortega L. (2000). Mercury toxicity due to the use of a cosmetic cream. *Journal of Occupational and Environmental Medicine 42:* 4-7.

Pérez-Peña, R. (2003). Dominican-made powder remedy is poisonous, health officials say. *The New York Times,* November 6. Available at: www.nytimes.com.

Pontifex AH, Garg AK. (1985). Lead poisoning from an Asian Indian folk remedy. *Canadian Medical Association Journal 133:* 1227-1228.

Schaumburg HH, Berger A. (1992). Alopecia and sensory polyneuropathy from thallium in a Chinese herbal medication. *Journal of the American Medical Association 268:* 3430-3431.

Weldon MM, Smolinski MS, Maroufi A, Hasty BW, Gilliss DL, Boulanger LL, Balluz LS, Dutton RJ. (2000). Mercury poisoning associated with a Mexican beauty cream. *Western Journal of Medicine 173:* 15-18.

Chapter 21

Andres E, Loukili NH, Noel E, Kaltenbach G, Abdelgheni MB, Perrin AE, Noblet-Dick M, Maloisel F, Schlienger JL, Blickle JF. (2004). Vitamin B12 (cobalamin) deficiency in elderly patients. *Canadian Medical Association Journal 171:* 251-259.

Basara LR, and Montagne M. (1994). *Searching for Magic Bullets: Orphan Drugs, Consumer Activism, and Pharmaceutical Development.* Binghamton, NY: Pharmaceutical Products Press.

Bleich S, Degner D, Sperling W, Bonsch D, Thurauf N, Kornhuber J. (2004). Homocysteine as a neurotoxin in chronic alcoholism. *Progress in Neuro-Psychopharmacology & Biological Psychiatry 28:* 453-464.

Brantigan CO. (1997). Folate supplementation and the risk of masking vitamin B12 deficiency. *Journal of the American Medical Association 277:* 884-885.

Dalton K. (1985). Pyridoxine overdose in premenstrual syndrome. *Lancet* 1168-1169.

Doran M, Rassam SS, Jones LM, Underhill S. (2004). Toxicity after intermittent inhalation of nitrous oxide for analgesia. *British Medical Journal 328:* 1364-1365.

Fairfield KM, Fletcher RH. (2002). Vitamins for chronic disease prevention in adults: Scientific review. *Journal of the American Medical Association 287:* 3116-3126.

Fletcher RH, Fairfield KM. (2002). Vitamins for chronic disease prevention in adults: Clinical applications. *Journal of the American Medical Association 287:* 3127-3129.

Gerriot S, Bente L. (n.d.). Nutrient content of the U.S. food supply, 1909-1997. U.S. Department of Agriculture, Center for Nutrition Policy and Promotion. Home Economics Report #54. Available at: www.usda.gov/cnpp/Pubs/Food%20Supply/foodsupplyrpt.pdf.

Jacobs EJ, Connell CJ, Chao A, McCullough ML, Rodriguez C, Thun MJ, Calle EE. (2003). Multivitamin use and colorectal cancer incidence in a US cohort: Does timing matter? *American Journal of Epidemiology 158:* 621-628.

Kenny AM, Biskup B, Robbins B, Marcella G, Burleson JA. (2003). Effects of vitamin D supplementation on strength, physical function, and health perception in older, community-dwelling men. *Journal of the American Geriatrics Society 51:* 1762-1767.

Kinsella LJ, Green R. (1995). "Anesthesia paresthetica": Nitrous oxide-induced cobalamin deficiency. *Neurology 45:* 1608-1610.

Kizer KW, Fan AM, Bankowska J, Jackson RJ, Lyman DO. (1990). Vitamin A—A pregnancy hazard alert. *Western Journal of Medicine 152:* 78-81.

Lasagna L. (1994). Over-the-counter niacin. *Journal of the American Medical Association 271:* 709-710.

Lewis JH. (2002). The rational use of potentially hepatotoxic medications in patients with underlying liver disease. *Expert Opinion on Drug Safety 1:* 159-172.

Lindenbaum J, Healton EB, Savage DG, Brust JCM, Garrett TJ, Podell ER, Marcell PD, Stabler SP, Allen RH. (1988). Neuropsychiatric disorders caused by cobalamin deficiency in the absence of anemia or macrocytosis. *New England Journal of Medicine 318:* 1720-1728.

Linus Pauling Institute (2005). Micronutrient information center. Available at: www.lpi.oregonstate.edu/infocenter/vitamins.html.

Malabanan AO, Holick MF. (2003). Vitamin D and bone health in postmenopausal women. *Journal of Women's Health 12:* 151-156.

Malterud K. (2001). The art and science of clinical knowledge: Evidence beyond measures and numbers. *Lancet 358:* 397-400.

McKenney JM, Proctor JD, Harris S, Chinchili VM. (1994). A comparison of the efficacy and toxic effects of sustained- vs immediate-release niacin in hypercholesterolemic patients. *Journal of the American Medical Association 271:* 672-677.

McLean RR, Jacques PF, Selhub J, Tucker KL, Samelson EJ, Broe KE, Hannan MT, Cupples LA, Kiel DP. (2004). Homocysteine as a predictive factor for hip fracture in older persons. *New England Journal of Medicine 350:* 2042-2049.

Melhus H, Michaelsson K, Kindmark A, Bergstrom R, Holmberg L, Mallmin H, Wolk A, Ljunghall S. (1998). Excessive dietary intake of vitamin A is associated with reduced bone mineral density and increased risk for hip fracture. *Annals of Internal Medicine 129:* 770-778.

Morris MC, Evans DA, Bienias JL, Scherr PA, Tangney CC, Hebert LE, Bennett DA, Wilson RS, Aggarwal N. (2004). Dietary niacin and the risk of incident Alzheimer's disease and of cognitive decline. *Journal of Neurology Neurosurgery and Psychiatry 75:* 1093-1099.

Moss RW. (1987). *Free radical: Albert Szent-Gyorgyi and the battle over vitamin C.* New York: Paragon House.

Rim EB, Stampfer MJ, Curham GC. (2004). Folate intake lowers women's risk of high blood pressure. Presented at the American Heart Association's Council for High Blood Pressure Research Annual Conference, October, 2004, Chicago, Illinois. Available at: http://www.americanheart.org/presenter.jhtml?identifier=3025283.

Saul A. (2003). *Doctor Yourself: Natural Healing That Works.* North Bergen, NJ: Basic Health Publications.

Schaumburg H, Kaplan J, Windebank A, Vick N, Rasmus S, Pleasure D, Brown MJ. (1983). Sensory neuropathy from pyridoxine abuse. A new megavitamin syndrome. *New England Journal of Medicine 309:* 445-448.

Seeman E, Melton LJ, III, O'Fallon WM, Riggs BL. (1983). Risk factors for spinal osteoporosis in men. *American Journal of Medicine 75:* 977-983.

Tang AM, Graham NM, Semba RD, ND Saah AJ. (1997). Association between serum vitamin A and E levels and HIV-1 disease progression. *AIDS 11:* 613-620.

van Meurs JB, Dhonukshe-Rutten RA, Pluijm SM, van der Klift M, de Jonge R, Lindemans J, de Groot LC, Hofman A, Witteman JC, van Leeuwen JP, et al. (2004). Homocysteine levels and the risk of osteoporotic fracture. *New England Journal of Medicine 350:* 2033-2041.

Verlangieri AJ, Bush MJ. (1992). Effects of d-a-tocopherol supplementation on experimentally induced primate atherosclerosis. *Journal of the American College of Nutrition 11:* 131-138.

Verlangieri AJ, Kapeghian JC, el-Dean S, Bush MJ. (1985). Fruit and vegetable consumption and cardiovascular mortality. *Medical Hypotheses 16:* 7-15.

Chapter 22

AREDS (2001). Age-Related Eye Disease Study Research Group. A randomized, placebo-controlled, clinical trial of high-dose supplementation with vitamins C and E, beta-carotene, and zinc for age-related macular degeneration and vision loss. *Archives of Ophthalmology 119:* 1417-1436.

Bazzano LA, He J, Ogden LG, Loria C, Vupputuri S, Myers L, Whelton PK. (2001). Dietary potassium intake and risk of stroke in US men and women: National Health and Nutrition Examination Survey I epidemiologic follow-up study. *Stroke 32:* 1473-1480.

Cho E, Smith-Warner SA, Spiegelman D, Beeson WL, van den Brandt PA, Colditz GA, Folsom AR, Fraser GE, Freudenheim JL, Giovannucci E, et al. (2004). Dairy foods, calcium, and colorectal cancer: A pooled analysis of 10 cohort studies. *Journal of the National Cancer Institute 96*(13): 1015-1022.

Davis WM. (1993) The truth about mighty minerals. *Drug Topics 137*(15): 56-66.

de Jong N, Gibson RS, Thomson CD, Ferguson EL, McKenzie JE, Green TJ, Horwath CC. (2001). Selenium and zinc status are suboptimal in a sample of older New Zealand women in a community-based study. *Journal of Nutrition 131:* 2677-2684.

Dean C. (2003). *The Miracle of Magnesium.* New York: Ballantine Books.

Dunea G. (2001). Au zinc. *British Medical Journal 322:* 117.

Glick JL. (1990). Dementias: The role of magnesium deficiency and an hypothesis concerning the pathogenesis of Alzheimer's disease. *Medical Hypotheses 31:* 211-225.

Green DM, Ropper AH, Kronmal RA, Psaty BM, Burke GL. (1979). Serum potassium level and dietary potassium intake as risk factors for stroke. *Neurology 59:* 314-320.

Jiang R, Ma J, Ascherio A, Stampfer MJ, Willett WC, Hu FB. (2004). Dietary iron intake and blood donations in relation to risk of type 2 diabetes in men: a prospective cohort study. *American Journal of Clinical Nutrition 79*(1): 70-75.

Makrides M, Crowther CA, Gibson RA, Gibson RS, Skeaff CM. (2003). Efficacy and tolerability of low-dose iron supplements during pregnancy: A randomized controlled trial. *American Journal of Clinical Nutrition 78:* 145-153.

McElroy BH, Miller SP. (2002). Effectiveness of zinc gluconate glycine lozenges (Cold-Eeze) against the common cold in school-aged subjects: A retrospective chart review. *American Journal of Therapeutics 9:* 472-475.

McElroy BH, Miller SP. (2003). An open-label, single-center, phase IV clinical study of the effectiveness of zinc gluconate common cold in school-aged subjects. *American Journal of Therapeutics 10:* 324-329.

Mercola J. (2002) How to diagnose iron overload. Available at: www.mercola .com/2002/ dec/18/iron_diagnosis.htm.

Mossad SB, Macknin, ML, Medendorf SV, Mason P. (1996). Zinc gluconate lozenges for treating the common cold. A randomized, double-blind, placebo-controlled study. *Annals of Internal Medicine 125:* 81-88.

Piotrowski AA, Kalus JS. (2004). Magnesium for the treatment and prevention of atrial tachyarrhythmias. *Pharmacotherapy 24:* 879-895.

Prasad AS. (1993). Clinical spectrum of human zinc deficiency. In AS Prasad (ed.), *Biochemistry of Zinc*. New York: Plenum, pp. 219-258.

Prasad AS. (1996). Zinc: The biology and therapeutics of an ion. *Annals of Internal Medicine 125:* 142-144.

Prasad AS. (2003). Zinc deficiency. *British Medical Journal 326:* 409-410.

Sharma VR, Brannon MA, Carloss EA. (2004). Case report: Effect of omeprazole on oral iron replacement in patients with iron deficiency anemia. *Southern Medical Journal 97:* 887-889.

Song Y, Manson JE, Buring JE, Liu S. (2004). Dietary magnesium intake in relation to plasma insulin levels and risk of type 2 diabetes in women. *Diabetes Care 27: 59-65.*

Sullivan JL. (1981). Iron and the sex difference in heart disease risk. *Lancet i-1981:* 1293-1294.

Swanson DR. (1988). Migraine and magnesium: Eleven neglected connections. *Perspectives in Biology & Medicine 31:* 526-557.

Vincent JB. (2003). The potential value and toxicity of chromium picolinate as a nutritional supplement, weight loss agent and muscle development agent. *Sports Medicine 33:* 213-230.

Vincent JB. (2004). Recent developments in the biochemistry of chromium (III). *Biological Trace Element Research 99:* 1-16.

Worthington-Roberts B. (1985). The role of nutrition in pregnancy course and outcome. *Journal of Environmental Toxicology, Pathology, and Oncology 5:* 1-80.

Chapter 23

Anonymous. (2003). Methylsulfonylmethane (MSM). Monograph. *Alternative Medicine Review 8:* 438-441.

Barrager E, Veltmann JR, Jr., Schauss AG, Schiller RN. (2002). A multicentered, open-label trial on the safety and efficacy of methylsulfonylmethane in the treatment of seasonal allergic rhinitis. *Journal of Alternative & Complementary Medicine 8:* 167-173.

Berkson B. (1998). *The Alpha Lipoic Acid Breakthrough.* New York: Prima Publishing, p. 15.

Blaylock RL. (1997). *Excitotoxins: The Taste That Kills.* Santa Fe, NM: Health Press.

Bonhaus DW, Huxtable R. (1984). Seizure susceptibility and decreased taurine transport in the genetically epileptic rat. *Neurochemistry International 6:* 365-368.

Braverman, ER, Pfeiffer CC, Blum K, Smayda R. (2003). *The Healing Nutrients Within,* Third Edition. North Bergen, NJ: Basic Health Publications.

Castelo-Branco C, Casals G, Haya J, Cancelo MJ, Manasanch J. (2004). Efficacy and safety of ibuprofen arginine in the treatment of primary dysmenorrhoea. *Clinical Drug Investigation 24:* 385-393.

Davis WM. (1987). Secret drugs: The pharmacology and therapeutic role of amino acids. *Bulletin of the Bureau of Pharmaceutical Services, University of Mississippi 23*(2): 1-6.

Davis WM. (1991). Use of amino acids in neuropsychopharmacology. *Pharmacy Times 57*(9): 124-135.

Ebisuzaki K. (2003). Aspirin and methylsulfonylmethane (MSM): A search for common mechanisms, with implications for cancer prevention. *Anticancer Research 23*(1A): 453-458.

Fisman EZ, Tenenbaum A, Shapiro I, Pines A, Motro M. (1999). The nitric oxide pathway: Is L-arginine a gate to the new millennium medicine? A meta-analysis of L-arginine effects. *Journal of Medicine 30:* 131-148.

Food and Drug Administration (FDA) (2003). Phosphatidylserine and cognitive dysfunction and dementia (Qualified health claim: Final decision letter). Office of Nutritional Products, Labeling, and Dietary Supplements, May 13, 2003. Available at: http://www.cfsan.fda.gov/~dms/ds-ltr36.html.

Horvath K, Noker PE, Somfai-Relle S, Glavits R, Financsek I, Schauss AG. (2002). Toxicity of methylsulfonylmethane in rats. *Food & Chemical Toxicology 40:* 1459-1462.

Hucker HB, Ahmad PM, Miller EA, Brobyn R. (1966). Metabolism of dimethyl sulphoxide to dimethyl sulphone in the rat and man. *Nature 209:* 619-620.

Jacob SW, Appleton J. (2003). *MSM: The Definitive Guide.* Topana, CA: Freedom Press.

Lindenbaum J, Healton EB, Savage DG, Brust JCM, Garrett TJ, Podell ER, Marcell PD, Stabler SP, Allen RH. (1988). Neuropsychiatric disorders caused by cobalamin deficiency in the absence of anemia or macrocytosis. *New England Journal of Medicine 318:* 1720-1728.

Muscaritoli M, Micozzo A, Conversano L, Martino P, Petti MC, Cartoni C, Cascino A, Rossi-Fanelli F. (1997). Oral glutamine in the prevention of chemotherapy-induced gastrointestinal toxicity. *European Journal of Cancer 33:* 319-320.

Packer L. (1998). α-Lipoic acid: A metabolic antioxidant which regulates NFκ-B signal transduction and protects against oxidative injury. *Drug Metabolism Reviews 30:* 245-275.

Packer L, Colman C. (1999). *Antioxidant Miracle: Put Lipoic Acid, Pycnogenol and Vitamins E and C to Work for You.* New York: John Wiley & Sons, Inc.

Packer L, Witt EH, Tritschler HJ. (1995). Alpha-lipoic acid as a biological antioxidant. [Review.] *Free Radical Biology and Medicine 19:* 227-250.

Parcell S. (2002). Sulfur in human nutrition and applications in medicine. *Alternative Medicine Review 7:* 22-44.

Rozen TD, Oshinsky ML, Gebeline CA, Bradley KC, Young WB, Shechter AL, Silberstein SD. (2002). Open label trial of coenzyme Q10 as a migraine preventive. *Cephalalgia 22:* 137-141.

Santaella ML, Font I, Disdier OM. (2004). Comparison of oral nicotinamide adenine dinucleotide (NADH) versus conventional therapy for chronic fatigue syndrome. *Puerto Rico Health Sciences Journal 23:* 89-93.

Tran MT, Mitchell TM, Kennedy DT, Giles JT. (2001). Role of coenzyme Q10 in chronic heart failure, angina, and hypertension. *Pharmacotherapy 21:* 797- 806.

Tsai G, Yang P, Coyle JT. (1998). D-Serine added to antipsychotics for the treatment of schizophrenia. *Biological Psychiatry 44:* 1081-1089.

Chapter 24

Agarwal S, Rao AV. (2000). Tomato lycopene and its role in human health and chronic diseases. *Canadian Medical Association Journal 163:* 739-744.

Baht KPL, Pezzuto JM. (2002). Cancer chemoprotective activity of resveratrol. *Annals of the New York Academy of Sciences 957:* 210-229.

Borrelli F, Capasso R, Russo A, Ernst E. (2004). Systematic review: Green tea and gastrointestinal cancer risk *Alimentary Pharmacology & Therapeutics 19:* 497-510.

Committee on Comparative Toxicity of Naturally Occurring Compounds. (1996). *Carcinogens and Anticarcinogens in the Human Diet.* Washington, DC: National Academy Press.

Crowell JA, Korytko PJ, Morrissey RL, Booth TD, Levine BS. (2004). Resveratrol-associated renal toxicity. *Toxicological Sciences 82:* 614-619.

de la Taille A, Hayek OR, Burchardt M, Burchardt T, Katz AE. (2000). Role of herbal compounds (PC-SPES) in hormone-refractory prostate cancer: Two case reports. *Journal of Alternative & Complementary Medicine 6:* 449-451.

Eng J, Ramsum D, Verhoef M, Guns E, Davison J, Gallagher R. (2003). A population-based survey of complementary and alternative medicine use in men recently diagnosed with prostate cancer. *Integrative Cancer Therapies 2:* 212-216.

Gann PH, Ma J, Giovannucci E, Willett W, Sacks FM, Hennekens CH, Stampfer MJ. (1999). Lower prostate cancer risk in men with elevated plasma lycopene levels: Results of a prospective analysis. *Cancer Research 59:* 1225-1230.

Jang M, Cai L, Udeani GO, Slowing KV, Thomas CF, Beecher CWW, Fong HHS, Farnsworth NR, Kinghorn AD, Mehta RG, et al. (1997). Cancer chemopreventive activity of resveratrol, a natural product derived from grapes. *Science 10:* 218-221.

Jang M, Pezzuto JM. (1999). Cancer chemopreventive activity of resveratrol. *Drugs Under Experimental and Clinical Research 25:* 65-77.

Kaegi E. [on behalf of the Task Force on Alternative Therapies of the Canadian Breast Cancer Research Initiative]. (1988). Unconventional therapies for cancer: 2. Green tea. *Canadian Medical Association Journal 158:* 1033-1035.

Katz AE. (2002). Flavonoid and botanical approaches to prostate health. *Journal of Alternative & Complementary Medicine 8:* 813-821.

Kim L, Rao AV, Rao LG. (2002). Effect of lycopene on prostate LNCaP cancer cells in culture. *Journal of Medicinal Food 5:* 181-187.

Klein SL, Wisniewski AB, Marson AL, Glass GE, Gearhart JP. (2002). Early exposure to genistein exerts long-lasting effects on the endocrine and immune systems in rats. *Molecular Medicine 8:* 742-749.

Kris-Etherton PM, Keen CL. (2002). Evidence that the antioxidant flavonoids in tea and cocoa are beneficial for cardiovascular health. *Current Opinion in Lipidology 13:* 41-49.

Lewis R. (2003). Preventing cancer supplement: The unraveling of the genetic roots of cancer highlights more controllable risk factors. *The Scientist 17* (Suppl. 2): S6-S7.

McElderry MQB. (1999). Grape expectations: The resveratrol story. September 1. Available at: www.quackwatch.com/01QuackeryRelatedTopics/DSH/resveratrol .html. Accessed April 23, 2002.

Pervaiz S. (2001) Resveratrol—From the bottle to the bedside? *Leukemia & Lymphoma 40:* 491-498.

Putter M, Grotemeyer KH, Wurthwein G, Araghi-Niknam M, Watson RR, Hosseini S, Rohdewald P. (1999). Inhibition of smoking-induced platelet aggregation by aspirin and pycnogenol. *Thrombosis Research 95:* 155-161.

Schoonen WM, Salinas CA, Kiemeney LA, Stanford JL. (2005). Alcohol consumption and risk of prostate cancer in middle-aged men. *International Journal of Cancer 113:* 133-140.

Stocker R, O'Halloran RA. (2004). Dealcoholized red wine decreases atherosclerosis in apolipoprotein E gene-deficient mice independently of inhibition of lipid peroxidation in the artery wall. *American Journal of Clinical Nutrition 79:* 123-130.

Tedeschi E, Menegazzi M, Yao Y, Suzuki H, Förstermann U, Kleinert H. (2004). Green tea inhibits human inducible nitric-oxide synthase expression by down-regulating signal transducer and activator of transcription-1 activation. *Molecular Pharmacology 65:* 111-120.

Wang HK, Xia Y, Yang ZY, Natschke SL, Lee KH. (1998). Recent advances in the discovery and development of flavonoids and their analogues as antitumor and anti-HIV agents. *Advances in Experimental Medicine and Biology 439:* 191-225.

Wilt TJ, Ishani A, Stark G, MacDonald R, Lau J, Mulrow C. (1998). Saw palmetto extracts for treatment of benign prostatic hyperplasia: A systematic review. *Journal of the American Medical Association 280:* 1604-1609.

Yang J, Meyers KJ, van der Heide J, Liu RH. (2004). Varietal differences in phenolic content and antioxidant and antiproliferative activities of onions. *Journal of Agricultural and Food Chemistry 52:* 6787-6789. Available at: www.pubs.acs .org/journals/jafcau/index.html.

Chapter 25

Bram S, Froussard P, Guichard M, Jasmin C, Augery Y, Sinoussi-Barre F, Wray W. (1980). Vitamin C preferential toxicity for malignant melanoma cells. *Nature 284:* 629-631.

Cameron E, Campbell A. (1991). Innovation vs. quality control: An "unpublishable" clinical trial of supplemental ascorbate in incurable cancer. *Medical Hypotheses 36:* 185-194.

Cameron E, Pauling L. (1973). Ascorbic acid and the glycosaminoglycans: An orthomolecular approach to cancer and other diseases. *Oncology 27:* 181-192.

Cameron E, Pauling, L. (1976). Supplemental ascorbate in the supportive treatment of cancer: Prolongation of survival times in terminal human cancer. *Proceedings of the National Academy of Sciences USA 73:* 3685-3689.

Cameron E, Pauling L. (1978). Supplemental ascorbate in the supportive treatment of cancer: Reevaluation of prolongation of survival times in terminal human cancer. *Proceedings of the National Academy of Sciences USA 75:* 4538-4542.

Cameron E, Pauling L. (1979). Ascorbic acid as a therapeutic agent in cancer. *Journal of the International Association of Preventive Medicine 5:* 8-29.

Cameron E, Pauling L, Leibovitz B. (1979). Ascorbic acid and cancer: A review. *Cancer Research 39:* 663-681.

Casciari J, Riordan N, Schmidt T, Meng X, Jackson J, Riordan H. (2001). Cytotoxicity of ascorbate, lipoic acid and other antioxidants in hollow fiber *in vitro* tumors. *British Journal of Cancer 84:* 1544-1550.

Cathcart RF. (1984). Vitamin C in the treatment of acquired immune deficiency syndrome (AIDS). *Medical Hypotheses 14:* 423-433.

Cathcart RF. (1985). Vitamin C: The nontoxic, nonrate-limited, antioxidant free radical scavenger. *Medical Hypotheses 18:* 61-77.

Cathcart RF. (1991). A unique function for ascorbate. *Medical Hypotheses 35:* 32-37.

Goodwin JS, Goodwin JM. (1984). The tomato effect. Rejection of highly efficacious therapies. *Journal of the American Medical Association 251:* 2387-2390.

Kalokerinos A, Dettman I, Dettman G. (1982a). Ascorbate—The proof of the pudding! A selection of case histories responding to ascorbate. *Australasian Nurses Journal 11:* 18-21.

Kalokerinos A, Dettman I, Dettman G. (1982b). How much vitamin C should I take? *Australasian Nurses Journal 11*(6): 8-9, July.

Kurl S, Tuomainen TP, Laukkanen JA, Nyyssonen K, Lakka T, Sivenius J, Salonen JT. (2002). Plasma vitamin C modifies the association between hypertension and risk of stroke. *Stroke 33:* 1568-1573.

Levy TE. (2002). *Vitamin C, Infectious Diseases, and Toxins.* Princeton, NJ: Xlibris Co.

Ling L, Zhao SP, Gao M, Zhou QC, Li YL, Xia B. (2002). Vitamin C preserves endothelial function in patients with coronary heart disease after a high-fat meal. *Clinical Cardiology 25:* 219-224.

Prasad KN, Prasad CP. (2001). *Fight Cancer with Vitamins and Supplements.* Rochester, VT: Healing Arts Press.

Riordan NH, Riordan HD, Casciari JP. (2000). Clinical and experimental experiences with intravenous vitamin C. *Journal of Orthomolecular Medicine 15:* 201-213.

Rossig L, Hoffmann J, Hugel B, Mallat Z, Haase A, Freyssinet JM, Tedgui A, Aicher A, Zeiher AM, Dimmeler S. (2001). Vitamin C inhibits endothelial cell apoptosis in congestive heart failure. *Circulation 104:* 2182-2187.

Saul A. (2003). *Doctor Yourself: Natural Healing That Works.* North Bergen, NJ: Basic Health Publications.

Scott P, Bruce C, Schofield D, Shiel N, Braganza JM, McCloy RF. (1993). Vitamin C status in patients with acute pancreatitis. *British Journal of Surgery 80:* 750-754.

Smith AF. (1991). Tomato pills will cure all your ills. *Pharmacy in History 33:* 163-177.

U.S. Preventive Services Task Force. (2003). Routine vitamin supplementation to prevent cancer and cardiovascular disease: Recommendations and rationale. *Annals of Internal Medicine 139:* 51-55, 56-70.

Chapter 26

Atherton P. (1998). Aloe vera: Myth or medicine? *Nursing Standard 12:* 49-52, 54. Available at: www.dspace.dial.pipex.com/town/road/ymp93/doctors/atherton.htm.

Blitz JJ, Smith JW, Gerard JR. (1963) Aloe vera gel in peptic ulcer therapy. Preliminary report. *Journal of the American Osteopathic Association 62:* 731-735.

Coats BC [with Robert Ahola]. (1984). *The Silent Healer: A Modern Study of Aloe Vera,* Second Edition. Garland, TX: Author.

Coats BC, Ahola R. (2003). *Aloe Vera the New Millennium: The Future of Wellness in the 21st Century.* Lincoln, NE: iUniverse, Inc.

Collins CE, Collins C. (1935). Roentgen dermatitis treated with fresh whole leaf of aloe vera. *American Journal of Roentgenology 33:* 396-397.

Danhof IE, McAnally BH. (1983). Stabilized aloe vera: Effects on human skin cells. *Drug and Cosmetic Industry 133:* 52-56.

Davis RH. (n.d.) Whole leaf aloe vera—Polysaccharides and wound healing. Available at: www.wholeleaf.com/aloeverainfo/aloeverapolysaccharide.htlm.

Ikeno Y, Hubbard GB, Lee S, Yu BP, Herlihy JT. (2002). The influence of long-term aloe vera ingestion on age-related disease in male Fischer 344 rats. *Phytotherapy Research 16:* 712-718.

Rowe TD, Lovell BK, Parks LM. (1941). Further observations on the use of aloe vera leaf in the treatment of third-degree x-ray reactions. *Journal of the American Pharmaceutical Association 30:* 266-269.

Strickland FM, Pelley RP, Kripke ML. (1994). Prevention of ultraviolet radiation-induced suppression of contact and delayed hypersensitivity by *Aloe barbadensis* gel extract. *Journal of Investigative Dermatology 102:* 197-204.

Vogler BK, Ernst E. (1999). Aloe vera: A systematic review of its clinical effectiveness. *British Journal of General Practice 49:* 823-828.

Wright CS. (1936). Aloe vera in the treatment of roentgen ulcers and telangiectasis. *Journal of the American Medical Association 106:* 1363-1364.

Chapter 27

AREDS (2001). A randomized, placebo-controlled, clinical trial of high-dose supplementation with vitamins C and E, beta carotene, and zinc for age-related macular degeneration and vision loss. *Archives of Ophthalmology 119:* 1417-1436.

Brown L, Rimm EB, Seddon JM, Giovannucci EL, Chasan-Taber L, Spiegelman D, Willett WC, Hankinson SE. (1999). A prospective study of carotenoid intake and risk of cataract extraction in U.S. men. *American Journal of Clinical Nutrition 70*(4): 431-432.

Chasan-Taber L, Willett WC, Seddon JM, Stampfer MJ, Rosner B, Colditz GA, Speizer FE, Hankinson SE. (2000). A prospective study of alcohol consumption and cataract extraction among U.S. women. *Annals of Epidemiology 10*(6): 347-353.

de La Marnierre E, Guigon B, Quaranta M, Mauget-Faysse M. (2003). Phototoxic drugs and age-related maculopathy. [In French.] *Journale Francais de la Ophtalmologie 2:* 596-601.

Fraunfelder FW. (2004). Ocular side effects from herbal medicines and nutritional supplements. *American Journal of Ophthalmology 138:* 639-647.

Gao X, Talalay P. (2004). Induction of phase 2 genes by sulforaphane protects retinal pigment epithelial cells against photooxidative damage. *Proceedings of the National Academy of Science USA 101:* 10446-10451.

Klein R, Klein BE, Tomany SC, Moss SE. (2002). Ten-year incidence of age-related maculopathy and smoking and drinking: The Beaver Dam eye study. *American Journal of Epidemiology 156:* 589-598.

Nestle M. (1997). Broccoli sprouts as inducers of carcinogen-detoxifying enzyme systems: Clinical, dietary, and policy implications. *Proceedings of the National Academy of Sciences USA 94:* 11149–11151.

Rennie IG. (1993). Clinically important ocular reactions to systemic drug therapy. *Drug Safety 9:* 196-211.

Semba RD, Dagnelie G. (2003). Are lutein and zeaxanthin conditionally essential nutrients for eye health? *Medical Hypotheses 61:* 465-472.

van Leeuwen R, Vingerling JR, Hofman A, de Jonge PTVM, Stricker BHC. (2003). Cholesterol lowering drugs and risk of age related maculopathy: Prospective cohort study with cumulative exposure measurement. *British Medical Journal 325:* 255-256.

Wang L, Del Priore LV. (2004). Bull's-eye maculopathy secondary to herbal toxicity from uva ursi. *American Journal of Ophthalmology 137:* 1135-1137.

Wilson HL, Schwartz DM, Bhatt HR, McCulloch CE, Duncan JL. (2004). Statin and aspirin therapy are associated with decreased rates of choroidal neovascularization among patients with age-related macular degeneration. *American Journal of Ophthalmology 137:* 615-624.

Chapter 28

Casto BC, Kresty LA, Kraly CL, Pearl DK, Knobloch TJ, Schut HA, Stoner GD, Mallery SR, Weghorst CM. (2002). Chemoprevention of oral cancer by black raspberries. *Anticancer Research 22*(6C): 4005-4015.

Jepson RG, Mihaljevic L, Craig J. (2000a). Cranberries for preventing urinary tract infections. *Cochrane Database of Systematic Reviews* (2): CD001321.

Jepson RG, Mihaljevic L, Craig J. (2000b). Cranberries for treating urinary tract infections. *Cochrane Database of Systematic Reviews* (2): CD001322.

Kontiokari T, Sundqvist K, Nuutinen M, Pokka T, Koskela M, Uhari M. (2001). Randomized trial of cranberry-lingonberry juice and Lactobacillus GG drink for the prevention of urinary tract infections in women. *British Medical Journal 322:* 1571.

Lampe JW. (1999). Health effects of vegetables and fruit: Assessing mechanisms of action in human experimental studies. *American Journal of Clinical Nutrition* 70 (Suppl. 3): 475S-490S.

Maurer HR. (2001). Bromelain: Biochemistry, pharmacology and medical use. *Cellular & Molecular Life Sciences 58:* 1234-1245.

Patel N, Daniels IR. (2000). Botanical perspectives on health: Of cystitis and cranberries. *Journal of the Royal Society of Health 120:* 52-53.

Stacewicz-Sapuntzakis M, Bowen PE, Hussain EA, Damayanti-Wood BI, Farnsworth NR. (2000). Chemical composition and potential health effects of prunes: A functional food? *Critical Reviews in Food Science & Nutrition 41:* 251-286.

Thompson J. (2002). Be afraid . . . be very afraid. Part II. Available at: www .HSIResearch@healthiernews.com.

Verlangieri AJ, Kapeghian JC, el-Dean S, Bush M. (1985). Fruit and vegetable consumption and cardiovascular mortality. *Medical Hypotheses 16:* 7-15.

von Woedtke T. (1999). Aspects of the antimicrobial efficacy of grapefruit seed extract and its relation to preservative substances contained. *Die Pharmazie 54:* 452-456.

Youdim KA, Joseph JA. (2001). A possible emerging role of phytochemicals in improving age-related neurological dysfunctions: A multiplicity of effects. *Free Radical Biology & Medicine 30:* 583-594.

Zhaov C, Giusti MM, Malik M, Moyer MP, Magnuson BA. (2004). Effects of commercial anthocyanin-rich extracts on colonic cancer and nontumorigenic colonic cell growth. *Journal of Agricultural and Food Chemistry 52:* 6122-6128.

Chapter 29

Breckenridge A. (1999). Renal failure associated with aristolochia in some Chinese herbal medicines. Press release, July 27, 1999. Available at: http://www.info.doh.gov.uk/doh/embroadcast.nsf/0/33d8946ea66f1fec80256dad004541da?OpenDocument.

Chen JK. (2000). Nephropathy associated with the use of *Aristolochia. HerbalGram 48:* 44-45.

Cronin AJ, Maidment G, Cook T, Kite GC, Simmonds MS, Pusey CD, Lord GM. (2002). Aristolochic acid as a causative factor in a case of Chinese herbal nephropathy. *Nephrology Dialysis Transplantation 17:* 524-525.

Food and Drug Administration (FDA). (2001). Letter to industry associations regarding safety concerns related to the use of botanical products containing aristolochic acid. Office of Nutritional Products, Labeling, and Dietary Supplements, April 9, 2001. Available at: http://www.cfsan.fda.gov/~dms/ds-botl4.html.

Frasca T, Brett AS, Yoo SD. (1997). Mandrake toxicity: A case of mistaken identity. *Archives of Internal Medicine 157:* 2007-2009.

Gold LS, Slone TH. (2003). Aristolochic acid, an herbal carcinogen, sold on the Web after FDA alert. *New England Journal of Medicine 349:* 1576-1577.

Greensfelder L. (2000). Herbal product linked to cancer. *Science 288:* 1946.

Hoffer E. (1998). *The Passionate State of Mind*. Cutchogue, NY: Buccaneer Books.

Kessler DA. (2000). Cancer and herbs. *New England Journal of Medicine 342:* 1742-1743.

Lord GM, Hollstein M, Arlt VM, Roufosse C, Pusey CD, Cook T, Schmeiser HH. (2004). DNA adducts and p53 mutations in a patient with aristolochic acid-associated nephropathy. *American Journal of Kidney Diseases 43:* e11-e17.

Mason RG, Donaldson D. (2002). Chinese herbal nephropathy and urothelial malignancy. *Journal of the Royal Society of Health 122:* 266-267.

Nortier JL, Martinez M-CM, Schmeiser HH, Arlt VM, Bieler CA, Petein M, Depierreux MF, De Pauw L, Abramowicz D, Vereestraeten P., et al. (2000). Urothelial carcinoma associated with the use of a Chinese herb *(Aristolochia fangchi). New England Journal of Medicine 342:* 1686-1692.

Schmeiser HH, Bieler CA, Wiessler M, van Ypersele de Strihou C, Cosyns JP. (1996). Detection of DNA adducts formed by aristolochic acid in renal tissue from patients with Chinese herbs nephropathy. *Cancer Research 56:* 2025-2028.

Stengel B, Jones E. (1998). End-stage renal insufficiency associated with Chinese herbal consumption in France. *Nephrologie 19*(1): 15-20.

Vanhaelen M, Vanhaelen-Fastre R, But P, Vanherweghem JL. (1994). Identification of aristolochic acid in Chinese herbs. *Lancet 343:* 174.

Vanherweghem LJ. (1998). Misuse of herbal remedies: The case of an outbreak of terminal renal failure in Belgium (Chinese herbs nephropathy). *Journal of Alternative & Complementary Medicine 4:* 9-13.

Vanherweghem J-L, Depierreux M, Tielemans C, Abramowicz D, Dratwa M, Jadoui M, Richard C, Vandervelde D, Verbeelen D, Vanhaelen-Fastre R, et al. (1993). Rapidly progressive interstitial renal fibrosis in young women: Association with slimming regimen including Chinese herbs. *Lancet 341:* 387-391.

Chapter 30

AHK Israel Newsletter (2004). Humana to compensate Remedia baby formula victims' families. *AHK Israel Newsletter,* September. Available at: http://www.ahkisrael.co.il/newsletter/newsletter_september04.htm.

Anonymous. (1996). Eosinophilia-myalgia syndrome: Review and reappraisal of clinical, epidemiologic and animal studies, Symposium. Washington, DC, December 7-8, 1994; Proceedings. *Journal of Rheumatology 46*(Suppl.): 1-110.

Criswell LA, Pincus T. (1996). Eosinophilia-myalgia syndrome. Status of patients at onset and after four years of disease. *Advances in Experimental Medicine & Biology 398:* 371-372.

Das YT, Bagchi M, Bagchi D, Preuus HG. (2004). Safety of 5-hydroxy-L-tryptophan. *Toxicology Letters 150:* 111-122.

Food and Drug Administration (FDA) (2001). Center for Food Safety and Applied Nutrition, Information paper on L-tryptophan and 5-hydroxy-L-tryptophan, February. Available at: www.cfsan.fda.gov/~dms/ds-tryp1.html. Accessed September 17, 2003.

Johnson KL, Klarskov K, Benson LM, Williamson BL, Gleich GJ, Naylor S. (1999). Presence of peak X and related compounds: The reported contaminant in case related 5-hydroxy-L-tryptophan associated with eosinophilia-myalgia syndrome. *Journal of Rheumatology 26:* 2714-2717.

Lecos C. (1990). Recall of L-tryptophan. FDA press release. Available at: http://www.fda.gov/bbs/topics/news/new00064.html.

Pollins DA, Kaufman LD, Masur DM, Krupp LB. (1998). Pain, fatigue, and sleep in eosinophilia-myalgia syndrome: Relationship to neuropsychological performance. *Journal of Neuropsychiatry & Clinical Neurosciences 10:* 338-342.

Sternberg EM. (1996). Pathogenesis of L-tryptophan eosinophilia myalgia syndrome. *Advances in Experimental Medicine & Biology 398:* 325-330.

Sullivan EA, Kamb ML, Jones JL, Meyer P, Philen RM, Falk H, Sinks T. (1996). The natural history of eosinophilia-myalgia syndrome in a tryptophan-exposed cohort in South Carolina. *Archives of Internal Medicine 156:* 973-979.

Sullivan EA, Staehling N, Philen RM. (1996). Eosinophilia-myalgia syndrome among the non-L-tryptophan users and pre-epidemic cases. *Journal of Rheumatology 23:* 1784-1787.

Williamson BL, Johnson KL, Tomlinson AJ, Gleich GJ, Naylor S. (1998). On-line HPLC-tandem mass spectrometry structural characterization of case-associated contaminants of L-tryptophan implicated with the onset of eosinophilia myalgia syndrome. *Toxicology Letters 99:* 139-150.

Williamson BL, Klarskov K, Tomlinson AJ, Gleich GJ, Naylor S. (1998). Problems with over-the-counter 5-hydroxy-L-tryptophan. *Nature Medicine 4:* 983.

Chapter 31

Carper J. (1997). *Miracle Cures: Dramatic New Scientific Discoveries Revealing the Healing Powers of Herbs, Vitamins, and Other Natural Remedies.* New York: Harper Perennial.

Williams MH. (1992). Ergogenic and ergolytic substances. *Medicine & Science in Sports & Exercise 24* (Suppl. 9): S344-S348.

Chapter 32

Anonymous. (n.d.). Dietary supplements: Buyers beware. Available at: www.sciencedaily.com/releases/2000/11/001116080726.htm.

Miller M. (2003). About the CODEX. (The Health Letter of the Foundation for the Advancement of Innovative Medicine.) *Innovation,* Spring, p. 31.

Moss RW. (2001). Complementary and alternative medicine *Lancet 357:* 803.

Tyler V. (1993). *The Honest Herbal,* Third edition. Binghamton, NY: The Haworth Press.

Chapter 33

Brain M. (2006). How laughter works. Available at: http://science.howstuffworks.com/laughter.htm.

Cousins N. (1979). *Anatomy of an Illness As Perceived by the Patient: Reflections on Healing and Regeneration.* New York: Norton.

Cousins N. (1983). *The Healing Heart: Antidotes to Pain and Helplessness.* New York: Norton.

Davis WM. (2002). What pharmacists should know about West Nile virus—The newest arbovirus to cause encephalitis in the USA. Available at: rxed.org/umce/.

Davis WM, Wellwuff HG, Garew L, Kidd OU. (1992). Psychopharmacology of lycanthropy. *Canadian Medical Association Journal 146:* 1191-1197.

Douglas WC. (2003) *Daily Dose* (e-newsletter). Available at: www.realhealthnews.com/ dailydose/freecopy.html.

Fry WF, Jr. (1977). The respiratory components of mirthful laughter. *Journal of Biological Psychology 19:* 39-50.

Fry WF, Jr. (1992). The physiological effects of humor, mirth and laughter. *Journal of the American Medical Association 267:* 1857.

Fry WF, Jr., Savin WM. (1988). Mirthful laughter and blood pressure. *Humor 1:* 49-62.

Fry WF, Jr., Stoft PE. (1971). Mirth and oxygen saturation levels of peripheral blood. *Psychotherapy and Psychosomatics 19:* 76-84.

Golub ES. (1997). *The Limits of Medicine: How Science Shapes Our Hope for the Cure.* Chicago: University of Chicago Press.

Huxtable RJ. (1992). The myth of beneficent nature: The risks of herbal preparation. *Annals of Internal Medicine 117:* 129-132.

Herber D. (2002). *What Color Is Your Diet?* New York: Regan Books.

Herber D. (2004). Vegetables, fruits and phytoestrogens in the prevention of diseases. *Journal of Postgraduate Medicine 50:* 145-149.

Joseph JA. (2003). *The Color Code: A Revolutionary Eating Plan for Optimum Health.* New York: Hyperion.

Lloyd EL. (1938). The respiratory mechanism in laughter. *Journal of General Psychology 10:* 179-189.

McGuire FA, Boyd RK, James A. (1992). *Therapeutic Humor with the Elderly.* Binghamton, NY: The Haworth Press.

McDonald FA, Boyd RK, James A. (1992). *Therapeutic Humor with the Elderly.* Binghamton, NY: The Haworth Press, Inc.

Miller M. (2000). Laughter is good for your heart, according to a new University of Maryland Medical Center study. Available at http://www.sciencedaily.com/releases/2000/11/001116080726.htm.

Neuberger J. (2000). The educated patient: New challenges for the medical profession. *Journal of Internal Medicine 247:* 6-10.

Saul A. (2003). *Doctor Yourself: Natural Healing That Works.* North Bergen, NJ: Basic Health Publications. [e-newsletter, available at updatesubscribe@doctor yourself.com.]

Chapter 34

Astin JA, Harkness E, Ernst E. (2000). The efficacy of "distant healing": A systematic review of randomized trials. *Annals of Internal Medicine 132:* 903-910.

Barnes PM, Powell-Griner E, McFann K, Nahin RL. (2004). Complementary and alternative medicine use among adults: United States 2002. *Advance Date from Vital and Health Statistics,* no. 343. Hyattsville, MD: National Center for Health Statistics.

Braverman ER (1994). *What's Your Spiritual Health? Diagnosing This Critical Component of Your Total Health.* Princeton, NJ: Publications for Achieving Total Health.

Carnegie D. (1984). *How to Stop Worrying and Start Living,* Revised edition. New York: Simon and Schuster.

Cherry RB. (2002). What about prayer for healing? In J. Wilhout (ed.), *The Personal Handbook on Prayer.* Nashville, TN: Thomas Nelson, Inc., pp. 137-139.

Colbert D. (2001). *Toxic Relief: Restore Health and Energy Through Fasting and Detoxification.* Lake Mary, FL: Siloam Press.

Frank JD. (1975) The faith that heals. *Johns Hopkins Medical Journal 137:* 127-131.

Gardner R. (1983). Miracles of healing in Anglo-Celtic Northumbria as recorded by the Venerable Bede and his contemporaries: A reappraisal in the light of 20th century experience. *British Medical Journal 287:* 1927-1933.

Gundersen L. (2000). Faith and healing. *Annals of Internal Medicine 132:* 169-172.

Kowey PR, Friehling TD, Marinchak RA. (1986). Prayer meeting cardioversion. *Annals of Internal Medicine 104:* 727-728.

Larson D. (1997). *Scientific Research on Spirituality and Health. A Consensus Report.* Rockville, MD: National Institute on Healthcare Research.

Lerner B. (2003). *Body by God: The Owner's Manual for Maximized Living.* Nashville, TN: Thomas Nelson Publisher.

MacLean CD, Susi B, Phifer N, Schultz L, Bynum D, Franco M, Klioze A, Monroe M, Garrett J, Cykert S. (2003). Patient preference for physician discussion and practice of spirituality. *Journal of General Internal Medicine 18:* 38-43.

McCaffrey AM, Eisenberg DM, Legedza AT, Davis RB, Phillips RS. (2004). Prayer for health concerns: Results of a national survey on prevalence and patterns of use. *Archives of Internal Medicine 164:* 858-862.

McCord G, Gilchrist VJ, Grossman SD, King BD, McCormick KF, Oprandi AM, Schrop SL, Selius BA, Smucker WD, Weldy DL, et al. (2004). Discussing spirituality with patients: A rational and ethical approach. *Annals of Family Medicine 2:* 356-361.

National Center for Health Statistics, Centers for Disease Control and Prevention. (2004, May). Available at: www.eurekalert.org/images/05.

Peteet JR. (1993). A closer look at the role of a spiritual approach in addiction treatment. *Journal of Substance Abuse Treatment 10:* 263-267.

Poloma MM. (1993). The effects of prayer on mental well-being. *Second Opinion 18:* 37-51.

Poloma MM and Gallup GH, Jr. (1991). *Varieties of Prayer: A Survey Report 1991.* Philadelphia: Trinity Press International.

Post SG, Puchalski CM, Larson DB. (2000). Physicians and patient spirituality: Professional boundaries, competency, and ethics. *Annals of Internal Medicine 132:* 578-583.

Rubin JN. (2004). *The Maker's Diet.* Lake Mary, FL: Siloam Press.

Sapolsky RM. (1996). Why stress is bad for your brain. *Science 273:* 749-750.

Schaefer J, Nierhaus KH, Lohff B, Peters T, Schaefer T, Vos R. (1998). Mechanisms of autoprotection and the role of stress-proteins in natural defenses, autoprotection, and SALUTOGENESIS. *Medical Hypotheses 51*(2): 153-163.

Segerstrom SC, Miller GE. (2004). Psychological stress and the human immune system: A meta-analytic study of 30 years of inquiry. *Psychological Bulletin 130:* 601-630.

Selye H. (1956). *The Stress of Life.* Columbus, OH: McGraw-Hill.

Selye H. (1975). *Stress without Distress.* New York: Signet.

Shedd OL, Sears SF Jr, Harvill JL, Arshad A, Conti JB, Steinberg JS, Curtis AB. (2004). The World Trade Center attack: Increased frequency of defibrillator shocks for ventricular arrhythmias in patients living remotely from New York City. *Journal of the American College of Cardiology 44:* 1265-1267.

Steinberg JS, Arshad A, Kowalski M, Kukar A, Suma V, Vloka M, Ehlert F, Herweg B, Donnelly J, Philip J, et al. (2004). Increased incidence of life-threatening ventricular arrhythmias in implantable defibrillator of patients after the World Trade Center attack. *Journal of the American College of Cardiology 44:* 1261-1264.

Thomas CB, McCabe OL. (1980). Precursors of premature disease and death: Habits of nervous tension. *The Johns Hopkins Medical Journal 147:* 137-145.

Index

Page numbers followed by the letter "f" indicate exhibits; those followed by the letter "t" indicate tables.

Consumer's Guide to Dietary Supplements and Alternative Medicines

doi:10.1300/5698_39

Order a copy of this book with this form or online at:
http://www.haworthpress.com/store/product.asp?sku=5698

CONSUMER'S GUIDE TO DIETARY SUPPLEMENTS AND ALTERNATIVE MEDICINES

Servings of Hope

_______in hardbound at $89.95 (ISBN-13: 978-0-7890-3040-5; ISBN-10: 0-7890-3040-3)

_______in softbound at $49.95 (ISBN-13: 978-0-7890-3041-2; ISBN-10: 0-7890-3041-1)

503 pages plus index • Includes photos and illustrations

Or order online and use special offer code HEC25 in the shopping cart.

COST OF BOOKS________

POSTAGE & HANDLING________
(US: $4.00 for first book & $1.50 for each additional book)
(Outside US: $5.00 for first book & $2.00 for each additional book)

SUBTOTAL________

IN CANADA: ADD 6% GST________

STATE TAX________
(NJ, NY, OH, MN, CA, IL, IN, PA, & SD residents, add appropriate local sales tax)

FINAL TOTAL________
(If paying in Canadian funds, convert using the current exchange rate, UNESCO coupons welcome)

☐ **BILL ME LATER:** (Bill-me option is good on US/Canada/Mexico orders only; not good to jobbers, wholesalers, or subscription agencies.)

☐ Check here if billing address is different from shipping address and attach purchase order and billing address information.

Signature________________________

☐ **PAYMENT ENCLOSED:** $________________

☐ **PLEASE CHARGE TO MY CREDIT CARD.**

☐ Visa ☐ MasterCard ☐ AmEx ☐ Discover
☐ Diner's Club ☐ Eurocard ☐ JCB

Account # ________________________

Exp. Date________________________

Signature________________________

Prices in US dollars and subject to change without notice.

NAME________________________

INSTITUTION________________________

ADDRESS________________________

CITY________________________

STATE/ZIP________________________

COUNTRY________________ COUNTY (NY residents only)________________

TEL________________ FAX________________

E-MAIL________________________

May we use your e-mail address for confirmations and other types of information? ☐ Yes ☐ No We appreciate receiving your e-mail address and fax number. Haworth would like to e-mail or fax special discount offers to you, as a preferred customer. **We will never share, rent, or exchange your e-mail address or fax number.** We regard such actions as an invasion of your privacy.

Order From Your Local Bookstore or Directly From

The Haworth Press, Inc.

10 Alice Street, Binghamton, New York 13904-1580 • USA
TELEPHONE: 1-800-HAWORTH (1-800-429-6784) / Outside US/Canada: (607) 722-5857
FAX: 1-800-895-0582 / Outside US/Canada: (607) 771-0012
E-mail to: orders@haworthpress.com

For orders outside US and Canada, you may wish to order through your local sales representative, distributor, or bookseller.
For information, see http://haworthpress.com/distributors

(Discounts are available for individual orders in US and Canada only, not booksellers/distributors.)

PLEASE PHOTOCOPY THIS FORM FOR YOUR PERSONAL USE.

http://www.HaworthPress.com BOF06